Harriet Meyer

GAYELORD HAUSER'S
NEW
TREASURY OF SECRETS

Also by Gayelord Hauser

BE HAPPIER, BE HEALTHIER

DIET DOES IT

THE GAYELORD HAUSER COOKBOOK

LOOK YOUNGER, LIVE LONGER

MIRROR, MIRROR ON THE WALL

NEW GUIDE TO INTELLIGENT REDUCING

GAYELORD HAUSER'S NEW TREASURY OF SECRETS

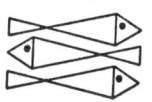

FARRAR, STRAUS AND GIROUX • NEW YORK

A completely revised and updated edition,
with a new preface by Gaylord Hauser
Copyright © 1951, 1952, 1955, 1961, 1963, 1974
by Gayelord Hauser
All rights reserved
Printed in the United States of America
First printing, 1974
Published simultaneously in Canada
by Doubleday Canada, Ltd., Toronto
Designed by Dorris Huth

Library of Congress Cataloging in Publication Data

Hauser, Benjamin Gayelord.
   Gayelord Hauser's new treasury of secrets.

   Edition of 1963 published under title: Treasury of secrets.
   Includes indexes.
   1. Hygiene.   2. Diet.   I. Title.   II. Title: New treasury of secrets.
RA776.H357   1974   613.2   74-22102

Preface

Over fifty years have passed since I first started teaching people the inestimable value of fresh, living foods, and in those fifty years, many of the old, outworn notions about food have passed also. I'm pleased that I have had some small part in bringing people to healthy food awareness, and I think people today—especially young people—are more willing to consider new ideas. These people are seeking simpler, more natural prescriptions for living—natural looks, natural fashions, and natural foods. They are more willing to avoid buying fruits and vegetables sprayed with chemical fertilizers and pesticides, foods processed with bleaches, preservatives, emulsifiers, and other artificial additives, and meats and poultry shot full of hormones and dyes. These people are learning the million-dollar secret of *fresh, vital foods*—a secret I want to pass on now to everyone, whether young or old, healthy or sick: fresh food, the fresher the better, contains all the living elements! And only living food can build a living body. Every one of our daily meals should give our bodies living food: the freshest milk, cheese, and eggs; lean meat, fish, liver, and other organ meats; and always, the freshest green and yellow vegetables and fresh fruits. And above all else, eating these foods should be a *pleasure*—to the eye and mind as well as to the palate! A regime of vitamins and minerals will not profit anyone for long if it is a duty grudgingly undertaken and then ignored. It is never too late to try! Living foods are foods to be enjoyed thoroughly, and mealtimes are times of the day when the mind can relax and absorb with delight the company of one's family or the comfort of one's surroundings.

These are some of my million-dollar secrets, which, of course, rightfully belong to everyone. Since that time more than fifty years ago, I have seen thousands of people eat their way to health and vitality. I am more convinced than ever that a good diet can cure many of the world's ills.

But, one may ask, *are* the foods we eat as unhealthy as all that? Let me give you some facts.

In the early sixties, while food manufacturers and nutrition "experts" were telling us we were the best-fed nation in the world, our President announced to a nationwide television audience: "To get two men today, the United States Army must call seven men. Of the five rejected, three are turned down for physical reasons and two for mental disabilities . . . and the rejection rate is increasing each year."

If we are so well fed, why then are we so unhealthy? The answer lies not in the amount of food we consume but in the quality of our food. The advances and possibilities of modern technology are worthless if we sacrifice nutrition for the sake of production.

Dr. E. V. McCollum, of the famous Johns Hopkins Hospital, expressed the problem in a few words when he said: "Eat only food that decays or spoils easily, but eat it before it does."

How many foods did you eat today that spoil easily? Most of the foods we eat keep indefinitely. They have been peeled, pickled, chemicalized, and embalmed for the manufacturers who want a long shelf life for their products. In this way, the manufacturers have traded a long shelf life for our own long lives.

In Russia I found tremendous interest in better nutrition. There are posters everywhere telling people to eat fresh food, to gather herbs, to take vitamins—especially vitamin C, for which they especially cultivate rose hips. According to our standards, food in Russia is monotonous; but it is much more earthy and natural.

While interviewing some of their nutritionists, I was asked bluntly, "Why have you so many sick people in your rich country? Why have you so many deaths from atherosclerosis and heart attacks?"

I could not deny that we in the United States have a high death rate from circulatory disease, for statistics prove it. But I did say proudly that more and more people are now using sunflower, safflower, peanut, corn, sesame, and olive oils and are becoming more aware of the healthy effects of sound nutrition and daily exercise. Perhaps the sprouting of many health-food stores and health farms all across the nation, and indeed all over the Western world, testifies to a new awareness, a new desire to "return to nature." For example, people from all over the world travel to Zurich, Switzerland, to take a *Frischkost* diet at the Bircher-Benner Sanatorium; hundreds of patients who were given up by their physicians have found new health. Yet the diet is a simple one, consisting entirely of such living foods as green salads, fresh vegetables and vegetable juices, milk, and the famous Bircher apple muesli. For many years I knew the beloved physician Dr. Bircher-Benner, and I listened to many of his lectures (given at six o'clock in the morning). Fresh food had saved his life, and fresh food was his favorite subject. He often spoke of "sun-cooked food," especially green leaves, which are saturated with sun energy and therefore have the most potent health-giving properties.

For half a century I have been advancing Dr. Bircher-Benner's findings, along with those of many other health pioneers. I have taught nutrition in all parts of the world—the United States, Europe, Australia, and Japan. In schools and clinics, in laboratories and sanatoriums, I have asked thousands of questions, made tests, and always offered myself as an experimental guinea pig to demonstrate my conviction that with good nutrition comes a good life. I have always taken great pride in interpreting the complicated and confusing technical language of the latest scientific discoveries into plain everyday speech. I saw what modern nutrition could do and wrote a book called *Be Happier, Be Healthier* about good food and good health, and how it affects our happiness and *joie de vivre*. Later I wrote *The New Guide to Intelligent Reducing*, giving the harassed overweighters fundamental reducing secrets without gimmicks. It quickly became a best seller and was translated into French, German, Swedish, and Italian. When many requests came from England and France, I finally wrote *Mangez pour être belle,* or *Eat and Grow Beautiful,* showing how a cosmetic diet creates an inner vitality and the kind of beauty that does not come off at night. This book created a sensation in France.

My most popular book was *Look Younger, Live Longer.* Almost overnight I became a hero. With it came offers for radio and television; King Features Syndicate serialized the book in every large city; it was condensed in *The Reader's Digest; The Saturday Evening Post* and many other magazines featured stories about me and my Wonder Foods. The book has been translated into twenty-seven languages.

I learned an important lesson during those hectic days. Wherever I went, I found one common problem: people were hungry. They were not particularly interested in me, nor were they hungry for more food. They were hungry for more life, for better health, for younger bodies and keener minds. And only because I could satisfy this hunger, and teach them the secret of eating for health, good looks, and high vitality, did they become my devoted friends and followers.

My publishers have now asked me to revise and update my *Treasury of Secrets,* a book that brought together the most valuable materials from my books and nutrition classes. It is time to tell of all the new and exciting discoveries made in the field of health and nutrition in the past ten years, of the incredible findings and facts about ourselves. I hope this book will succeed in being the most helpful one in your library—a book that will answer the thousand and one questions I am constantly asked.

Before I end, I would like to tell you a personal story.

A boy lay dying in a hospital in Chicago. He had undergone many operations and countless injections, and still his tubercular hip refused to heal. Finally the doctors decided, "Send this boy home. There is nothing more we can do for him."

The unhappy boy was sent home to die in the serenity of the Swiss mountains. One morning the boy was having his usual breakfast of coffee, rolls, and marmalade, when an old man, a family friend who had spent his life as a missionary, said to him, "If you keep on eating such dead foods, you will die. Only living foods can make a living body."

"What are living foods?" asked the boy.

The gentle old man described them: "Fresh young growing things, especially green and yellow garden vegetables, saturated with earthy elements; lemons, oranges, and other tree fruits, full of sunshine and living juices."

The sick boy listened thoughtfully. From that day on, he began to eat enormous amounts of fresh living foods. And wonder of wonders, the hip that had defied all treatment now slowly but surely healed. Through this amazing recovery, I discovered for the first time what fresh food can do. Yes, food saved my life —for I was that boy.

And now all the million-dollar secrets I learned from that wise old Swiss man, and have learned since that time, I pass on to you. They are all in this book. I know that if you apply them faithfully, they can bring to you a new vitality and a joy in living worth more than money.

For even the greatest wealth is worthless without health, and joy in living is more precious than gold.

GAYELORD HAUSER

August 1974
New York

Contents

One LOOK YOUNGER, LIVE LONGER

1. PASSPORT TO A NEW WAY OF LIFE 3
   You Can Forget Your Age 6
   Eat Vital Foods for Longer Life 8

Two YOU ARE WHAT YOU EAT

2. NATURAL, WHOLESOME FOODS 15
   Proteins for Body Building, Repairing, and
     Rejuvenation 16
   The Carbohydrates—Quick-Energy Foods 21
   The Good Fats—for Sustained Energy and
     Smaller Waistlines 23
   Meet the Wonder Foods 26

3. VITAMINS AND MINERALS FOR LONGER LIFE 33
   Vitamin A 33
   Those Important B Vitamins 35
   The Lesser-Known B Vitamins 38
   Vitamin C—Ascorbic Acid 45
   Vitamin D 48
   Vitamin E 49

Vitamin "F" 51
Vitamin K 51
Minerals for Maximum Nutrition 51

4. HIGH-VITALITY MEAL PLANNING 60
   Eat a Protein Breakfast 60
   Make Lunchtime Salad Time 64
   Your Midafternoon Vitality Lift 67
   Dinnertime Is Relaxing Time 67
   Recipes and Menus to Guide You 69
   The High-Vitality Diet—Breakfasts, Luncheons,
     and Dinners 73

5. EATING—THE PLEASURE PRINCIPLE 76
   Lean Cookery 77
   Short-Cook Your Vegetables 79
   Finger Salad and Fresh Juices 81
   Fruit for Dessert 82

6. LET'S DINE OUT 84
   Chicago—the Pump Room 85
   New York—"21" 86
   New York—Mercurio 86
   Buenos Aires—the Alvear Palace Hotel 87
   London—Restaurant Caprice 88
   Paris—Maxim's 88
   Venice—Taverna della Fenice 89
   Dining with Friends 90

Three YOUR GOOD HEALTH

7. BODY WORKS 93
   Your Body Architecture 93
   Your Muscular Body 96
   Your Digestive Laboratory 97
   Your Circulatory System 101
   Your Respiratory System 103
   Your Nervous System 106

8. RESISTANCE TO DISEASE — 108

Infections — 108
Diabetes — 112
Hypoglycemia—Low Blood Sugar — 113
Cancer — 117
Kidney Disease — 118
Urinary Troubles — 119
Gallstones — 120
Anemia — 121
Varicose Veins — 122
Mental Disturbances — 124
Allergies, Hay Fever, and Asthma — 126
Psychosomatic Difficulties — 128
Arthritis — 129
Sex and Menopause Problems — 130
Take Care of Your Glands — 132
Megavitamin Therapy—the New Science — 139

9. FIGHT FATIGUE WITH EXERCISE AND RELAXATION — 142

The Million-Dollar Secret of Relaxation — 142
The Magic Yoga Slant — 145
Midriff Flattener—the Stomach Lift — 146
Muscular Joy — 148
Walk Your Way to a Longer Life — 150
Sleep — 151

10. KEEP YOUR BODY YOUNG — 155

Smokers Need More Vitamin C — 155
Excessive Drinking Destroys Vitamins — 156
Prevent Brittle Bones — 157
Ward Off Hardening of the Arteries — 158
Your Heart and Your Diet — 162
Lecithin Combats Cholesterol Build-up — 165
Vitamin P and Your Capillaries — 168
Problems with Digestion and Elimination? — 169
Natural Laxatives — 174
The Niehans Cellular Therapy — 175

Four YOUR GOOD LOOKS

11. EAT AND GROW BEAUTIFUL — 179
- Your Eyes — 179
- New Ways to Hear Better — 185
- Your Teeth — 186
- Your Hair — 191
- Your Skin — 194
- Lines and Wrinkles Tell a Story — 201
- Psycho-Cosmetics — 202
- Three Ways to Lift Your Face — 203
- Your Feet — 205

12. TREAT YOURSELF TO BEAUTY — 207
- Bathe Yourself to Health and Beauty — 207
- Superfluous Hair and Moles — 213
- The Case for Plastic Surgery — 213
- More Beauty Secrets — 215

13. THE BEAUTY FARM — 227
- Mealtimes at the Beauty Farm — 228
- Have Your Own Beauty Farm — 230
- Foods Fit for My Garbage Can — 234
- Clean Out Your Pantry — 236
- Just One Day a Week — 237
- Take Care of the Inner Self — 241
- Visit a Beauty Farm — 242

Five YOUR GOOD LIFE

14. YOU ARE WHAT YOU THINK AND FEEL — 247
- A Philosophy of Life — 247
- Laugh and Be Healthy — 248
- The Joy of Participation — 250
- The Secret Ingredient — 250

15. MEET SOME OF MY PEOPLE — 252
- Ann Astaire — 255
- Albert Schweitzer — 257
- Fulfillment in Later Life — 258

	The Fabulous Lady Mendl	260
	Today's Beautiful People	263
16.	MAKE YOUR CHILDREN BEAUTIFUL	265
	Your Infant	265
	Your Growing Child	268
	Your Teen-ager	269
17.	THE MAN IN THE FAMILY	271
	Three Gifts Every Man Wants	273
	The Epidemic of Heart Disease	273
	The Sedentary Man	274
	Million-Dollar Secrets for the Kitchen	275
	How to Fight Baldness	276
	Ancient Secrets for Sexual Strength	277
	A Man-Size Diet	280
	A Malnourished President	280

Six INTELLIGENT DIETING

18.	REDUCE AND REJUVENATE	285
	Make Reducing a Pleasure	285
	Nonregimented Reducing Regimen	293
	Sample Menus for Reducing	296
19.	REDUCING PLANS FROM ALL OVER THE WORLD	298
	How the French Reduce without Tears	298
	The Truth about Cellulite	303
	How the Russians Fight Bulging Waistlines	303
	The Thrifty Swiss Apple Diet	306
	The Japanese Way to Health and Longevity	311
20.	MY SEVEN-DAY ELIMINATION DIET	314
21.	MORE MILLION-DOLLAR SECRETS	320
	Purely Personal	320
	A Few Reducing Tips	322
	Advice from Doctors and Researchers around	
	the World	323
	Follow the Stars	326

Seven RECIPES AND FORMULAS

22. FABULOUS PROTEINS BUILD BEAUTIFUL BODIES 331
    Learn to Like Liver 332
    Beef—a Favorite Protein 336
    Veal 338
    Chicken at Its Best 339
    Eat Fish and Live Longer 341
    Delicious Meatless Protein Dishes 343
    The Wonder Vegetable 346
    Grow Your Own Vitamins 347
    Eggs—a Wonder Food 350
    Protein Soups—a Meal in a Cup 351

23. SUNLIT FOOD 355
    Sunlit Food Needs Little Cooking 360
    Leafy Vegetables 361
    Delightful Chinese Dishes 363

24. THE GOOD CARBOHYDRATES 367
    A New Look at Bread 367
    Natural Cereals and Other Grains 373
    Potatoes Can Be Good for You 375

25. HEALTHY, HEALING VEGETABLE JUICES 378
    How to Make Fresh Vegetable Juices 380
    Liquid Salads—If Chewing Is a Problem 383
    Eat, Drink, and Be Beautiful! 384

26. DELIGHTFUL DESSERTS 385
    Do Something New with Fresh Fruit 385
    You Can Make Gelatin Doubly Nutritious 389
    Sherbets, Custards, and Other Desserts 390

27. COFFEE OR TEA 394
    Coffee for Connoisseurs 394
    Tea for Connoisseurs 397

28. MILK AND MILK FOODS 399
Hi-Vi Milk 400
Fortified Milk for Reducers 400
Special Formulas for Reducers 404
Yogurt Means Long Life 406

APPENDIX: The New 1973 Recommended
Dietary Allowances 412

INDEXES 415

ONE

LOOK YOUNGER, LIVE LONGER

1

Passport to a New Way of Life

For those people who are interested in lists and charts—who want merely a prescription for better health, not a passport to a new way of life—here is a quick summary of what you need each day.

>Sufficient calories to maintain your ideal body weight
>
>At least 2 tablespoons of liquid vegetable oil
>
>At least 1 gram of protein for each 2.2 pounds of your ideal body weight
>
>At least 1 gram of carbohydrate for each 3 pounds of your ideal body weight (but remember, don't overdo; carbohydrate consumption is wildly high)

And sufficient amounts of the following:

>Vitamin A
>
>The B-complex vitamins (B_1, thiamine; B_2, riboflavin; niacin; B_6, pyridoxine; B_{12}; pantothenic acid; biotin; folic acid; choline; inositol; para-aminobenzoic acid)
>
>Vitamin C (ascorbic acid)
>
>Vitamin D
>
>Vitamin E

Vitamin K

Minerals (calcium, phosphorus, iodine, iron, magnesium, zinc)

Trace minerals (sodium, potassium, chromium, manganese, cobalt, selenium, molybdenum, and others)

Essential fatty acids (linoleic, linolenic, arachidonic, etc.)

Essential amino acids (lysine, valine, leucine, threonine, isoleucine, tryptophan, phenylalanine, methionine)

And the "nonessential" amino acids

Doesn't that sound boring? Overwhelming? Well, I have good news for you. If you eat natural, unprocessed foods—organically grown if they are available—and use the few diet supplements I suggest in the following chapters, you will come as close as one can get to the ideal nutritional regime. Your diet will be a natural, healthful, high-protein, medium-fat, low-carbohydrate regimen, and all you need do is follow my menu plans and learn to enjoy unprocessed foods.

Of course, you should know about the nutrients listed above and you should have some idea of how they are used in the body. For this you should read carefully chapters 2 and 3. But once you have learned about these vital factors, put yourself in my hands and let me show you how to get all these nutrients without sentencing yourself to a daily dose of dozens of vitamin pills and capsules. I refuse to reduce the joy of good eating to fine measurements. It discourages the busy person whose table is not set with a balance scale along with a knife and fork.

So this book is not an ordinary book on nutrition, exercise, and health. It is a passport, an invitation to a journey of discovery—the discovery of a new way of life.

Like any journey, this one requires a certain amount of courage at the outset—the courage to do new things, keep an open mind, consider new ideas (some of which may surprise you), and, hardest of all, let go of old ideas and old ways. Like any journey, again, this one invites at the outset a certain excitement. But unlike most other journeys, this one will cost you no extra money— it might, in fact, save you money by giving you the good health that is your right.

Before we start, you should know who I am, since I am to be

your guide on this journey. I am a doctor, not of medicine, but of natural science. I have taken my inspiration from the teachings of Hippocrates, Paracelsus, Father Kneipp, Hindhede, Bircher-Benner, and other great teachers of ancient, medieval, and modern times.

I have three special qualifications for teaching people how to live longer. One is my own great relish for living. I find it very good and very satisfying to be alive. Each year on May 17 I celebrate my birthday. I like to receive the good wishes of my friends and the good thoughts of my students, but I refuse to get older. I celebrate each birthday not just as the end of another good and satisfying year of life but as the beginning of a new year of exciting work, travel, and accomplishment.

My second qualification is my great relish for meeting people. As a dietician, nutritionist, lecturer, and writer, I travel constantly. Wherever I go, I meet more and more People (with a capital *P*), and many become my good friends. I meet them on trains, ocean liners, and airplanes, at Hollywood parties, and in drawing rooms in New York, London, Paris, and Rome. I meet them in the learned circles of Vienna, Copenhagen, and Tokyo, and in the crowds that gather around my lecture platform from Boston to Seattle.

I meet People in another place, too—on the shelves of the nearest library, wherever I happen to be, for my appetite for reading about People is almost as great as my appetite for knowing the People themselves.

My third qualification is my own great relish for the idea of longevity. I have always devoured everything bearing upon the subject of longevity—in the fields of nutrition, endocrinology, surgery, biology, biochemistry, osteopathy, naprapathy, chiropractic naturopathy, psychiatry, philosophy, physical culture—wherever I could find it. I have visited many of the famous watering places in Europe, the United States, and Japan and tested their special diets and regimes. I have visited doctors in their offices and sanatoriums, research scientists in their laboratories, and many health resorts and beauty farms. I have assembled rooms full of books and filing cabinets full of pamphlets, reprints, and clippings dealing with my favorite subject. I have inquired into and experimented with or speculated upon everything I could find that anyone has said, thought, written, discovered, developed, invented, promised, prophesied, or dreamed of that had to do with living a long life.

Why?

Because I want to live for one hundred years. Don't you?

I know what you are thinking. "This man is mad! Suppose I can live to be one hundred. Who wants to hang on to life—frail, dried-up, useless—just for the sake of proving it can be done?"

Who indeed! Not I. You are thinking in old terms. Haven't I told you that this book is a journey requiring the courage to consider new ideas? And that includes seeing yourself at one hundred, still of definite use in the world—*without* aches and pains or skin like a dried-up apple.

In this book, this journey that we are taking together, I will teach you how to eat not merely to satisfy hunger but for health, good looks, youth, vitality, the joy of living. I will show you that you are not old at forty, fifty, sixty, seventy. That you need not be old at eighty, ninety—shall I go on?

Certainly I shall. I am now eighty years old. I've enjoyed every moment of those years to its fullest, and I plan to continue to do so. I have arrived at my principles and beliefs through study, research, and experiment. However, many of my friends and students who have passed seventy, eighty, even ninety years of age arrived at their understanding of health intuitively. It has been their lifelong habit to eat a balanced diet, keep their bodies in shape, and maintain a cheerful, positive frame of mind. They know instinctively that it is better to undereat than to overeat. And they know a secret that is harder than any other to pass on—the secret of complete body relaxation. You are soon to meet these wonderful people and share their secrets.

You Can Forget Your Age

Now, put this book down for a moment. Say to yourself, "I—this person sitting here in this chair—I can live to be one hundred years old." Say it aloud. Listen to your words. Repeat them.

This idea is new to you. It is a new kind of thinking. Take your time with it. Accept the idea of living to be one hundred. Think what the world will probably be like, what new, interesting, unheard-of things will probably be happening. Say to yourself, "I shall be alive then. I can be alive in the year ——."

Accept those years. They are yours. This is not wishful thinking or idle daydreaming. It is simple acceptance of scientific fact. Science has increased your life-span beyond your wildest expectations.

Instead of telling yourself despondently, "I am *forty*," try an optimistic "I am *only* forty." Whatever your present age, you are *young*.

There is a biologic limitation on the age to which each individual can aspire; however, if he is assured a life reasonably free from tension and is fed an ideal diet rich in every vital necessity, his chances of living a full, complete life are great.

The world over, scientists studying the extension of life are finding more and more evidence that the fountain of youth is *good nutrition*. Dr. Henry C. Sherman of Columbia University believes that good nutrition can greatly extend life and, perhaps more importantly, can make later life more worth living.

What is meant by good nutrition? First, it is adequate nutrition, giving the individual cells of the body not only the quantity but the quality of nourishment they require. Second, it is balanced nutrition, supplying the body cells with vital nutrients in the proper proportion. Scientists are unanimous in agreeing that over-nutrition, through excess calories stored as fat, contributes materially to physical deterioration and the aging process.

As a simplified, perhaps crude, illustration, think of your body as a motor car. It is made of protein, inside and out. Arteries, glands, colon, connective tissue; muscles, skin, bones, hair, teeth, eyes: all contain protein and are maintained and rebuilt with protein. Fats and carbohydrates are your body's oil and gasoline; they are burned together to produce energy. Vitamins and minerals are its spark plugs, essential to the utilization of food and its assimilation into the blood stream.

It is a marvelously sturdy motor car, this body of yours—marvelous in its ability to maintain and rebuild itself. Given care, consideration, and respect, it will function smoothly, on and on. Provided that none of its important organs has been allowed to break down, it can and will heal and regenerate itself at any age. It cannot be neglected or abused. It must be fed and cared for faithfully. When it does not hit on all cylinders, it must be examined by an expert mechanic who can not only find out what is wrong but also detect hidden weaknesses, forestall serious breakdowns. Even when it is functioning adequately it should have regular over-all checkups, preferably always at the same "machine shop" where its history is known and its special characteristics and needs are understood. Headed by the Mayo Clinic in Rochester, Minnesota, Johns Hopkins Hospital in Baltimore, Maryland, and the Scripps Clinic in La Jolla, California, where I go, human "machine shops" are springing up all over America. These clinics study the *whole* patient, not just the complaint.

I am convinced that with our growing knowledge of preventive health care, plus the immense progress the science of nutrition is making, America can lead the world into a new era, a Look Younger, Live Longer era.

Your body may seem much the same to you as it was a year ago, plus or minus a few pounds or inches, but . . . in a single year, 98 percent of the old atoms will be replaced by the new atoms which we take into our bodies from the air we breathe, the food we eat, and the water we drink.

Dr. Paul G. Aebersold
Former head of the Atomic Energy Commission
Washington, D.C.

Eat Vital Foods for Longer Life

Age is a physiological and psychological matter. Examination of men and women over one hundred years of age at some of our famous clinics revealed that they had four outstanding qualities:

>   Strong digestive juices
>   A slow, rhythmic heartbeat
>   Good elimination
>   Happy dispositions

Let me tell you a story about a woman whom I first met thirty years ago. She had worked with Wallace Beery, Sonja Henie, Charles Laughton, Don Ameche, Bette Davis, James Stewart, and a dozen others, but I did not know that. To me she was one of the hundreds of people who had crowded into a large auditorium in Los Angeles to hear me lecture.

I had never seen her before, but I recognized her at once. She was one of my People. I knew by the way she sat—erect and disciplined, her shining white hair, her head resting proudly on straight shoulders. I knew by her face—strong as well as sweet, revealing inner beauty as well as beauty of line and feature.

She was a Person, no question about it. After my lecture I saw her among the crowd gathering around the platform to meet me. We shook hands, and then I realized that she was an actress, too.

"Tell me," she said, her eyes sparkling with humor, her trained, resonant voice carrying clearly. In mock despair she put her hands on her stomach, which was perhaps not quite so flat as it might have been. "Tell me—*what* am I going to do about this *jelly belly?*"

Of course she brought the house down.

Adeline De Walt Reynolds was born in 1862. At the age of sixty-five, she told me, having raised four children and helped raise a raft of grandchildren, she had decided to go to college. At sixty-nine she was graduated from the University of California. Then Hollywood discovered her and the new star "Grandma Reynolds" was born. When I met her, at the age of eighty-two, with thirteen years of stardom behind her, she saw no limit to the years of stardom ahead. *If* she could get rid of her "jelly belly."

That was not difficult. With a lifelong habit of regular exercise, a natural talent for relaxation, and the drive that comes from sheer zest for living, she had long since made of her body a well-trained, responsive instrument. Her basic dietary habits were already good; I advised only such changes as would make sure that her diet contained many of the good proteins needed to rebuild tissue more firmly and strengthen the natural "muscular corset" that has been given to all of us to protect the abdomen, the most vital and vulnerable region of the body. I added brewers' yeast, yogurt, and cottage cheese to her diet and taught her the one exercise I consider indispensable—the stomach lift. She bought herself two yoga slant boards—one a plain board, the other with a motor attached, which mildly rocked her to sleep after a hard day's work at the studio. (I shall have more to say about the stomach lift and about yoga slant boards later.)

Six months passed. I lectured again in Los Angeles. Again Grandma Reynolds was in the audience. She was at my elbow the minute my lecture was over.

Her head was prouder than ever; her eyes were full of excitement and delight. She had just begun work on a new picture, she told me. It was the best role she had had yet. She was appearing with Bing Crosby in *Going My Way*.

The "jelly belly"?

Neither of us even mentioned it. Grandma Reynolds was as flat across the midriff as I am.

At the ripe young age of ninety-six, Grandma was still starring on television. What was her secret for long life, good health, and happiness? She herself could not have told you. She had a strong constitution, she had always loved life, and she believed in living each day to the full. She did not know her own secret. She had never analyzed it. But her secret was that all of her life she followed *instinctively* the basic principles of the Look Younger, Live Longer program.

What you eat between the ages of forty and sixty largely determines how you feel, look, and think at seventy and eighty. But it is never too late. Now is the time to take stock of yourself. Now is the time to discard myths of "age," and concentrate on agelessness. Now is the time to discard careless habits and swing into the Look Younger, Live Longer way of life. *The body can be rebuilt at any age. Well and wisely fed, the body and all its organs are capable of reaching a greater age than most of us ever before dared hope for.*

ENJOY YOUR FOOD

Food is made for man. By all means, let us enjoy it. I believe in eating all kinds of good food, either fresh or cooked (never overcooked) in infinite variety. I believe in spiking meats and sauces with herbs and fragrant spices, as the French do. I believe that everyone should not only consider a large, crisp salad as an important part of the main meal but *eat it as the first course of the meal, when appetite is keenest.* Fruit should become the favorite dessert, either fresh or stewed with honey. (Recipe for Lady Mendl's Honey Compote in chapter 26; see index.)

The secret of longevity largely lies in eating intelligently. Learn to like foods that are health-giving. This becomes easy as you learn about food values and also the values of vitamins and minerals. It is exciting to think of yourself as a kitchen chemist rather than a kitchen slave.

Looking back over all the years I have studied and taught nutrition, I realize that one of the most important factors is the *satisfaction center.* Certainly eating should be a pleasure. But too many people—especially people who are not happy—try to use rich, fattening foods as a substitute for other pleasures. And often these foods are eaten absent-mindedly or bolted hurriedly, with a minimum of satisfaction. If you will choose wholesome, natural foods, eat them slowly, chewing them twice as long as you now do, you will feed your satisfaction center. You will eat half as much and enjoy it many times more. Then you can throw away your calorie charts, throw away your diets, and never again overeat. You can have a slim, healthy, attractive body for the rest of your long life.

The most important thing is to eat fresh, unprocessed foods. Ever since we learned to refine and "preserve" food, we have begun to eliminate vital nutrients. What science has accomplished in combating disease is nearly offset by the outrages done to our food by the processors. Only a small percentage of foods in our super-duper markets contains the good nutrients that our forefathers enjoyed in their simple, home-cooked meals. Today, when overrefined foods are the rule rather than the exception, we should rely primarily on the finest fresh foods available and supplement the diet with the wonder foods (see chapter 2) and the best vitamin concentrates available.

It is my belief that, because man has long been adapted to foods as produced in nature, he should eat *natural* foods. I advocate the use of whole-grain flour and cereals instead of refined products, even the so-called enriched variety. For by means of what is termed "enrichment," the processors put back only a fraction of what has been taken out. In the lost portion are vital nutritive factors that, in the earlier days of nutritional science, were brushed off with the claim that "their need in human nutrition has not been established." Today we are learning of more and more essential food factors. It behooves us to keep our knowledge of nutrition up to date.

I hope to see the day when all of us, especially growing children and persons over forty, will eat intelligently, consuming foods adequate to our bodily needs for vital factors. If these vital factors can't be supplied by diet alone, then supplements must be used.

> *I believe that a well-fed body is the best defense against the tensions of modern living.*

How Much Shall I Eat

That is a question that I am frequently confronted with. First, we must eat to satisfy our energy requirements. Physical hunger—not to be confused with emotional cravings for food, sometimes caused by frustrations and tensions—is generally a good guide to the amount of food we need for energy; certainly, to the person who is at all observant, experience, together with honest hunger, is an ample guide to how much to eat. It is too bad that we do not also have a mechanism that tells us about the hidden hunger of the cells for vital nutritive factors. However, we are endowed with intelligence and we are supposed to use it. But you cannot use your brains until you know a little about nutrition, and that's where this book comes in.

Just remember that wholesome, natural food gives much greater appetite satisfaction, tastes better, and is better for you. Let's make that step one on your road to a better life.

TWO

YOU ARE WHAT YOU EAT

Natural, Wholesome Foods

Man has been asking for trouble ever since he began tampering with the quality of nature's foodstuffs. Our bountiful grains are denatured in the milling process—stripped of vitamins and minerals—and the bleached-out leftovers are processed into soft, fluffy white breads. Sugar is refined and bleached. Most fats and oils are overrefined and hydrogenated to negative value. Fruits and vegetables are sprayed with poisonous insecticides. Finally, the valuable food elements we don't overlook and throw away we overcook.

Of course, I know that life can no longer be lived as naturally and as simply as in our forefathers' day, but even in our technological age there is much we can do to protect ourselves nutritionally. If we are to keep our bodies slim, fit, and wholly alive, we must have more wholesome food—food that is 100 percent nourishment, as nature intended it to be. It can be had in lean meats, crisp and tasty salads, tender, well-scrubbed, briefly cooked vegetables, ripe fruit, fruit and vegetable juices, natural sugar with all its vitamins and minerals intact, and breads that retain the "staff of life," nutrients of the original grain.

Good, nourishing meals mean much more than a certain quota of calories. They mean balanced proportions of the BIG THREE (proteins, carbohydrates, and fats), along with the "hidden" food elements (the vitamins, minerals, enzymes, and many as yet undiscovered food factors). The last word in nutrition has not yet been spoken, but this much we do know: people do not get an excess of proteins, vitamins, and minerals; they overdo starches, sugars, and hard fats.

Proteins for Body Building, Repairing, and Rejuvenation

Proteins are of first importance for growth, development, and maintenance of life. They are *protective foods*. They satisfy hunger, stick to the ribs, nourish, and keep the body young and elastic.

In addition to building and repairing body tissue, protein is used in making hemoglobin, the iron-containing substance of the red blood corpuscles. Hormones are made of proteins. All of the enzymes in the body, which aid in the production of energy, the digestion of foods, the building of new tissue, and the tearing down of worn-out tissue, are made of protein. Proteins in the blood are responsible for the collection of urine and waste from the tissues. Proteins also help prevent the blood and tissues from becoming either too acid or too alkaline. They are important in making possible the clotting of the blood. Proteins even form substances known as antibodies, which combine with and render harmless the bacteria, bacterial toxins, and other foreign materials that act as poisons in the blood. When proteins are not supplied to carry on these many functions, the body is susceptible to sickness and even premature death.

Protein is an "active" nutrient, busily employed in repairing the daily wear and tear. Nutritionists agree that every man and woman should have, daily, about one gram of first-class protein for each 2.2 pounds of body weight. (This means your real weight, not overweight: the right weight for a person of your height, bone structure, and sex. See the chart on page 293 if you are not certain, or let the doctor help you.) A woman weighing 120 pounds should have 54 or 55 grams of protein a day; a man weighing 150 pounds should have about 68. Since round figures are easier to work with and to remember, and since extra protein in your diet is all to the best, I shall use the recommendation of

60 to 70 grams of protein per day for the average woman and man. Many people ignore this important point, and without sufficient proteins they feel weak, tired, and irritable, and their best plans go overboard. Also, protein foods are not the lowest in cost—and this cost factor is one of the reasons why I introduced the "life-saving" proteins of powdered skim milk, brewers' yeast, soya flour, and wheat germ, which are excellent fortifiers for those who cannot afford the more expensive forms of protein foods.

First-class proteins contain the eight essential amino acids: lysine, leucine, isoleucine, tryptophan, phenylalanine, threonine, methionine, and valine. These eight amino acids (out of about twenty) are the ones that cannot be manufactured by the body, so we must have them in our daily food. A detailed discussion of the whole theory of balancing amino acids (for those who are fascinated by the chemistry of all this) can be had in Frances Moore Lappe's *Diet for a Small Planet* (Ballantine Books). For the rest of us, however, it is not necessary to fuss over those strange-sounding names; the important thing to remember is that all eight can be obtained from the following *first-class protein foods:* eggs, cheese, milk, yogurt; the glandular and organ meats such as liver, kidney, heart, brain, sweetbreads; and, of course, roasts, chops, steaks, poultry, and fish. Organ meats are most highly preferred because they are also richest in essential vitamins and minerals. Only a few vegetables contain first-class proteins; they are soybeans, nuts, some seeds, and fresh wheat germ. *Second-class proteins* are found in dried beans, lentils, corn, rye, and other grains, and gelatin. Because they do not contain all eight essential amino acids, they should always be combined with a first-class protein.

First-Class Proteins

Eggs	Soybeans
Cheese	Nuts
Milk and yogurt	Fresh wheat germ
Meat and fish	Some seeds

Glandular and organ meats—richest in essential vitamins too!

Second-Class Proteins

Dried beans and peas   All grains
Peanuts   Gelatin
Lentils

From long experience I have found that meals including both animal and vegetable proteins are the best insurance of a firm and healthy body. The average man should eat not less than 70 grams of protein, the average woman not less than 60 grams (28 grams are about 1 ounce), each and every day. Protein foods are the most expensive part of our daily diet, and for that reason I recommend the fortification of ordinary foods with dried skim milk, brewers' yeast, wheat germ, seeds, and soya products—all of them protein-filled bargains. Doctors often recommend extra amounts of the first-class protein foods before or after surgery, or in cases of burns or ulcers. Otherwise, make it a habit to eat not less than 60 to 70 grams a day for the rest of your life.

Here, then, is a check list of good protein foods. May I suggest that you check your protein intake for the last twenty-four hours? You may be surprised.

FRESH MEATS AND FOWL	AMOUNT	GRAMS PROTEIN
beef, lean	1 serving *	20
chicken	1 serving	23
ham	1 serving	20
heart, beef	1 serving	19
kidney, lamb's	1 serving	18
lamb chop	1 medium	14
liver, calf's	1 serving	21
sausage, bologna	5 slices	12
steak	1 serving	21
turkey	1 serving	22

FRESH DAIRY PRODUCTS		
cheese, American	2 x 1 x 1 inches	14
cottage	3 tablespoons	10
cream	1½ tablespoons	0.6

* The average serving is usually considered to be about ¼ pound of meat or fish.

cream soups	¾ cup	4
egg	1 large	8
milk		
whole	1 quart	34
powdered skim	½ cup, level	20
skim	1 quart	34
yogurt	1 cup	9

FRESH FISH AND SEAFOOD

clams	6	14
fish, average	1 serving	21
oysters	7 medium	12
salmon, canned	⅓ cup	11
shrimp	6 medium	8
tuna	⅓ cup	12

NUTS

almonds	10 medium	6
peanuts	2 tablespoons	8
peanut butter	2 tablespoons	9
pecans	10 large	3
walnuts	½ cup	8

VEGETABLES

beans		
lima (green)	½ cup	6
navy	½ cup	6
soya, dry	½ cup	36
soya grits	½ cup	25
soya flour	1 cup	40
corn, fresh or canned	⅓ cup	3
lentils	½ cup	10
peas		
dried, cooked	½ cup	6
fresh	½ cup	5
potato		
white	1 medium	3
sweet	1 medium	3
yeast, brewers'	1 level tablespoon	8

GRAIN PRODUCTS

barley, whole, cooked	½ cup	8
bread, whole-wheat	1 slice	3
buckwheat, whole (dark)	⅓ cup	5
oatmeal, cooked	½ cup	3
rice, brown or white	¾ cup	3
shredded wheat	1 biscuit	3
spaghetti	¾ cup	3
wheat germ	½ cup	14

The average serving of many vegetables contains only 1 gram of protein. This amount is so small and the protein so inferior that it is best not to consider it. You will notice that I haven't listed the protein content of special health foods now on the market. There really isn't any need to, as the nutritional content is prominently listed on the labels. If you want to add to your protein intake, why not try one of the following.

FORTIFY YOUR MEALS WITH EXTRA PROTEIN

1. Make your own Hi-Vi milk. Mix 1 cup of powdered skim milk with 1 quart of fresh skim milk. Believe it or not, you have about 74 grams of protein—a whole day's supply of first-class protein in a single bottle. Keep this in the refrigerator and use any time during the day.
2. Add one or more tablespoonfuls of brewers' yeast to all stews and gravies.
3. Add ½ cup of fresh wheat germ to meat loaves and hamburgers, and sprinkle wheat germ over cereals.
4. Use yogurt in place of sour cream.
5. Learn to use soya flour and soya grits in your cooking and baking. Two tablespoons can be added to your favorite recipes for waffles and biscuits. Remember, just 1 cup of soya flour gives you 40 grams of good protein.

The Carbohydrates—Quick-Energy Foods

The chief function of carbohydrates in nutrition is to provide energy for the body (especially for brain function) and for muscular exertion, and to assist in the digestion and assimilation of other foods. In moderation, they are indispensable to the metabolic processes. Taken in excessive quantities, such as when gorging oneself with sweets, pastries, and starchy foods, the carbohydrates cannot be used up by the body and are stored as fat—in the double chin, potbelly, and buttocks. Carbohydrates, as they are broken down by the body, eventually form pyruvic acid, which not only inhibits the disposal of body fat but is actually converted into more fat. It can safely be said that most people overeat on overprocessed, empty carbohydrates.

Another minus factor of excessive carbohydrate intake is that it causes B vitamin deficiency. In an effort to burn up the necessary carbohydrates, the body uses extra B vitamins—which are rarely sufficient for other metabolic needs.

Unfortunately, most Americans eat as much as 20 percent of their daily calories in sugar. White sugar, which is 99.96 percent sucrose, is an empty and problem-causing food. I say it is an empty food because it has no vitamins, no minerals, no protein, no fat—nothing in it has any use except for energy, and the body can draw energy from other, better food sources. Beyond this, sucrose contributes to tooth decay. (More accurately, it is the acids formed from the breakdown of sucrose that cause tooth decay.) And finally, because sugar satisfies hunger, the sugar-eater is often uninterested in foods that might actually provide nutrients. The average consumption of sugar in this country is 102 pounds per person per year. This is the number one vitamin-depleting factor in modern diets.

The best carbohydrates, with all their important vitamins and other nutrients intact, are found chiefly in the whole-grain flours and cereals (maltose), fresh fruits (fructose), fresh vegetables and their juices (fructose and glucose). Nutritionists suggest that at least 1 gram of carbohydrate daily for each 3 pounds of ideal body weight is the absolute minimum necessary for proper body function. This would come to about 40 grams for a 120-pound woman and 50 grams for a 150-pound man. But you would be out of the ordinary if you could keep your carbohydrate consumption this low. For example, many fruit juices contain high amounts of carbohydrates. A cup of grapefruit juice has 23 grams; a cup of fresh orange juice, 26 grams. It would help if you made part of your juice consumption a tall glass of delicious carrot juice (13 grams), tomato juice (10 grams), or sauerkraut juice (6 grams).

For a normal diet, you should allow no more than one third of your calorie intake to come from carbohydrates (1 gram of carbohydrates = 4 calories). The "low-carbohydrate" reducing diet calls for 60 grams of carbohydrates a day, at which rate you would lose weight rather quickly. If you are like most Americans in your consumption of sweets, you will probably have to lower your carbohydrate intake drastically. I strongly urge you to do away with your white-sugar bowl and in its place get one of those nondrip honey jars, especially if you have to feed a large family. Honey is one of our finest natural sweets, containing its own vitamins and minerals.

You never need to worry about not getting enough sugar. You may be surprised to know how many other sources of sugar there are. Practically every mouthful of fruit and vegetables you eat contains sugar. All breads, cereals, dried beans, and other starchy vegetables are changed to sugar in the process of digestion. Even meat and liver contain some starch, which is changed into sugar—and listen to this: about 10 percent of the fats you eat yield glycerin, when digested, and this in turn becomes glucose. In fact, about 65 percent of the food you put into your body is turned to sugar.

Yes, you can get your full quota of sugar without your beloved sugar bowl, and I can promise you that your craving for sweets will become less and less strong as you eat more natural foods. If you crave sweets, you can satisfy that hunger with honey, molasses, sweet fruits, or fruit drinks.

Here is a list of the wholesome carbohydrates you can use with good conscience.

Your Best Carbohydrates

Wheat, rye, barley	Briefly cooked vegetables
Brown rice	Fresh vegetable juices
Whole-grain breads	Fresh fruits
Whole-grain cereals	Fresh fruit juices

Your Best Sweets, If You Must

Honey, unheated	Brown sugar, natural
Unsulphured molasses	Dried fruit, unsulphured
Maple sugar	Carob powder, in place of chocolate

The Good Fats—for Sustained Energy and Smaller Waistlines

Fat is used as a source of sustained energy, as heat insulation under the skin, as a padding for the framework, and to round out the contours of the body. Fat foods supply more than twice the number of calories available from the same amount of protein or carbohydrate. Meals containing some fat have greater "staying power" because fat is more slowly digested and absorbed than all other foodstuffs. This aspect is an important point for those wishing to reduce; it means that the stomach feels full and contented for a longer time.

When liquid vegetable fats are used in normal amounts—never less than 2 tablespoonfuls a day (even on reducing diets)—they are completely and easily digested. Unfortunately, with increased prosperity, Americans, instead of using 25 percent fat in their daily meals, today consume 40 to 50 percent of their calories in hard fats. No wonder Carl Sandburg, our beloved poet, said: "We are dripping in fat." The unsuspecting public doesn't know that so many foods such as crackers, cakes, and cookies are often saturated with the wrong kind of fat (which, incidentally, needn't be animal fat; coconut oil is particularly bad).

In recent years the danger of excess animal fat in the diet has been brought to our attention. The debate regarding the relationship between large amounts of cholesterol in the blood and heart attacks goes on, but the fact remains that hard animal fats do create a high cholesterol level in the blood. The liquid golden vegetable oils do not. In fact, Dr. Bronte Stewart's experiments done in the 1950's showed that when he gave his patients oil instead of animal fat, he actually brought about a rapid decrease in their blood cholesterol.

All animal fats, including cream, butter, lard, and all meat fat, are frequently guilty of contributing to overweight, hardening of the arteries, heart trouble, gallstones, and many other diseases. There are those who say that tension and stress and strain can also create excessive amounts of cholesterol. No doubt that is also true, but diet can be much more easily controlled than one's emotions.

Liquid vegetable oils contain the unsaturated fatty acids—especially linoleic acid, which is so important not only for good health but for good looks. A German chemist, in his experiments with animals, proved that when he deprived his animals of linoleic acid, their skin became dry and scaly and their hair became dry and thin. As soon as the important linoleic acid was returned to the diet, the skin and hair again became normal.

Last, and most important, the vegetable oils, with their rich supply of unsaturated fatty acids, actually stimulate (via the pituitary) the burning of stored fat. Thus you never need to be afraid of these oils—they are not weight adders; instead, they even help to burn up excessive fat deposits.

However, given our modern propensity for processing foods, you should look out for the *kind* of vegetable oil you use. Most oils prepared for commercial consumption are heated and hydrogen is pumped through them (hence, "hydrogenation") to keep them from becoming rancid. The process solidifies oils (giving us margarine). Liquid vegetable oils are so overprocessed that they are not only purged of many nutrients but also pumped with additives, some of which can be harmful. The high heat used to extract these oils destroys amino acids, lecithin, and vitamin E. Besides, hydrogenated oils have just as bad an effect on cholesterol as does animal fat.

It is almost impossible to find fresh crude oil. The next-best thing is "cold-pressed oils," available in health-food stores. "Cold-pressed" is a misleading term because even these oils have been heated to some degree and some nutrients have been lost.

Buy cold-pressed or crude oils (these will be clearly labeled) and keep them refrigerated. These oils will not have chemical additives; they must be carefully kept so they don't turn rancid.

Here is your choice of liquid vegetable oils, with their approximate percentages of the valuable linoleic acid. (Linoleic acid is the major unsaturated acid in these oils. The higher the percentage of linoleic acid, therefore, the more unsaturated the substance.)

Safflower	75	Sesame	43
Sunflower	68	Avocado	39
Poppyseed	62	Peanut	31
Corn	57	Flaxseed	20
Cottonseed	54	Olive	15
Soybean	50	Sardine	15
Wheat-germ	50	Coconut	2

You should be wary of coconut oil, which contains only 2 percent linoleic acid. This makes it what could almost be termed "supersaturated" (butter and lard have something like 4 and 12 percent linoleic acid respectively, putting them higher on the scale toward unsaturatedness). No one uses coconut oil for cooking, but, because of its "better than butter" saturatedness, it turns up in unexpected places—crackers and nondairy coffee creamers. If you want to add a milk product to your coffee when you eat out, why not carry a little packet of powdered milk with you. You'll be better off doing this than trusting chance in some restaurants.

Sunbutter

Many who object to the taste of margarine like the delightful combination of highly unsaturated sunflower oil and fresh butter. Here you have both the health benefits of sunflower oil, with its valuable unsaturated fatty acids, and the excellent taste and vitamins of fresh dairy butter. My cook in Sicily first made a combination of one pound of fresh butter with one cup of olive oil. It is delicious. Of course, Sicilians love the strong olive-oil flavor. However, sunflower oil is cheaper and, from the point of view of saturated fats, better for you. For an all-around delightful buttery combination, on toast or sandwiches and over cooked vegetables, use butter mixed with one of the milder oils; cold-pressed sunflower oil makes the best-tasting combination. It is most important, when using oils, that they be absolutely fresh. Sunflower oil stays fresh much longer than safflower oil and is ideal for our sunbutter:

Sunbutter

1 pound fresh dairy butter
1 cup sunflower oil
Season to taste

Place fresh butter in bowl and whip until soft and smooth. Gradually add sunflower oil, and mix thoroughly. When blended, put mixture in square butter dish or small cake pan and place in refrigerator until hard enough to be cut into squares or pats.

For variety, spike mixture with vegetable salt, your favorite herbs, or fresh garlic. Keep refrigerated at all times.

Food cooked with sunbutter will delight a gourmet!

Meet the Wonder Foods

There are certain foods I call "wonder foods" because they are so full of concentrated goodness, so inexpensive, so readily available, that they are indeed wonderful. They provide excellent quantities of many of the hard-to-get B vitamins; or they are rich in easily digested protein—and ease of digestion is of great importance, especially in the second half of life. They also provide generous quantities of calcium and iron, two minerals that become more and more difficult to obtain from ordinary foods. These wonder foods can also easily be eaten every day without becoming tiresome, and they can be mixed with other foods to add valuable nutritive factors. I talk a great deal about them, for I am convinced that if they are used generously, they will so improve the nutritive quality of the diet that your health is bound to be benefited. Wonder foods can also help you to look younger and live longer.

Brewers' Yeast

This wonder food has been found to contain 17 different vitamins, including all of the B family; 16 amino acids; and 14 minerals, including the "trace" minerals, held to be essential. It also contains 36 percent protein (sirloin steak, not counting the bone, may contain as little as 23 percent protein). Brewers' yeast contains only 1 percent fat, whereas sirloin steak contains 22 percent!

The calorie requirement of the average woman is about 2,000 per day. One tablespoonful of brewers' yeast adds up to only one-hundredth of this calorie requirement, but it provides over one third of my generous daily allowance of vitamin B_1 (thiamine) and very nearly one fifth each of the vitamin B_2 (riboflavin) and niacin allowances.

Remember, the amount of brewers' yeast we are talking about is just *one tablespoonful*—8 grams, only 22 calories! Think how easy it is to add to your B vitamins and iron. To be sure that you get a true abundance, simply stir a tablespoonful of brewers' yeast into a glass of tomato juice, fruit juice, or buttermilk, or sprinkle it over your salad or your whole-grain cereal.

The figures given here are derived from ordinary brewers' yeast. Specially cultured strains, sometimes referred to as food yeast, are even richer in B vitamins. When you purchase brewers' yeast, examine the label carefully. It should always give you in 8 grams (a little over one-fourth ounce) not less than 0.78 milligram of vitamin B_1, 0.44 milligram of vitamin B_2, and 2.9 milligrams of niacin. Do not be confused if the label states the quantity in micrograms. There are 1,000 micrograms in one milligram; therefore, 0.78 milligram would be 780 micrograms. If you encounter micrograms and want to transpose them into milligrams, just move the decimal point three places to the left. The food yeasts, which are richer in vitamins than ordinary brewers' yeast, cost only a little more and are cheaper in the long run because they give you more vitamins. Moreover, they are more convenient to store, since you need a smaller quantity. If you do not care for the flavor of ordinary brewers' yeast, you can obtain it in a pleasantly flavored form.

I use the terms *brewers' yeast* and *food yeast* because these indicate a palatable form of yeast. Many kinds of yeast are produced, primarily for baking, that have an unpleasant, bitter taste. If you have trouble finding brewers' yeast, any diet or health-food shop will have it on hand. *Under no circumstances should you ever eat fresh yeast, which is intended for baking.*

If you have never supplemented your diet with brewers' yeast or food yeast, start slowly. Many poorly nourished people lack the enzymes necessary to digest yeast, and may be troubled with indigestion and bloating. If you are a beginner, start slowly with a very small amount, a half teaspoon or less, and gradually work up to the full tablespoon as your body responds.

Powdered Skim Milk

Powdered skim milk has many properties that cause me to classify it as a wonder food. First and foremost, it gives you protein of high biologic quality, practically free from fat, and in combination with rich quantities of calcium and riboflavin (vitamin B_2). Moreover, its vital nutritive factors are in a form readily available to the body and easily digested. Of secondary importance is its convenient physical form; being a dry powder, it can be kept on hand at all times. It is well to store it in an airtight container, preferably a metal one with a screw-on closure provided with a rubber liner. This will exclude the moisture of the air and light, prevent the product from "staling" or becoming lumpy, and also preserve its riboflavin content.

Add powdered skim milk (also called instant nonfat dry milk) to fresh milk, sauces, soups, custards, waffles, muffins, and all breads; no change of recipe is necessary. It is also delicious whipped into potatoes.

A nourishing beverage for everyone—youngsters and oldsters alike—can be made by mixing one-half cup of powdered skim milk into a quart of whole or skimmed fluid milk. If whole milk is used, the calories are increased by only about 20 percent, whereas the vital food factors are increased by the following percentages: protein, 62.3; calcium, 62.5; iron, 50; vitamin B_1, 60; vitamin B_2, 100; niacin, 63.

YOGURT

Yogurt is an important wonder food because it is an excellent source of easily assimilated, high-quality protein and contributes significant quantities of calcium and riboflavin to the diet. Yogurt fills a need that has long existed—for that between-meal or bedtime snack when so many people eat what I call "foodless foods" —devil's food cakes, or cinnamon toast made with white bread lavishly sprinkled with white sugar. A taste for yogurt is acquired quickly; you will become fonder and fonder of it as time goes on. It is a good hunger satisfier and, most important of all, contributes much-needed vital food factors with every mouthful. A cup of yogurt fortified with powdered skim milk provides only about 7 percent of the calories for a 2,000-calorie-a-day diet; at the same time it provides, in terms of my generous daily allowances: protein, 17.5 percent; calcium, 50 percent; and vitamin B_2, 30 percent.

Yogurt and the acidophilus cultured milks have undergone many ups and downs in popularity. They have been advocated for everything from "that tired feeling" to typhoid fever. My interest in yogurt is wholly concerned with *nutrition,* and from a nutritional point of view it is tops.

Bulgarians are credited with retaining vigor, vitality, and the characteristics of youth to an extremely advanced age; their longevity is traditional. Yogurt and certain cultured milks constitute a major item of diet for the Bulgarian peasant. To state that all of these virtues stem solely from the consumption of yogurt is to treat the subject most superficially; climate, heredity, and other factors must be considered. But clearly the Bulgarians have established the nutritional excellency of yogurt. That, and that alone, first attracted me to yogurt and caused me to investigate and study it. Its superior nutritive qualities caused me to recommend it to my students, and my faith in it has been justified in every respect. The extent to which the bacteria present in yogurt may reach the colon is to me of incidental interest only. They are "friendly" and helpful bacteria, active in the synthesis of certain B vitamins, and the acid they produce from milk sugar tends to suppress the activities of pathogenic and putrefactive types of organisms. If yogurt eaters receive these benefits in any measure at all, they are just that much ahead.

While excellent yogurt can be purchased in dairy and food stores, the homemade variety is far less expensive and can be made with inexpensive skim milk. With the growing popularity of the home yogurt-maker, there has been a growing sophistication about the taste of good, fresh yogurt. A recipe for my own favorite yogurt appears in chapter 28 (see index).

Yogurt can be eaten plain, seasoned with chives or other herbs, served with fresh or canned fruits, or made into a sundae with maple syrup, honey, or molasses. Real yogurt connoisseurs prefer it plain! I'm indeed sorry that many dairies now sell "jazzed-up" yogurt, loaded with white sugar and glucose preserves. Buy it plain or—better still—make your own.

The World's Best Cereal—Fresh Wheat Germ

Fresh wheat germ is worth its weight in gold. It takes its place on my list of wonder foods as an outstanding source of vitamin B_1. One-half cup provides about three and a half times my generous daily allowance of this important vitamin.

Fresh wheat germ should be sprinkled over hot or cold cereals. Excellent hot cakes, waffles, muffins, and breads can be prepared by substituting from one-half to one cup of wheat germ for an equivalent quantity of flour. If you own an electric blender, you can make delicious drinks with a pint of any fruit juice, a small section of banana, and half a cup of wheat germ.

Wheat germ also contains vitamin E. Man, over centuries of time, became adapted to the consumption of whole cereal grains, including the germ. He cannot now lightly drop the germ from his diet. Many modern processes of refining natural foods have led to a number of dietary deficiencies, some of them dramatically clear-cut, others more subtle and difficult to identify.

If at all possible, do get the fresh wheat germ. If you live near a mill that produces it, by all means buy it directly. If not, you will find it on sale at your local health-food shop. Not only is the fresh wheat germ better for you but it will cost about half as much as the processed toasted wheat germ. Stored in a tight can or jar in a cool place, it will keep its freshness for a month. And above all, avoid the "processed" wheat germ that has other ingredients added—especially foodless white sugar. The best wheat germ is made in France. There the Moulin de Paris exposes the freshly milled wheat germ to the rays of a powerful ultraviolet lamp, which adds sweetness and brings out the natural flavor of the "heart of the wheat." In chapter 24 you will find a recipe for making your own Honeyed Wheat Germ (see index).

UNSULPHURED MOLASSES

For many years I have advocated the use of blackstrap molasses because it is an unusually rich source of iron and the B vitamins. The late Dr. Tom Spies, of Hillman Hospital in Birmingham, Alabama, first told me of the wonders he performed with it. It has long been an important staple in the diets of many Southerners in the United States. However, because of its unusual taste, it invokes in most people a strong *yes* or *no*—and, unfortunately, more often *no* than *yes*. So, if you are one of those who say *no* to blackstrap molasses, use instead the darkest molasses you can find, or mix a little blackstrap in with your regular molasses, which should be the unsulphured kind. Molasses is made from the residue left from making sugar out of sugar cane. "Sulphured" molasses is bleached with potassium to make it more attractive. This process, of course, destroys important nutrients.

Molasses is an excellent source of nutritionally available iron. Moreover, it is the best source of natural sugar, and it also provides significant quantities of thiamine and riboflavin.

I list it as a wonder food primarily for its rich iron content. It lends itself in dozens of ways to the preparation of foods; added to muffins, waffles, spiced cookies, and the like, it enriches them significantly with much-needed iron. Milk is poor in iron, yet the growing youngster requires three or four glasses a day; a tablespoonful of molasses stirred into each glass turns an iron-poor food into an iron-rich one, providing from 50 to 75 percent of the daily iron allowance. Used in place of table syrups, which for the most part are nascent sugar solutions, its nutritional superiority is undoubted.

Six-Course Dinner Growing on One Tree

Mother Nature put many of her best ingredients into a fruit-vegetable that grows on a tree—the avocado. In each avocado (or alligator pear) are combined the proteins of meat, the fat of butter (unsaturated, as an extra bonus), the vitamins and minerals of vegetables, and the flavor of nuts. You might say that the avocado is a complete meal from soup to nuts.

The protein content of the avocado is the equal of many kinds of meat; when fully ripe, the fruit contains little starch and practically no sugar. It offers generous quantities of calcium, magnesium, potassium, sodium, copper, phosphates, manganese, and iron. It is loaded with vitamins A, B_1, B_2, and C and has some vitamins D and E.

About one fourth of the avocado consists of fat or oil. What makes avocado oil so valuable is its high percentage of polyunsaturated fatty acids. This oil gives the avocado its mellow texture and nutlike flavor. The Mexicans call the soft green pulp "butter growing on trees"; and they spread it generously on their tortillas. A very ripe, soft avocado, mashed with a few drops of lemon juice and spiked with herbs, makes an utterly delicious dressing over fruit and vegetable salads. Because the vegetable oils are easily burned by the body, even overweighters can enjoy this "green butter."

Vitamins and Minerals for Longer Life

Dr. H. C. Sherman, in his longevity experiments at Columbia University, pointed out again and again that more vitamins are necessary for a long and healthy life. He insisted that the ideal intake of vitamins should be four times the recommended maintenance amount. I couldn't agree more and make the same recommendation to my students.

Today, 80 percent of the foods available to us have been meddled with to prevent them from spoiling; a great deal of their important nutrients are lost. For this and many other reasons, intelligent people the world over have learned to fortify and supplement their diets with extra vitamins and minerals. In the next few pages I shall list the foods and nutrients that help fortify and supplement the average diet. Do not hesitate to use extra vitamin concentrates, but *not* at the expense of the good basic foods—these must always come first.

Vitamin A

Dr. Sherman particularly stresses an abundance of vitamins A and C, together with the B vitamins. First, we shall deal with vitamin A, which is important for good eyesight and healthy skin. In the interests of a longer and healthier life, your daily diet should provide you with about 15,000 to 20,000 units (following Dr. Sherman's rule of four times the minimum requirements). The following table gives you the best sources of vitamin A. The values given are generally for cooked foods, unless the foods are commonly eaten raw, as is fruit.

Foods for Vitamin A

RICH SOURCES	SERVING	UNITS
*Liver, lamb's	3 ounces	42,930
Dandelion greens	1 cup	27,310
Spinach	1 cup	21,200
*Liver, calf's	3 ounces	19,130
Carrots, diced	1 cup	18,130
Turnip greens	1 cup	15,370
Collards	1 cup	14,500
Squash, Hubbard	1 cup	12,690
Sweet potato	1 medium	11,410
Beet greens	1 cup	10,790
Mustard greens	1 cup	10,050
Kale	1 cup	9,220
Pumpkin	1 cup	7,750
Cantaloupe	½ medium	6,190
Broccoli	1 cup	5,100
GOOD SOURCES		
Apricots	3 whole fruit	2,990
*Kidney, lamb's	3 ounces	980
Tomato	1 medium	1,640
Cheese, American	2 x 1 x 1 inches	740
Peas, green	1 cup	1,150
*Egg	1 large	550
*Butter	1 tablespoon	460
Peach, fresh	1 medium	880
Beans, green	1 cup	830
Asparagus	6 stalks	760
Corn, yellow	1 med. ear	500

*These foods contain actual vitamin A, which is about twice as effective in the body as carotene (provitamin A), provided by foods not marked with an asterisk.

Here's how to fortify your daily meals with more vitamin A:

1. A cup of finely chopped carrots added to your green-salad bowl gives you an added 13,000 units of vitamin A.
2. A piece of inexpensive lamb's liver, about 4 ounces, ground up with your meat loaf or hamburger, fortifies it with about 57,000 units of vitamin A.
3. Adding just 1 cup of finely chopped spinach, turnip tops, or parsley to stews or soups fortifies them with thousands of additional units of vitamin A.
4. Use an egg yolk for thickening gravies instead of pasty white flour. Each egg yolk gives you an additional 500 units of vitamin A.
5. The richest source of vitamin A is fish-liver oils, which doctors and dietitians recommend for extra fortification. Because vitamin A is fat-soluble and is not readily excreted, it, unlike most other vitamins, can be stored in the body. In rare instances, overdoses have been reported. Because of fear of this, small fish-liver-oil vitamin capsules containing 25,000 units, which have been available until recently, are now off the market by order of the F.D.A. (The F.D.A. has restricted capsule dosage to 10,000 units.) At the moment the National Health Foundation has brought a suit against the F.D.A., and hopefully this miserable law will be reversed. In the meantime, I simply take two capsules, right after meals, for a total of 20,000 units.

Those Important B Vitamins

The B vitamins represent an extensive family; its many members play a wide variety of roles in the economy of the body. The maintenance requirements of the three best-known members of the family—thiamine (B_1), riboflavin (B_2), and niacin—are well established and agreed upon by the authorities. These three B vitamins are all important for energy metabolism. Beyond that, thiamine is best known for its ability to prevent beriberi, a nerve disease. Niacin is important in the treatment of pellagra, whose symptoms are described as the three D's: dermatitis, diarrhea, and dementia. Riboflavin is not associated with any one disease, but mild deficiencies may result in light sensitivity and dimness of vision. Maintenance requirements suffice only to protect the body against deficiency diseases and should not be confused with the requirements for buoyant health and longevity. My generous daily allowance for a total of 100 percent (see chart below) of these three B vitamins significantly exceeds the maintenance requirement.

Here's how to fortify your meals with the vitamin B family foods:

1. Sprinkle fresh wheat germ or corn germ over green salads, over hot or cold cereals; also add 1 tablespoonful to every cup of flour in all your baking.
2. Use fresh wheat germ in place of bread crumbs to coat fish or veal chops.
3. Eat several cups of yogurt a day, and use it in place of sour cream.
4. Add a tablespoon of food yeast to all gravies, stews, and tomato juice.
5. Have broiled liver at least twice a week. The less-expensive beef or lamb's liver is just as rich as calf's liver.
6. Use molasses or honey for sweetening instead of white sugar.
7. If you eat out a lot, it is wise to take a high-potency all-in-one vitamin capsule right after your meal.

To render the table as informative as possible, the values for the three B vitamins are given in milligrams and in percentages of my generous allowance. The table is compiled in descending order of the percent of thiamine present, as adequate quantities of thiamine are the most difficult to obtain of the three.

You can see from the table opposite that these three vitamins are much harder to get than, for example, vitamins A and C. The B vitamins are present in foods in much smaller amounts than vitamins A and C.

In addition, diets high in sugar (in other words, the average American diet) burn up the B vitamins at a fast rate, thus making it necessary to supply even higher quantities. Better yet, why not reduce your sugar intake.

No single food will provide 100 percent of a generous requirement of *thiamine* in an ordinary serving. Of the twenty-eight foods listed, only five provide between 25 and 39 percent, and eighteen of the twenty-eight foods provide less than 10 percent per serving. For *riboflavin*, only three foods, all of which are

Food for Thiamine, Riboflavin, and Niacin*

FOOD	SERVING	B_1 THIAMINE MGS.	% HDR	B_2 RIBO-FLAVIN MGS.	% HDR	NIACIN MGS.	% HDR
Brewers' yeast	1 tablespoon	.78	39	.44	17.6	2.9	19.3
Peas, split, raw	½ cup	.76	38	.28	11.1	3.15	21.0
Wheat germ	½ cup	.7	35	.27	10.8	1.6	10.6
Soybean flour, low-fat	½ cup	.55	27.5	.18	7.2	1.45	9.7
Heart, beef, raw	3 ounces	.5	25	.75	30.0	6.6	44.0
Flour, whole-wheat	½ cup	.33	16.5	.07	2.8	2.6	17.3
Rice, brown, raw	½ cup	.33	16.5	.05	2.0	4.8	32.0
Kidney, beef	3 ounces	.32	16.0	2.16	87.0	5.5	36.0
Flour, white, enriched	½ cup	.24	12.0	.145	5.8	1.9	12.6
Skim milk, dry	½ cup	.21	10.5	1.175	47.0	0.7	4.65
Liver, calf's	3 ounces	.18	9.0	2.65	106.0	13.7	93.0
Liver, beef	2 ounces	.15	7.5	2.25	90.0	8.4	56.0
Lamb, leg	3 ounces	.12	6.0	.21	8.4	4.4	29.4
Oatmeal	½ cup	.11	5.5	.025	1.0	0.4	2.66
Peanuts	¼ cup	.105	5.25	.05	2.0	6.0	40.0
Turkey	4 ounces	.1	5.0	.16	6.4	9.1	60.0
Turnip greens	1 cup	.09	4.5	.59	23.5	1.0	6.7
Chicken	4 ounces	.09	4.5	.18	7.2	9.1	60.0
Bacon, medium-fat	2 slices	.08	4.0	.05	2.0	0.8	5.3
Kale	1 cup	.08	4.0	.25	10.0	1.9	12.6
Peanut butter	¼ cup	.08	4.0	.08	3.2	10.4	69.5
Bread, whole-wheat	1 ½-inch slice	.07	3.5	.03	1.2	.7	4.65
Molasses	1 tablespoon	.06	3.0	.05	2.0	.4	2.66
Beef, sirloin	3 ounces	.06	3.0	.16	6.4	4.1	27.4
Rice, converted	½ cup	.05	2.5	.01	0.4	.95	6.3
Egg	1 medium	.05	2.5	.14	5.7	—	—
Salmon, red	3 ounces	.03	1.5	.14	5.7	6.2	41.4
Cheese, American	2x1x1 inches	.02	1.0	.24	9.6	—	—

* In the tables, you will find "% HDR"—that is, percentage of Hauser's Daily Requirement in the right-hand column. These figures will give you a generous amount of the vitamins, far above the recommended daily doses.

organ meats, provide between 87 and 106 percent. One-half cup of skim milk provides 47 percent, and another food (another organ meat) provides 30 percent. All the rest provide less than 25 percent, with the majority falling below 10 percent. *Niacin* is a little more richly distributed; however, no single food provides

100 percent of Hauser's Daily Requirement (HDR) per serving, and only one as much as 90 percent.

The Lesser-Known B Vitamins

The lesser-known B vitamins, even though they have been known (and synthesized) for years, still labor under the legend "Their need in human nutrition is not yet established." That appears on the label of all vitamin concentrates containing these lesser-known B vitamins. As the legend is misunderstood by many people, let's talk about what it might mean.

It is required by law that the above statement about nutrition be placed on the label of all products containing the lesser-known B vitamins, if the claim is made that they are present. The purpose of the law is to protect the public against imposition, and it is laudable in every respect, since the law was made at a time when there were virtually no data to indicate that such vitamins were needed by humans. You see, in general these vitamins display a subtle and diffused effect in the body. Whereas thiamine deficiency, for example, causes the disease beriberi, which can be reversed by the administration of adequate amounts of the vitamin, the lesser-known B vitamins do not appear to be associated with such clear-cut deficiency diseases. For example, choline and inositol, either separately or in combination, have been found to play a role in preventing and relieving atherosclerosis, or "fatty" hardening of the arteries (see chapter 10). However, as the condition involved is slow in developing, requiring a good portion of a lifetime, the shortage of these vitamins does not display its effect so quickly or dramatically as a shortage of thiamine or niacin.

Discoveries like these have led some leading nutritional authorities to make recommendations as to the desirable quantity of certain lesser-known B vitamins in the diet. As expressed by these authorities: ". . . In some cases where there *may* be no nutritional requirement under normal circumstances, it is nevertheless suggested that a level of these vitamins be provided in the diet as a precaution, in view of our lack of knowledge regarding the subject."

PYRIDOXINE—VITAMIN B_6

Vitamin B_6 is an important factor in the breakdown of unsaturated fatty acids and in the use of protein by the body. It also stimulates the production of antibodies (which are proteins, after all) and thus aids in fending off disease. Claims have been made for its usefulness in treating anemia, Parkinson's disease, cerebral palsy, and other nerve problems. Suffice it to say, it's a necessary part of your diet. It is especially important to get good amounts of it during pregnancy.

Foods for Pyridoxine—B_6

FOOD	SERVING	PERCENT HDR
Beef liver	4 ounces	60
Banana	1 medium	27
Lima beans, dry	1 cup	26
Sweet potato	1 medium	26
Cabbage, cooked	1 cup	24
Chicken, broiled	8 ounces	20
Cabbage, raw, shredded	1 cup	19
Brewers' yeast	1 heaping tablespoon	18
Lettuce	½ head	11
Irish potato, baked	1 medium	11
Spinach, cooked	1 cup	10
Turnips, diced, cooked	1 cup	9
Beef heart, cooked	3 ounces	9
Halibut	4 × 3 × ½ inches	7
Veal cutlet, no bone	3 ounces	7
Peanuts, roasted	¼ cup	7
Beef, round steak, no bone	4 ounces	6
Green peas	1 cup	5
Cantaloupe	½ large	4
Dark molasses	1 tablespoon	4
Apple	1 average	4
Wheat germ	1 tablespoon	2
Cauliflower, cooked	1 cup	2
Cheese, American	1 1-inch cube	1
Whole milk	1 cup	1
Egg	1 medium	1

CALCIUM PANTOTHENATE

This B vitamin has been shown to stabilize the adrenal glands and in this way is thought to help keep the natural color of our hair. Also, it has been shown to be an important nutrient for the nervous system.

Foods for Pantothenic Acid

FOOD	SERVING	PERCENT HDR
Beef liver	4 ounces	58
Broccoli	1 cup	21
Chicken, broiled	8 ounces	12–20
Mushrooms	10 large	17
Beef heart, lean	3 ounces	17
Whole wheat	1 cup	15
Beef brains	3 ounces	15
Wheat bran	1 cup	14
Wheat germ	1 cup	13
Egg	1 medium	13
Oysters	1 cup, 13–19 medium	12
Sweet potato	1 medium	11
Cauliflower, cooked	1 cup	11
Soybeans, dry	¼ cup	10
Green peas	1 cup	9–16
Cauliflower buds, raw	1 cup	9
Roasted peanuts	¼ cup	9
Orange	1 medium	8
Lima beans, dry, cooked	1 cup	7
Whole milk	1 cup	7
Salmon	½ cup	6–11
Lamb, leg	3 ounces	5
Rolled oats, cooked	1 cup	5
Ham, smoked	4 ounces	4–7
Irish potato	1 medium	4–6
Cheese, American	1 1-inch cube	1–3
Bacon, broiled	4 slices	1–3
Veal cutlet	3 ounces	1–2
Whole-wheat bread	1 ½-inch slice	1

INOSITOL

The effect of this B vitamin, together with another B vitamin, choline, is that of protecting against fatty hardening of the arteries. Choline and inositol function in this way by maintaining cholesterol in solution, in other words, by keeping it from forming deposits in the arteries. Inositol has also been reported to aid in utilization of vitamin E.

Foods for Inositol

FOOD	SERVING	PERCENT HDR
Orange	1 large	49
Wheat germ	1 cup	48
Grapefruit	½ medium	40
Watermelon	¹⁄₁₆ melon 16 × 10 inches	30
Peas, green	1 cup	26
Beef heart, lean	3 ounces	22
Cantaloupe	½ medium	22
Whole wheat	1 cup	20
Peas, dry	⅓ cup	20
Beef brains	3 ounces	17
Lima beans, dry	1 cup	15
Cabbage, cooked	1 cup	13
Lettuce	½ head, medium	12
Cauliflower, cooked	1 cup	11
Peaches, frozen	4 ounces	11
Chicken, broiled	½ bird, 8 ounces	11
Oysters, raw	1 cup (13–19 medium)	10
Onion, dry	1 medium	10
Cauliflower buds, raw, diced	1 cup	9
Cabbage, raw, shredded	1 cup	9
Strawberries	1 cup	9
Sweet potato, baked	1 medium	8
Tomato, raw	1 medium	7
Roasted peanuts	¼ cup	6
Turnips, diced	1 cup	6
Beef liver	4 ounces	6
Corn meal, white	1 cup	5

Lamb, leg	3 ounces	5
Raisins	¼ cup	5
Spinach	1 cup	5
Banana	1 medium	4
Whole milk	1 cup	4
Ham	4 ounces	3–6
Apple	1 medium	3
Veal cutlet	3 ounces	3
Irish potato	1 medium	3
Carrot	1 medium	2
Halibut	4 × 3 × ½ inches	2
Mushrooms	10 large	2
Salmon	½ cup	2
Egg	1 medium	2
Whole-wheat bread	1 ½-inch slice	1
Beef, round steak	4 ounces	1
Cheese, American	1-inch cube	1

BIOTIN

Man is less likely to be deficient of this B vitamin than any of the others, for it is made in appreciable amounts in the intestinal tract. It is essential to certain enzymes of the body fluids. Only very little is needed, about 0.15 to 0.3 milligrams per day. The best sources of biotin are beef liver, chicken, oysters, mushrooms, peanuts, lima beans, and eggs.

FOLIC ACID

This is an important B vitamin, essential to the proper formation of red blood (and therefore necessary for the prevention of anemia) and also important for the growth of cells. Like biotin, this can be synthesized in the intestines. The quantity required is again very little, about 0.2 milligrams a day. The best sources of folic acid are salmon, watermelon, oysters, spinach, lima beans, chicken, cantaloupe, and whole wheat.

CHOLINE

This, in partnership with inositol, performs a valuable service in keeping cholesterol from accumulating in the arteries. Choline, which is a part of lecithin (I will have much more to say about lecithin in a moment), is important for liver, kidney, brain, and nerve functions. The exact amount of choline required daily has not been established for man, but foods rich in choline should be used frequently in the diet.

Foods for Choline

FOOD	SERVING	MILLIGRAMS
Beef liver	4 ounces	790
Spinach	1 cup	425
Beans, green	1 cup	425
Cabbage, cooked	1 cup	420
Kidney, lamb's	3 ounces	306
Egg yolk	from 1 egg	289
Wheat germ	1 cup	272
Cabbage, raw, shredded	1 cup	250
Asparagus, cut tips	1 cup	227
Rolled oats, cooked	1 cup	222
Soybeans	¼ cup	185
Turnip, diced	1 cup	126
Whole wheat	1 cup	108
Beef	4 ounces	101
Irish potato	1 medium	99
Dried skim milk	½ cup	96
Lamb	3 ounces	94
Liver sausage	1 slice 3¼ × ¼ inches	73
Peanuts, roasted	¼ cup	60
Carrot, raw	1 medium	48
Sweet potato	1 medium	42
Corn on the cob	1 medium	37
Whole milk	1 cup	31
Bologna	1 piece, 2⅛-inch diameter × ½ inch	30
Cheese, American	1 ounce	14
Beets, diced	1 cup	13
Pecans, halves	¼ cup	11
Butter	1 tablespoon	8

CHOLINE AND INOSITOL PROMOTE LECITHIN PRODUCTION

Choline, inositol, and methionine (an amino acid that can be found in all complete proteins) all work together to promote the production of lecithin in the body. This invaluable substance can also be ingested. Dr. Lester M. Morrison, in his fine book *The Low-Fat Way to Health and Longer Life,* describes lecithin as one of the most important nutritional supplements developed in the last fifty years. I have known about lecithin since I was a schoolboy in Germany. Our family doctor insisted that we children, and especially my sisters, have it in its natural form of beaten egg yolk, in fruit juice or sherry wine; it was the only form in which we knew it then. In Germany at that time it was considered a very good food for the nerves.

Lecithin is better known now. We know today that it can be a lifesaver because it is a natural emulsifier of fat, and fat is the enemy of the heart, whether it is part of the added burden of overweight or a direct cause of high cholesterol in the arteries.

The Chinese and Japanese suffer very little heart disease. In their diet—which is so poor by our standards—the soybean has been the keystone. They call it their holy bean, their meat without a bone. It has been their flesh, fowl, milk, cheese, and oil for thousands of years. We now know that there is a likely connection. The soybean is one of the richest natural sources of lecithin. I beg you to use soybean oil; also try some of the soybean dishes I describe in the recipe section.

Mr. Edward R. Hewitt, who wrote that charming book *The Years Between 75 and 90,* learned about the tremendous benefits of lecithin while studying in Germany. Here is what he has to say: "Lecithin is well known to have a very great emulsifying action on fats. It is reasonable to suppose that it would have the same emulsifying action in the body . . . With older people the fats remain high in the blood for from 5 to 7 hours, and in some cases as long as 20 hours, thus giving the fats more time to become located in the tissues. If lecithin is given to older people before a fatty meal it has been found that the fats in the blood return to normal in a short time, in the same way they do in younger people . . . I myself also have observed that my memory is better than it was before I took lecithin regularly. My nervous reactions are still perfectly normal at 88. My hands are much steadier than those of any doctor who tested me." I leave it to you to decide how you want to add lecithin to your life—through soy products, eggs, or as a diet supplement—but don't neglect it in your plans for a healthier you.

B_{12}

A more recently discovered vitamin, B_{12}, has been shown to be necessary for the treatment of nerve damage associated with pernicious anemia. Vitamin B_{12} comes equipped with a mineral (cobalt) as part of its molecule—the only vitamin to have this feature. Sufficient daily doses of B_{12} are contained in milk and, of course, liver.

Vitamin C—Ascorbic Acid

Nobel Prize–winning scientist Dr. Linus Pauling says that large doses of vitamin C can prevent and treat the common cold. As a direct result of Dr. Pauling's work, many orthodox scientists and physicians, who in the past dismissed the use of vitamins to treat disease, have been stimulated to see for themselves the preventive and healing powers of ascorbic acid. In 1972, five studies were reported to show that high doses of vitamin C (at least one gram a day) reduce cold symptoms and occurrences. Other doctors have claimed that high doses produce bad side effects; I have yet to see this. The debate still goes on. If your family is plagued with colds, you might enjoy reading Dr. Pauling's exciting book *Vitamin C and the Common Cold.*

But vitamin C can do more for you than just help out with your occasional colds. It is necessary to prevent scurvy, for instance, and Dr. Sherman stresses the value of vitamin C in the retention of youthful characteristics and in lengthening the span of life—to add more youthful years.

There is no reason why anyone should fail to get an abundant supply of this very important vitamin from the diet. The generous use of citrus fruits, tomatoes, and green leafy vegetables is all that is required—but do use them generously.

In the table that follows, the rich and good food sources are listed. At least 100 to 150 milligrams of vitamin C per day are recommended for good health. If you smoke or if you feel a cold coming on, higher doses are in order.

Foods for Ascorbic Acid (Vitamin C)

FOOD	SERVING	MILLIGRAMS
Rose-hip powder	100 grams	500*
Orange juice	1 cup	122
Broccoli	1 cup	111
Grapefruit juice	1 cup	99
Strawberries	1 cup	89
Turnip greens	1 cup	87
Collards	1 cup	84
Pepper, green	1 medium	77
Mustard greens	1 cup	63
Brussels sprouts	1 cup	61
Cantaloupe	½ medium	59
Kale	1 cup	56
Spinach	1 cup	54
Cabbage, cooked	1 cup	53
Cabbage, raw, shredded	1 cup	50
Asparagus, cut spears	1 cup	40
Tomato juice	1 cup	38
Tomato	1 medium	35
Cauliflower	1 cup	34
Pineapple, fresh, diced	1 cup	33
Liver, calf's	3 ounces	30
Chard, leaves only	1 cup	30
Dandelion greens	1 cup	29
Sweet potato	1 medium	28
Tangerine	1 medium	25
Lima beans, immature	1 cup	24
Peas, green	1 cup	24
Beet greens	1 cup	22
Liver, beef	2 ounces	18
Endive	1 cup	18
Beans, green	1 cup	18

*Sometimes even more, depending on variety.

Here's how to fortify meals with extra vitamin C:

1. Have citrus fruit cups often, either as appetizers or for dessert. (Eating the fruit is preferable to drinking the juice for reducers. The pulp helps to prevent that hungry feeling.)
2. Add to salad dressing the juice of 1 lemon.
3. Sprinkle lemon juice and vegetable salt on all flat-tasting vegetables.
4. Drink at least 1 glass of fresh vegetable juice a day.
5. Fortify tomato juice with a tablespoon of lemon juice and spike with herbs.
6. Add ½ cup of chopped dark-green parsley to your stews, salads, dressings, hamburgers, mashed potatoes. Tastes wonderful; the vitamin C is free.
7. Serve pink rose-hip tea with meals, as they do in Switzerland. And serve rose-hip jam for breakfast, or use high-potency rose-hip tablets. (Those coming from the Scandinavian countries are the most potent.)

When taking high doses of vitamin C, it is best to drink milk or take calcium tablets with it to prevent stomach irritation.

In Northern Europe, where oranges and lemons are very expensive, many housewives have learned to grow their own inexpensive vitamin C. Some rose hips contain twenty times as much of this important vitamin as citrus fruit, and the wild Scandinavian varieties are even richer. Rose hips are easily grown, and the most nutritious variety can now be bought in the United States. The *Rosa rugosa* bushes grow the large, meaty variety, which can be used for jam, syrup, marmalade, and a delightful beverage—the pink rose-hip tea that is the great favorite at the famous Bircher-Benner Sanatorium in Switzerland. Even if you have only a small plot, plant some "vitamin roses," as the Russians call them.

Rose-Hip Marmalade: The ruby-red seed of the rose makes an excellent marmalade. If you have been to Switzerland or Sweden, you have probably enjoyed it for breakfast. Simply soak the cleaned rose hips for 2 hours in plain cold water; then let boil for 2 hours, and strain. Measure the purée, and add 1 cup of brown sugar to each cup of rose-hip purée. Let boil down to thick consistency, pour into sterilized glasses, and seal.

Vitamin D

Certain misunderstandings are current regarding vitamin D, to the effect that it is not needed by adults. Nothing could be further from the fact, and after forty it assumes an increased importance. There is need for an abundance of calcium all through life; and as we get older, for a variety of reasons, we do not absorb calcium as efficiently as we should. However, if vitamin D is present in the body in adequate amounts, the absorption of calcium is promoted (and also the absorption of phosphorus, which functions like calcium in the body but must be constantly replaced).

Almost no common foods contain vitamin D in significant amounts. The quantity present in butter, which is consumed daily in relatively small amounts, is so small that butter is out of consideration as a dietary source of vitamin D. Fortified whole milk provides 102 units of vitamin D per eight full ounces (a cup or drinking glass brimming full); thus four glasses, or a quart, would have to be consumed daily to meet requirements. Because of the fat in whole milk, this quantity amounts to 664 calories, which few adults can afford to use up solely on milk. Vitamin D is not present in skim milk or buttermilk.

Eggs vary in vitamin D content according to the diet of the hens. An egg will vary between 25 and 65 units. Clearly, eggs cannot be relied upon as the sole source of vitamin D in the body. Four ounces a day of tuna fish or Atlantic herring would provide adequate vitamin D, and four ounces per day of mackerel or canned salmon would go a long way toward supplying it; but obviously the daily consumption of these fish is impractical, not to say monotonously impossible.

Vitamin D is produced in the skin in the presence of sunlight through the conversion of cholesterol to vitamin D. An adult reasonably exposed to sunlight, in amounts sufficient to produce a reasonable tan every season, doubtless has sufficient vitamin D produced in the skin. However, persons who do not, or for any reason cannot, obtain adequate exposure to sunshine would do well to fortify their diet with fish-liver-oil concentrates of vitamin

D. The daily requirement for maintenance is set at 400 units, but after the age of forty, up to 1,000 units per day would be much better. Under no circumstances should infants get more than 400 units a day unless, of course, it is prescribed by a physician for a specific disorder. Expectant and nursing mothers should have up to 2,000 units a day. Even higher doses of vitamin D are used in therapy for the care of active rickets and for arthritis. But people should beware of abusing this valuable vitamin. Megadoses should be taken only with a doctor's approval. Large quantities of this vitamin can be toxic.

The F.D.A. ruling limiting the amount of vitamin A in one capsule also limits the dose of vitamin D to 400 units. Again, I simply take two capsules instead of one.

Here's how to fortify your meals with extra vitamin D:

1. Simply put your vegetable oil in the bright sunshine and irradiate it. This is how my cook in Sicily does it. She pours the oil in a flat tin pan, not more than ½ inch deep; then she puts the pan in the noonday sunlight for at least 2 hours. After that she pours this sun-drenched, vitaminized oil into dark bottles. This is the humble forerunner of the scientific irradiation process patented by the University of Wisconsin.
2. Orange, lemon, and grapefruit peelings also contain some vitamin D because the oil in the peel is constantly exposed to the sun. So instead of wasting this citrus peel, chop it and use it as often as possible in baking and cooking. It is delicious in stewed fruit.

Vitamin E

No other vitamin has ever provoked such controversy as vitamin E. It appears to act as a regulator of the metabolism of the nucleus of the cells, and it is reported to help prevent abortion. Authorities disagree as to the amount of vitamin E required, but a teaspoon of wheat-germ oil a day is often recommended.

A serious deficiency of vitamin E in the diet of the male leads to degeneration of the germinal epithelium; there is a tendency toward muscular wasting, an increased demand for oxygen by the tissues, and an improper use of phosphorus. The Drs. Shute, of Canada, have done extensive research with vitamin E; and according to Dr. Evan Shute, nothing has such a beneficial effect on the heart as concentrated vitamin E (or alpha-tocopherol, the most effective form of the tocopherol complex that makes up the vitamin).

For the last year I have taken 1,000 units of vitamin E with my other concentrates, with the result that after my last examination the doctor found my heart to be that of a young man. The Drs. Shute do not approve of self-medication; they insist on adjusting the proper dosage for each individual, as they did for me. I believe anyone with a heart problem should read Herbert Bailey's fascinating book *Vitamin E—Your Key to a Healthy Heart* (Arc Books).

The principal dietary sources of vitamin E are given in the following table.

Foods for Vitamin E

FOOD	SERVING	MILLIGRAMS
Wheat-germ oil	1 tablespoon	45.0
Corn oil	1 tablespoon	35.0
Soy oil	1 tablespoon	13–17
Cottonseed oil	1 tablespoon	11–13
Meats (average)	4 ounces	9.0
Kale	1 cup	8.0
Corn on the cob	1 medium	6.0
Wheat germ	¼ cup	4.6
Peanut oil	1 tablespoon	3.7–4
Spinach	1 cup	2.55
Carrots, diced	1 cup	2.1
Whole-wheat flour	½ cup	0.72–2.24
Egg	1 medium	1.5
Oatmeal	1 cup	0.5

Two scientists at the University of California, Dr. Lester Packer and Dr. James R. Smith, have recently disclosed (*The New York Times,* September 20, 1974) that vitamin E may be a key factor in increasing the life span of human cells in laboratory conditions. Although a person's increase in vitamin E intake could not "reverse the other important aging processes in the body," there is proof that vitamin E is fundamental in protecting living cells from too-high levels of oxidants, such as nitrogen dioxide and ozone, which are found in polluted areas. Moreover, "even if vitamin E can't turn a 40-year-old into a 14-year-old, it might prevent an early death, or brain disease, heart attacks or senility. Of course, we don't know these things at all, *yet*." (My emphasis added.)

Here's how to fortify your meals with the important vitamin E: add a tablespoonful of wheat-germ oil to any of the vegetable oils and use as a salad dressing. Eat all cereals (hot or cold) "à la mode," by sprinkling a heaping tablespoon of fresh wheat germ over them. You can also buy high-vitamin-E concentrates in capsule form.

Vitamin "F"

This unexpected letter in your vitamin alphabet stands for those essential unsaturated fatty acids; don't forget them.

Vitamin K

This vitamin is essential to the normal ability of the blood to clot. The daily need is very small. One or two milligrams per day is sufficient for normal nutrition. Larger amounts, from foods, are in no way harmful. The Japanese get extra amounts of vitamin K from the sea greens in their diet. You will find ample amounts of vitamin K in spinach, cabbage, cauliflower, uncooked tomatoes, and peas.

Minerals for Maximum Nutrition

Your body requires many minerals for maximum nutrition and high vitality. Minerals help to maintain in the body the amount of water necessary to the life processes. They keep blood and tissue fluid from becoming either too acid or too alkaline. They help draw chemical substances into and out of the cells. They influence the secretion of glands. They help set up conditions responsible for the irritability and contractility of muscle and tissue. And they are important in sending messages through the nervous system.

CALCIUM AND PHOSPHORUS

Calcium and phosphorus are necessary for maximum vigor. They are largely used in the body to give hardness to the teeth and bones. Although 99 percent of the calcium in the body is found in the bones and teeth, the remaining 1 percent plays an important role in regulating certain physiological functions. Calcium aids in the transmission of nerve messages and helps the nerves to be steady and relaxed. Conversely, a calcium-deficient person is inclined to be grouchy and irritable and to have a feeling of tenseness and uneasiness that quickly results in fatigue. Serving calcium-rich foods increases the efficiency, peace, and happiness of your family. A lack of calcium may also prevent a person from sleeping soundly. Needless dollars are spent each year for sleeping powders and tablets that could be replaced by calcium-rich foods.

Muscular cramps may also result from a lack of calcium. And abdominal cramps during menstruation are often caused by a decrease in blood calcium. This period is frequently accompanied by nervousness, headaches, mental depression, and other symptoms of calcium deficiency. An extra supply of calcium and vitamin D will usually cause these symptoms to disappear.

Calcium is also necessary for the clotting of blood; and a lack can lead to hemorrhage following the extraction of teeth or an accident, or during an operation. In treating hemorrhaging of any type, calcium—and vitamin D, necessary for the efficient absorption of calcium into the blood—should be given.

The best sources of calcium are milk, powdered skim milk, buttermilk, and yogurt. (Very fine bone flour or tablets are recommended for "milk haters.") Various types of cheese may be good or poor sources of calcium, depending on the way they are made. If the milk has been soured to develop flavor in the cheese, some calcium is lost. Commercial cottage cheese, for example, often contains little calcium; but if it is prepared at home it is an excellent source. (Recipe in chapter 28; see index.)

Calcium and phosphorus are used by the body in chemical combination with each other; one without the other is of little value. Good sources of phosphorus are meats, dairy products, all foods made from whole grains, and many vegetables. Phosphorus is used to build and maintain bones and teeth. It is also a part of each of the billions of cells in the body, and it is a constituent of all glandular secretions and all body fluids.

Vitamin D is necessary for the efficient use of calcium and phosphorus. It helps in their absorption into the blood and in depositing them in the bones and teeth. Most people get no more than 100 units of vitamin D daily, although about 1,000 units seems nearer the requirement. It is little wonder that people are nervous and tired, suffer from insomnia, and must resort to sleeping tablets.

Regardless of the amount of calcium and phosphorus in the diet, calcium and phosphorus are excreted daily in the urine and feces. If you are not getting enough of these minerals to supply the nerves, muscles, and body fluids, they are taken from the bones and teeth. On the other hand, if you receive an excess of calcium and phosphorus, the excess will be excreted.

Phosphorus is so readily available in many foods there is little danger of deficiency. Calcium, however, is more difficult to obtain. It can be furnished by one quart of milk, whole or skim, buttermilk, or yogurt. No other foods supply the amount of calcium needed daily.

As a correction for nervousness, and before operations of any kind, some doctors now recommend concentrated calcium such as dicalcium phosphate blended with very fine bone flour and fortified with vitamin D. Since calcium dissolves only in acids, it should be taken on an empty stomach, before meals or between meals, and preferably in or with citrus juice. Usually about a quarter teaspoonful of powdered dicalcium phosphate or two to four tablets daily are sufficient. Small amounts, taken frequently, can be absorbed more completely than a larger amount taken at one time.

Foods richest in calcium are:

Powdered skim milk	Molasses
Fresh milk	Almonds
Buttermilk	Sesame seeds
Yogurt	Turnip greens
Cottage cheese (homemade)	Broccoli

Also, in concentrates: very fine bone flour, dicalcium phosphate, and vitamin D in tablet form.

Iron

Iron is necessary to enable the blood to carry oxygen throughout the body; and it is also of great value in helping to remove carbon dioxide from the tissues. The number of red corpuscles in the blood varies widely with individuals, depending on their health. In addition to red corpuscles, each blood cell must contain a normal amount of hemoglobin, which actually carries the oxygen to every cell in the body.

Lack of iron in the diet—which I blame on the use of refined flour and white sugar—is the most common cause of anemia, a condition in which the body fails to produce either enough red corpuscles or enough hemoglobin. The anemic person is tired, listless, and lacking in endurance. (For a more complete discussion of this problem, see chapter 8.)

Iron is used more efficiently by the body in building blood if a trace of copper is present. Fortunately copper and iron occur together in several foods. The richest sources are liver, wheat germ, food yeast, and turnip greens. A good supply of whole-grain bread and natural sugars such as honey and dark molasses will supply additional iron.

Only about 50 percent of the iron in foods is freed during digestion to pass into the blood. The other 50 percent is lost in the feces. Thus, even though the diet may contain iron, if it does not reach the blood and bone marrow, anemia can exist. The quantity of iron in foods is less important than the actual amount that can be used by the body.

Fruits are not especially rich in iron, but most of the iron they do contain reaches the blood stream. Apricots are particularly valuable for correcting anemia. The iron in peanuts, celery, and carrots is well absorbed, as is that in molasses. Meats are rich sources of iron, especially liver and heart. Soybeans and eggs are also rich in easily assimilable iron.

Iron is dissolved only in acid, and unless it is dissolved it cannot pass through the intestinal walls. Normally the hydrochloric acid produced by a healthy stomach dissolves iron; but in many persons, especially those lacking the vitamins of the B family and those addicted to taking soda and alkalizers, sufficient acid is not present, and the end result is the same as if no iron were supplied by the diet.

It is by no means easy to plan a diet that supplies adequate iron. Average servings of the foods listed below furnish approximately the following amounts of iron, given in milligrams (20 milligrams a day are recommended for good health):

Foods for Iron

FOOD	SERVING	MILLIGRAMS
Turnip greens	½ cup	9
Liver, calf's	3 ounces	9
Wheat germ	½ cup	8
Yeast, brewers'	1 tablespoon	8
Molasses, dark	1 tablespoon	5
Beet tops	½ cup	4
Kidney	4 ounces	4
Wheat bran	½ cup	4
Dates, dried	4	4
Spinach	½ cup	4
Apricots	2	3
Eggs	2	3
Prunes	4	3
Chard	½ cup	3
Dandelion greens	½ cup	3
Raisins	⅔ cup	3
Muscle meat, fish, or fowl	4 ounces	3
Nuts	½ cup	3
Banana	1 large	2
Whole-wheat bread	1 ½-inch slice	1

There are many iron salts on the market, such as ferrous carbonate and ferrous sulphate, which are put up in tablets. These are inexpensive and are of great value in curing or preventing anemia. However, the tablets should not be used as an excuse for bad food habits. Deficiencies of protein, iodine, copper, and calcium, and of vitamins A, C, and those of the B family, particularly of vitamins B_6, B_{12}, folic acid, choline, and niacin, can also lead to anemia and tiredness.

One reason our forefathers were not so prone to developing anemia as we are is that they cooked their food in iron pots. Food absorbed iron from the pot and so supplied them with a daily supplement of this blood-strengthening element. Why not trade in your easy-clean, coated frypan for a healthy old-fashioned cast-iron skillet?

IODINE

Iodine forms part of the active substance thyroxine, produced by the thyroid gland. The iodine-containing thyroxine not only has a powerful effect on physical and mental development but gives the body its normal verve, its urge for work and play. A lack of iodine causes a corresponding lack of thyroxine and results in decreased stamina and vitality. A partial lack of iodine may cause goiter, an enlargement of the thyroid gland. See the section on the thyroid gland and goiters, under "Take Care of Your Glands," in chapter 8.

The amount of iodine in foods grown in this country varies widely; almost no food is a reliable source. The exceptions are ocean fish and seafoods, which are excellent sources. Many of my students use an iodized vegetable salt, which contains iodine from sea vegetables. It is a convenient way to get a small amount of iodine daily.

Many authorities believe that no salt should be sold except the kind that has iodine in it. Yet, although iodized salt has been on the market for almost half a century, only about 15 percent of the people use it. It is difficult to understand such indifference to health.

Foods richest in iodine:

Fish	Iodized vegetable salt
Shellfish	Sea water
Sea vegetables	

Also in concentrates made from sea greens; one single tablet contains the daily iodine ration.

Potassium

Even a partial deficiency of potassium leads to nervousness, constipation, gas distention, and sleeplessness. The heart beats slowly and irregularly, and the heart muscles become damaged. Potassium is also necessary for the normal contraction of all muscles. The green leafy vegetables and their juices are excellent sources of potassium, as well as of other minerals.

While whole-grain breads and cereals and molasses are extremely rich in potassium, three-fourths of this mineral is lost in refining grains; and white sugar contains none. In refining foods, practically all of the minerals are lost. A diet high in refined foods can cause a deficiency of a number of minerals.

Sodium and Chlorine

Sodium and chlorine are of tremendous importance in the body. Chlorine is used in the stomach to form hydrochloric acid, which is necessary for normal digestion of protein and the absorption of minerals into the blood. Many foods contain sodium and chlorine; and, of course, salt contains both of these minerals. Excessive amounts of salt are not needed, but it should never be entirely omitted except on the recommendation of your physician.

A healthy person who eats a reasonably varied diet runs little risk of a deficiency of sodium and chlorine. In extremely hot weather, particularly if the air is dry, so much salt can be lost through perspiration that death may result. In milder cases, a lack of sodium and chlorine can cause heat cramps or heatstroke. This condition is common among people who work in furnace rooms, in mines, or in any surroundings where the temperature is unusually high. Heatstroke is accompanied by nausea, dizziness, general exhaustion, and muscular cramps in the legs, back, and abdomen. People working under conditions of extreme heat should always be supplied with salt tablets.

Hot-weather fatigue is largely due to the loss of salt through perspiration. During very hot weather, keep on hand a supply of salty foods such as peanuts, popcorn, pretzels, or soybeans. At least one well-salted food should be served with each meal. In addition, the person who perspires freely and must work in the heat is wise to add a pinch of vegetable salt to each glass of water—actually, it makes a pleasant drink.

TRACE MINERALS

We do not know everything about trace minerals, but we do know that some of them are extremely important to our health and well-being. For example, when *magnesium* is omitted from the diet of experimental animals, their hearts beat with extreme rapidity, their blood vessels expand, and low blood pressure results; the animals are extremely irritable, and slight noises may cause them to go into convulsions.

The blood of some people suffering from extreme irritability has been found to be low in magnesium. It is possible that extreme irritability and even some types of mental disturbance may be connected with lack of magnesium. People who consume overrefined foods and neglect to eat green vegetables could easily become deficient in this mineral.

Aluminum is found in various parts of the human body. Whether its presence is necessary to health has not yet been determined.

Zinc is present in human tissues, especially in the thyroid and the sex glands. It is one of the constituents of insulin, which is necessary for the normal utilization of sugar. Liver and milk are good sources of zinc; people who avoid these foods might be deficient in this mineral.

Cobalt is also found in small amounts in most of the organs of the human body. It is a part of vitamin B_{12}. It appears to be related to the development of red corpuscles. In persistent anemia, doctors recommend cobalt, iron, and copper, with beneficial results. Liver of all kinds appears to be the best source of cobalt, iron, and copper.

Manganese is also necessary to human health, but its exact action is little understood. Manganese is found in green leaves and whole-grain breads and cereals.

Several other trace minerals seem to be essential to health. For example, *tin* is found in many human tissues, especially in the liver, brain, and thyroid gland. Relatively large amounts of *arsenic* are found in the liver; the concentration in the blood varies with glandular activity. *Bromine,* like arsenic, is best known as a drug and a poison; yet it is always in human blood. *Mercury* is found in the human liver; *nickel* is concentrated in the pancreas; *silver* occurs in the blood, liver, sex glands, heart, spleen, kidneys, and especially the thyroid and tonsils. However, the functions of these minerals are not well known.

Although a great deal is still to be learned about the exact role of trace minerals in human nutrition, they are undoubtedly of importance. Leafy vegetables, organ meats, and whole-grain breads and cereals should always be included in the diet to fulfill our needs in this respect. Since many of our minerals are washed into the oceans, thousands of people have learned to fortify their diets with sea vegetation and sea greens. These are extremely rich in many of the trace elements.

High-Vitality Meal Planning

If we relied on our *natural* appetites, we would never make a mistake in eating. In the brain there is a built-in regulator for thirst, hunger, appetite; and when the body needs a certain kind of food, that built-in regulator creates the appetite for that particular food.

Yes, nature would regulate our eating for us, if we would only allow her to do so. To get you started, come along with me and see how easy it is to arrange your meals so that you feel nourished and vital all day long.

Eat a Protein Breakfast

Breakfast is your vitality determinator for the day. Whether you start your day tired or glowing with energy is simple arithmetic.

When your blood sugar is at 90 milligrams per 100 cc. (approximately half a cup) of blood, you are comfortable. At 80, you are slowing down. At 70, you are hungry and your lassitude becomes fatigue. At 65, you are craving for sweets and your insides are grumbling, and if the level continues to drop you may suffer headache, weakness, wobbliness, heart palpitations, mental confusion, nausea, and worse. And your nerves, which feed only on the sugar supply in your blood, suffer first and most from this needless starvation!

Now let us see what happens when you begin your day with your habitual breakfast. It is about twelve hours since your last meal, and the average level of blood sugar after twelve hours of fasting is between 90 and 95. In a famous study which was reported some years ago by the United States Department of Agriculture, two hundred volunteers ate various kinds of breakfasts, from black coffee alone or "coffee-and" to a heavy breakfast of juice, oatmeal with sugar and cream, bacon, toast with butter and jam, coffee with sugar and cream.

With only coffee, the blood sugar went steadily down during the morning, and the volunteers became more and more irritable, nervous, headachy, and exhausted.

But for those who had taken a first-class protein with their breakfast, either eggs or fortified milk (recipe in chapter 28; see index), the blood sugar rose to a vigorous 120 and remained at that level through the morning hours.

Here is the most remarkable part of this remarkable story: all through the day, no matter what those volunteers ate, those who had eaten a breakfast without protein continued to have low blood sugar, with all its miseries. And those who had taken good protein with their breakfast enjoyed high blood sugar, high vitality, high efficiency, and high spirits all day long.

Now I know what you will say—I have heard it so many times: "But I *can't* eat such a big breakfast!" My answer to you is, you *will be able* to eat it, and enjoy it too. Begin by eating a bit less the night before, and in just a few days your natural morning hunger will return.

We have become upside-down people, giving our bodies the biggest load of food at night, before going to sleep, exactly when we need it least. And then we cheat ourselves at breakfast, just when we need food most and when calories can be worked off most easily.

Another argument I hear, especially from people who rush off to work each day, is "But I haven't got the time!" My answer is that it takes only five minutes to boil an egg and toast a piece of good bread, which with coffee and fresh fruit make an adequate breakfast. And it takes only another five or ten minutes to eat it and put the dishes in the sink. Isn't it worth getting up fifteen minutes earlier to function all morning in your most efficient way?

For small eaters, I offer this suggestion: if you really find it impossible to manage a substantial breakfast each day, then make sure to have a midmorning vitality booster that will keep your blood sugar at high level—not an empty, deceptive snack like coffee or cola and a doughnut, but a fortified milk drink, a bit of bread and cheese, a sweet fruit with a handful of nuts or a handful of sunflower seeds, which you can keep at the office.

BLUEPRINT FOR HIGH-VITALITY BREAKFASTS

First: Unsweetened fruit juice or whole fruit, preferably fresh

Second: Large helping of protein, not less than 20 grams

Third: Helping of whole-grain bread, gluten bread, or whole-grain cereal

Fourth: For enjoyment and more protein, have 1 or 2 cups of Swiss coffee (hot coffee mixed with an equal amount of foaming hot milk, with honey if you must have sweetening).

Now let us set a buffet on a big, long table so you can see the tremendous variety to choose from. I have listed the most popular breakfast dishes; you need not have ham and eggs every day of the week. They are a fine protein dish, but actually we need variety. The English like fish, South Americans eat steaks, the Swiss enjoy their famous cheese. These are all first-class breakfast proteins. If your pocketbook does not permit these proteins, then at least eat a whole-grain cereal, hot or cold, and fortify it with one or two tablespoons of wheat germ and lots of fortified skim milk.

Breads and cereals are disappointingly low in protein unless you fortify them with gluten flour, soya flour, powdered milk, or food yeast. But we *need* one good helping of carbohydrate to help keep energy and spirits high all day long.

I also urge you to learn to enjoy Swiss coffee in place of the health-destroying heavily sugared and creamed beverage. Swiss coffee for breakfast is much to be preferred to black coffee; the milk adds extra protein, plus milk sugar for extra morning energy. Some manufacturer could make a fortune by mixing instant coffee with dry milk powder. All we would have to do then is stir in hot water.

Fresh Things First

Each meal, make a fresh beginning. By this I mean, begin each meal with something fresh whenever you can.

Those of us who for many years have begun each meal with a fresh fruit or vegetable have always believed we were following the latest dictates of scientific nutrition—and so we were. But the truth of the matter is that, even without the aid of modern science, the wise Greeks practiced this rule four hundred years before the birth of Christ. More than two thousand years ago, the Greek physician Diocles, of Carystus wrote, "Eat your raw fresh foods first of all and follow with cooked food as your second course, and let fruit be the end of your meal." The lively fragrance and flavor refresh the taste buds, start the digestive juices, and set the body's wonderful chemistry going for the rest of the meal.

Today we know all this scientifically. One of the great scientists of the last century, Dr. Rudolf Virchow, discovered and proved that there are physiological reasons for eating fresh foods at the *beginning* of a meal. He observed that cooked food called up a great increase of white blood corpuscles in the blood, the same reaction that the body makes to disease germs and bacteria. This is the wonderful defense system of the body, the "immune reaction" that protects us against disease. But it was Virchow's astonishing discovery that the body makes this same defense against processed foods! Then he found that when he fed his patients fresh, unprocessed food *first*, this rise in white blood corpuscles did not occur. Even more important, his patients *then* could eat their cooked meal without causing this irritating reaction of the blood.

Fresh things, eaten at the beginning of the meal when appetite is keenest, satisfy that first sharp hunger and prevent overeating.

A salad, with its mildly acid dressing, also stimulates all the digestive processes and contributes bulk to encourage those muscular intestinal walls that might otherwise become lazy. Then, too, crisp fresh salads are our best vehicles to get valuable vegetable oils into our daily menus.

Make Lunchtime Salad Time

To save time and a lot of dishwashing, I have devised what I call a meal in just one bowl—tempting, compact, not too expensive, and, above all, nourishing enough to keep blood sugar at a high level all through the afternoon.

I am convinced that the eating of heavy and greasy luncheons causes much afternoon tiredness and mental letdown, which lead to short tempers and four o'clock letdowns, and cost big business millions. You can prevent this by forming the salad-lunch habit.

Whether you order this salad at your favorite restaurant or are lucky enough to have it at home, here are its essentials:

For a base, cut up the freshest, greenest, crispiest vegetables (at least a cupful); add to this a good portion, not less than twenty grams, of your favorite stick-to-the-ribs protein food (see list, page 18); and toss it all together with a vegetable-oil dressing of your choice (recipe for Fabulous Salad Dressing in chapter 23; see index).

On beauty farms, salads like this are served in great bowls with a choice of half a dozen different kinds of dressing. The salad itself can be different every day, with the endless variety of delicious fresh things we have to choose from all the year round. And there need never be monotony in the dressing with the many vegetable oils providing their different nuances of taste. I urge you to try them all, individually and in combination. Mix these oils, two or three different kinds in one dressing, the less expensive to extend the more costly ones, and by all means add a little of a good grade of olive oil. Olive oil is not rich in the polyunsaturated acids, but it is extremely rich in the monounsaturated acids (82 percent); it is far richer in flavor than any of the other oils, and it gives an elegance to salads that no other oil can.

Good oils deserve good vinegars, and again we have a wealth of them to choose from. Shun the white synthetic kind, which contributes neither goodness nor flavor but only an edge sharp as a knife. It is just as easy to use cider vinegar, with its mellowness of ripe apples; or if you have a French or Italian taste, flavorsome wine vinegar (but use it more sparingly), or, for something new, Japanese vinegar made from rice wine. A salad must never have an outright acid or sour taste; sheer sourness is so strong and dominating that it kills all other flavors. It is best to follow the classic French proportions of two-thirds oil and one-third vinegar.

For fresher and more exciting-tasting dressings use both lemon juice, rich in vitamin C, and vinegar; I know some excellent cooks who sprinkle a few drops of lemon juice over all salads, no matter what dressing they use. And to give their salads of all kinds a bit of mystery and to soften any sharpness in the dressing, they use their imagination and spike them with various flavors—vegetable salt, salad herbs, or something unexpected like a drop or two of honey, wonderful when fruits are in the salad. You can be a true gourmet and make your own delicately flavored herb vinegar, as is done in thousands of European homes. (Recipe for Swiss Herb Vinegar in chapter 23; see index.)

LEARN TO USE VEGETABLE OILS

No matter what you may have heard or read, take my word for it that vegetable oils are necessary at all times even when you are weight-watching. The excess of hard animal fats and of the many hydrogenated pure white and highly touted inert fats has given a bad name to all fats, including the oils that are so necessary to keep the body fires burning bright. The human body is not equipped to metabolize quantities of inert fats, so they are deposited where circulation is slowest—around the middle.

The unsaturated fatty acids in vegetable oils help burn up ugly fat deposits on the body. They keep cholesterol down, and they moisturize the skin from the inside—permanently, not just temporarily, as cosmetics do. Liquid oils are easier for the body to burn and they are not deposited as excess fat unless you are overeating generally.

So whether you are keeping your ideal weight or reducing, have not less than two tablespoons of your favorite oil a day, *every* day, in some form; use it in cooking, in plain salad dressing, or in your own delicious homemade mayonnaise. Real mayonnaise, made with unheated fresh oil, a fresh egg yolk, and a dash of vinegar, is a splendid food. The oil furnishes your body with the fatty acids; the fresh egg yolk contributes important lecithin and vitamin A; and the vinegar adds flavor and speeds digestion.

BLUEPRINT FOR HIGH-VITALITY LUNCHEONS

First: A fresh start with any and all fresh green salad vegetables, broken up or chopped, the more the merrier (at least a cup).

Second: Your favorite salad protein, at least 20 grams, never less than ½ cup. Have lean cottage cheese, shredded meat, eggs, or fish. Toss the salad with a vegetable-oil dressing or mayonnaise.

Third: A carbohydrate for prolonged energy. A muffin, a slice of protein, rye, or whole-wheat bread, lightly buttered or with mayonnaise.

Fourth: For enjoyment and stimulation, a cup of milk, yogurt, buttermilk, or your favorite beverage. No white sugar, please, or you'll have a letdown.

Proteins for Your Salad Bowl

Cottage cheese	Conch
Chicken	Tuna
American cheese	Eggs, hard-cooked
Lean ham	Leftover meat
Tongue	Soybean
Lobster	Gelatin meat or fish (aspic)
Shrimp	Fruits and nuts

Your Midafternoon Vitality Lift

One of my most difficult and fascinating Hollywood assignments was to keep the glamorous women from looking wilted by midafternoon. Making motion pictures is the cruelest, most strenuous kind of work; after a few hours of repetitious "takes" in stuffy air, under hot klieg lights, even the brightest of stars began to droop, and the sharpest of all eyes, the movie camera, caught every listless line.

Once, at the Hal Roach studio, my task was to sustain the gorgeousness of twelve showgirls who really deserved the word *gorgeous;* the picture was *The All-American Coed,* and Frances Langford was its lovely star. My answer was to set up a beauty bar, the first in Hollywood. At three o'clock sharp the cameras stopped turning, and all those beautiful girls came to the bar to replenish their beauty. For fifteen minutes, in their gold- and silver-lamé gowns, they sipped my booster cocktails and nibbled at the proteins laid out for them on platters.

They had their choice of these cocktails: orange juice with fresh egg yolk beaten into it; fortified skim milk flavored with orange-blossom honey; chilled yogurt fortified with dark molasses; or any Hi-Vi booster, cool glasses of lushly red tomato juice spiked with one or two heaping teaspoons of celery-flavored food yeast and a teaspoon of lemon juice. On the platters were the more solid Hi-Vi beauty treats: crisp whole-wheat crackers with cubes of cheese, nonhydrogenated peanut butter; avocado slices sprinkled with vegetable salt, spices, and lime juice; and that ever-wonderful, ever-popular standby, Hi-Vi cottage cheese with parsley, chives, basil, and all the fresh herbs we could find in the Farmer's Market.

After a few days of our beauty-bar refreshment, the girls and the director saw the difference. More important, the day's run of film showed the girls as fresh-looking and their dancing as crisp in the afternoon as in the morning.

Dinnertime Is Relaxing Time

Dinnertime is homecoming time, the end of the working day and the beginning of evening leisure; in many homes it is the one time when families can sit down together and eat in a peaceful atmosphere. The cocktail before dinner may be a custom, but it is too often misunderstood and abused. I am sorry to see people pickle their stomachs with martinis, killing their natural appetites and all sense of food taste. Instead, why not try nature's own cocktail, a tall glass of cool vegetable juice, spiked with fragrant garden herbs and spices, or that old standby—my Hi-Vi booster.

After a busy and perhaps a tense day, such a drink does wonderful things. It helps to unwind taut nerves; it quickly erases fatigue with its high content of natural sugars; most important, it raises the blood-sugar level to the point where you will have no wish to overeat.

Every dinner should be nutritious, light, and lean; about twenty to thirty grams of good protein in lean meat, fish, or fowl, with a short-cooked green vegetable, an occasional baked potato or kasha or brown rice, and always a crisp salad with vegetable-oil dressing. For pleasure and digestion, there is a bowl of fresh fruit or honey-sweetened compote, occasionally an open-face fruit pie, a custard, or a tangy cheese.

BLUEPRINT FOR HIGH-VITALITY DINNERS

Your choice of appetizers:

Fruit cup
Green salad
Finger salad
Vegetable juice
Hot or cold jellied broth occasionally

Your choice of protein dishes:

Lean meat
Liver
Lean fish
Nut loaf
Lean cheese
Eggs
Soybeans

Your choice:

> Short-cooked vegetables
> Baked potato
> Kasha
> Rice

Your choice of delightful desserts:

> Fresh fruit of the season
> Honey compote
> Gelatin with fruit
> Custard
> Open-face fruit pie
> Cheese
> Yogurt

Plus your favorite beverage

Recipes and Menus to Guide You

Sound nutrition demands that all the important nutrients for the entire body be eaten every day. Here follow some menus to guide you. If you like them, use them; or if you prefer, make up your own. Eating, as we have learned, should be fun and not regimented. I thoroughly agree with Dr. Margaret Mead when she says: "The present phase of American 'dieting' and 'slimming,' counting *calories,* has something of the same pathetic rigidity that accompanied early bottle feeding. Eventually bottle feeding was modified according to the needs of 'self-demand' or 'self-regulation.'"

It is this self-regulation we must strive for so that we can once and forever say goodbye to all diets, including those of Gaylord Hauser. For the present, all I ask of you is to remember that we cut down on all unfriendly hard fats, we eat fewer starches and sugars, but we eat more proteins and we include as many fresh fruits, vegetables, and unprocessed foods as possible.

Since protein foods are the most expensive of all foods, I suggest again that those of you with small budgets obtain a large part of your proteins from the inexpensive Hi-Vi lean milk, cottage cheese, or homemade cream cheese. Good bread—wheatgerm or soya or whole-wheat—can add another three to five grams of protein.

BETWEEN-MEAL VITALITY BOOSTERS UNLIMITED

There is exciting evidence coming from a famous nutrition laboratory that "nibbling" animals, who eat throughout the day, keep their vitality at a higher level than when given three square meals a day. So do not hesitate to nibble one of the between-meal vitality boosters should you feel hungry or have a sense of letdown. If you enjoy a coffee break, drink Swiss coffee. Remember it's the protein, and the protein alone, that gives a sustained lift, and the thrifty Swiss have known for years that their Swiss coffee sticks to the ribs.

Million-Dollar Eye-Opener

If you are a slow riser, or easily irritated, or just naturally mean in the morning, this eye-opener can help you to get going and be more amiable. The minute you get out of bed, drink a small glass of your favorite fruit juice. It must be naturally sweet, never sugared—orange, pineapple, apple, or papaya juice. The natural sugar in any unsweetened fruit juice, taken on an empty stomach, performs the magic.

Quick Hi-Vi Milk (Hot or Cold)

Put 4 tablespoons of instant dry milk into a glass of fresh skim milk. Waistline watchers can flavor this with a bit of instant coffee powder, vanilla, nutmeg, or cinnamon. Those with normal waistlines can add a little honey, molasses, carob powder, or frozen fruit juice. Or you can put 1 cup of dry milk into a quart of fresh milk and keep it in the refrigerator. This is a wonderful standby for busy mothers.

Hi-Vi Booster par Excellence

Beat 2 or 3 teaspoons of good-tasting brewers' yeast into a glass of chilled tomato juice; spike with a slice of lemon and a pinch of vegetable salt.

Hi-Vi Chocolaty Drink (Hot or Cold)

Stir 1 tablespoon of carob powder into a glass of skim milk. If necessary, sweeten with a little honey. Real chocolate prevents the calcium in milk from being assimilated and is especially undesirable for youngsters.

Hi-Vi Eat-and-Run Drink

Stir 1 fresh egg yolk into a glass of fresh orange juice; ½ teaspoon of honey gives added taste and very quick energy.

Hi-Vi Swiss Broth

Mix 1 tablespoon of dry skim-milk powder, 1 teaspoon food yeast, and ½ teaspoon dried herbs (savory, parsley, dill, tarragon, etc.). Stir into a cup of hot skim milk or tomato juice and season with vegetable salt. This instant Swiss broth is already available in health- and diet-food shops.

Hi-Vi Bomb

Into 1 cup of skim milk, stir 1 teaspoon *each* of golden honey, dark molasses, good-tasting food yeast, and carob powder. Can be taken hot or cold for a quick burst of vitality.

Hi-Vi Golden Drink

A favorite on beauty farms and with children. Mix ½ cup fresh cold milk with ½ cup freshly made carrot juice. Undernourished, finicky eaters thrive on this delicious combination.

> ### *Tranquilizing Nightcap*
>
> Mix 1 tablespoon of dry skim-milk powder into a cup of hot skim milk and flavor with a teaspoon of honey or molasses. Sip slowly. For more tranquilizing calcium and vitamin D, some nutritionists now recommend two calcium tablets to be taken with the hot milk instead of habit-forming sleeping tablets. Remember that hot milk drinks, sipped slowly at bedtime, are by far the best sleep inducers. The warm drink coaxes the blood away from the overactive brain—calcium is a great tranquilizer-relaxer—and before you know it, you're off to sleep.

Hi-Vi Egg Snack

Fresh hard-boiled eggs, when eaten very slowly, can sustain a high level of vitality. Contrary to public opinion, they are not hard to digest. Keep them in the refrigerator. Before eating, flavor them with herbs and a bit of vegetable salt. Hard-boiled eggs are especially valuable for reducers.

Hi-Vi Yogurt

Lean yogurt is extremely valuable. It supplies hard-working bacteria, useful acids, and easily digested protein. A cup of plain yogurt, or yogurt spiked with honey, molasses, or frozen fruit concentrate, makes an ideal between-meal boost.

Hi-Vi Cheese Spread

Two or three tablespoons of cottage or yogurt cream cheese (recipe in chapter 28; see index) mixed with chives, parsley, or green onions, seasoned with herbs and vegetable salt, and served with a slice of whole-wheat or gluten toast, are excellent for those wishing a more solid between-meal or bedtime snack.

Let these samples help you. There is really no limit to the delightful between-meal vitality boosters you can make. Let your imagination guide you.

Now, hold up your right hand and swear that, henceforth, you will not insult your body with empty coffee breaks, colas, pops, or other white-sugar concoctions that give you a swift lift and then a kick in the pants and drop you to an all-time low!

Protein Tablets

These tablets (available at any health-food store) are not meant to be a replacement for food, but in emergencies, when energy is low, they will give you a vitality boost. Keep some in your desk for that particularly harried day when you can't get to the real thing.

The High-Vitality Diet—Breakfasts, Luncheons, and Dinners

High-Vitality Vitamin Ritual

Don't forget your supplements! Make it a habit to take your vitamin and mineral concentrates with your breakfast and be fortified for the day ahead.

Menu One

Breakfast:	Fruit juice; scrambled eggs; 1 portion lean ham; 1 slice whole-wheat or gluten toast, lightly buttered; choice of beverage: coffee, tea, or milk; preferably Swiss coffee: half hot coffee and half hot foaming milk
Midmorning:	If hungry: your choice of between-meal vitality boosters

Luncheon: Salad bowl: cottage cheese on bed of dark-green lettuce; vegetable-oil dressing; 1 slice whole-wheat bread, buttered lightly; fresh or honeyed fruit, if desired; choice of beverage: tea, mint tea, papaya tea, coffee, milk, or yogurt

Midafternoon: If hungry: your choice of between-meal vitality boosters

Dinner: Mixed salad; vegetable-oil dressing; large lean hamburger, tenderized; steamed zucchini; apple snow or baked apple; choice of beverage: demitasse, milk, or tea

Before Retiring: If hungry: treat yourself to a between-meal snack or a hot tranquilizing nightcap

Menu Two

Breakfast: ½ grapefruit; your favorite hot or cold cereal à la mode (serve all cereals à la mode: topped with 2 tablespoons wheat germ, 1 teaspoon honey); serve with ½ cup Hi-Vi milk; 3 slices crisp lean bacon; choice of: coffee, tea, or milk (preferably Swiss coffee: half hot coffee and half hot foaming milk)

Midmorning: If hungry: your choice of between-meal vitality boosters

Luncheon: Salad bowl: ½ cup shrimp on bed of green leaves; vegetable-oil dressing; 1 wheat-germ muffin, buttered lightly; fresh or honeyed fruit, if desired; choice of: tea, mint tea, papaya tea, coffee, milk, or yogurt

Midafternoon: If hungry: your choice of between-meal vitality boosters

Dinner: Red-apple and red-cabbage salad; your favorite vegetable-oil dressing; lean pot roast; briefly cooked beets; kasha; fresh or stewed fruit; choice of: demitasse, milk, or tea

Before Retiring: If hungry: treat yourself to a between-meal snack or a hot tranquilizing nightcap

Menu Three

Breakfast: Applesauce, sprinkled with 1 tablespoon wheat germ and 1 teaspoon honey; chipped beef, simmered with Hi-Vi lean milk; served on whole-wheat toast; choice of: coffee, tea, or milk (preferably Swiss coffee: half hot coffee and half hot foaming milk)

Midmorning: If hungry: your choice of between-meal vitality boosters

Luncheon: Salad bowl: shredded Swiss cheese on bed of watercress and lettuce; vegetable-oil dressing; 1 slice rye bread, buttered lightly; fresh or honeyed fruit, if desired; choice of: tea, mint tea, papaya tea, coffee, milk, or yogurt

Midafternoon: If hungry: your choice of between-meal vitality boosters

Dinner: Raw tender spinach salad; vegetable-oil dressing; tender broiled liver; baked onions with orégano; broiled grapefruit; choice of: demitasse, milk, or tea

Before Retiring: If hungry: treat yourself to a between-meal snack or a hot tranquilizing nightcap

Eating—the Pleasure Principle

I shall never forget the favorite maxim of my favorite teacher, Ragnar Berg, the Swedish nutritionist: "There must be pleasure in eating." The pleasure principle is essential in the biological scheme of things.

Please, never think or speak of nutritious food as being "good for you" or let the family table be approached as though it were a prescription counter. Instead, you have to learn the joy of fresh, health-giving food—you'll never want to go back to your old ways once you do.

This is important: never eat when you are emotionally upset or overtired. Lie down before dinner, if possible (this is a perfect time for fifteen minutes on the yoga slant; see chapter 9). Half an hour or so before dinner, your whole family (I hope) enjoys a glass of refreshing fruit or vegetable juice, the natural appetite normalizer that is now part of your daily living. (See chapter 25.) I hope that you make this a leisurely get-together to which you all look forward, from which you go to dinner looking and feeling relaxed. I hope you indulge in a lot of conversational nonsense. Nonsense is the best thing I know to keep family machinery well oiled.

Overweighters especially are prone to be food-bolters and unconscious eaters; it is one reason why they have to eat more than they really need to feel satisfied.

Change family eating habits gradually and casually. Introduce new dishes as something novel and delicious that you dreamed up as a treat. If you are the one person in the family who is reducing, be nonchalant about your smaller portions or the foods you skip. Eat more slowly than the rest of the family, and nobody will know you are on a diet. If you truly want to trim down to better proportions, you are embarking upon the greatest adventure of your life—approach it in that spirit and your goal is half won. You are not depriving yourself. You are treating yourself to a new and interesting experience.

Lean Cookery

For years I have been advocating what I call *lean cookery*. Not just to help my students keep slender (this happens automatically) but to help them to keep healthy, stay youthful, live long, and enjoy all the best food in the world.

What is lean cookery? It means, first of all, using wholesome, natural, lean foods. It means no overcooking; food should be cooked as long as necessary for maximum goodness *and no longer;* in the case of almost all vegetables, this means only a few minutes. It means being miserly in the use of animal fats, sugars, and thickeners, wasting no time or money on pastries and rich sauces. Instead, we use our money for lean meats, lean fish, poultry, lean milk; for vegetable oils; for tasty, nourishing bread; for fresh vegetables and fruits. And these foods we do not spoil with rich additions, but we do make them tastier by spiking them with nonirritating spices, vegetable salt, sweet paprika, and all kinds of fragrant herbs. We use no synthetic sweeteners; instead, we use dark molasses, honey, natural brown sugar, and carob. I cannot conscientiously advocate synthetic sweeteners. Some have been suspected of causing disease, and I am happy to say at least one has been removed from the market. Hopefully, others will follow. I am convinced that only natural foods can help you retrain your appetite.

SALAD DAYS

Serving salad as the first course is not only the smart Continental and California way of dining, it is the smart way to eat anywhere, especially if you are reducing. But not a skimpy little dab of lettuce with perhaps a slice of tomato and a lot of thick dressing sloshed over it. That's a poor imitation of a salad. Make it a generous bowlful of live, crisp greens and vegetables, lovely to look at and delicious to eat. To help you get started on yours, you will find my favorite salads and lean salad dressings in chapter 23.

I know meat is expensive and becoming more costly every day. So let me tell you a secret. First, that the tough, muscular cuts of meat such as round steak, chuck, rump, and shoulder are more nourishing than the more expensive prime ribs, tenderloin steaks, and chops. Second, that these cheaper cuts of meat can be made tender enough to roast or broil (and in a matter of minutes) by using a natural meat tenderizer.

"Señor," said my Mexican cook in Taxco some years ago, when I protested because she brought home a tough old rooster, "this is a special bird, an educated bird, father of many chickens, full of nourishment and wisdom. Its muscles will make muscle and strength for Señor and his distinguished guests; its toughness I take away." And to my great surprise, she did. The educated old bird was tender and delicious (I did not taste the wisdom). I learned later that she had cut him up, wrapped bruised papaya leaves around each piece, and let it stand in a crockery jar overnight. I learned also that, for centuries, primitive cooks have been tenderizing their tough wild game by wrapping it in green leaves, especially papaya. No doubt they thought these leaves contained magic, but modern chemistry explains their tenderizing properties more prosaically by telling us that papaya leaves contain a digestive enzyme. Some of my California and Florida students have long been using papaya leaves for making digestive teas and for tenderizing tough meat; the only drawback was that the meat-tenderizing process took so long.

Nowadays this digestive enzyme has been extracted and put into all sorts of liquid sauces for tenderizing tough meats quickly. I find it easiest and most satisfactory to use a dry, sprinkle-on variety; there are many on the market. The one I use is a delicious blend of sea salt, vegetable extract, papaya, and some herbs for flavor. Sprinkle this on your meat before you broil, bake, or roast it.

Meat plays an important part in any scientific reducing program; we eat a good, lean portion at least once a day. Let us get all possible nourishment from it. Let us prepare it in the modern, healthful, and flavorsome way. Here are three things to remember:

First, always buy lean meat. Have the butcher remove all visible fat. Naturally there will be some invisible fat, which emerges as drippings during the cooking process.

Second, get rid of all these drippings. You have no use for them, no rich sauces or gravies to prepare.

Third, cook your meat correctly. This means broil steaks and chops. Larger cuts of meat should be roasted (meat should never be too well done, except for pork, of course) in a *slow* oven. Meat cookery experiments done by the U.S. Department of Agriculture showed that meat is juicier, tastier, and most healthful when roasted at a low temperature.

For a change of pace, eat fish. It is a wonder food containing first-class proteins and packed extra-generously with vitamins and minerals, especially iodine. When I lectured once in Buenos Aires, I gave my audience all these good reasons why, instead of concentrating on their Argentine beef, they should also take advantage of their bountiful fish supply. Nothing happened, until I told them that fish is one of the best foods for *"una bella figura."* Next day, the fish markets were sold out.

Short-Cook Your Vegetables

In lean vegetable cookery, just remember that the quicker vegetables are prepared and cooked, the better your family will like them. Also, the less is the loss of vitamins B, C, and P. These vitamins, like salt, dissolve in water; therefore we never pour off any vegetable water. Better still, we short-cook vegetables in such a way that all the goodness and nutrients remain. I have said it a thousand and one times and I'll say it again—when vegetables are cooked half an hour or more in pots full of water, you'd be wiser to throw out the dead vegetables and drink the water they were cooked in, for that's where the precious vitamins and minerals have gone.

> *Four Pointers for Vegetable Cookery*
> 1. Do not peel; instead, scrub thoroughly with a vegetable brush.
> 2. Boil or bake whole vegetables in their skins.
> 3. Short-cook sliced or shredded vegetables in the smallest amount of water or broth, and add a bit of vegetable salt *after* they are done.
> 4. If your family insists on a "buttery" taste, add a pat of sunbutter just before serving.

Any vegetable can be short-cooked in a matter of minutes. All you need is a heavy cooking utensil, preferably heavy enamelware, and one of those handy vegetable cutters. Or use an ordinary shredder (the coarse one). Or cut vegetables into thin slivers. Do your shredding or slivering as quickly as possible to prevent vitamin C loss.

Have your cooking pot piping hot; use a small one so it will be filled to the top; the less space for air, the better. In the bottom of the pot have three tablespoons of water; when this boils and the pot is filled with steam, put in your cut-up vegetables and cover the pot tightly. Let the vegetables cook on a low flame for two minutes; then shake the pot (without lifting the lid) so there is no possible chance of sticking. After about four minutes, remove the cover and taste one of the vegetable slivers; if it is soft but still a bit chewy, as the vegetables are in Chinese restaurants, it is at its best. Now all you add is a sprinkle of vegetable salt, some herbs, and a bit of vegetable oil; or, if you prefer, you may use half vegetable oil and half butter, as my Italian students do. Such short-cooked vegetables have a wonderful natural flavor and keep their attractive color. When you use vegetable salt last, the juices are not extracted during cooking.

For *extra*-lean short-cooking, here is a trick: instead of water, we steam the sliced vegetables in flavorsome broth—leftover "pot likker," Hauser Broth (see index), canned or dehydrated vegetable broth, or chicken or beef broth made with bouillon cubes.

Cooked this way, with the addition of vegetable salt and sprinkled with herbs, short-cooked vegetables can be enjoyed without the addition of extra fat.

Finger Salad and Fresh Juices

More and more smart hostesses are serving finger salad instead of (or in addition to) overrich canapés. I introduced the finger salad years ago in Paris and have been serving a big tray of these crisp vegetables at my parties ever since.

How to make finger salad? Simply cut up the youngest and tenderest vegetables you can find in your market. Everyone knows and likes crisp carrot sticks, chilled radishes, tender celery; in addition, try strips of green and red peppers, bits of fresh cauliflower, slices of cool, unpeeled cucumbers, nutlike kohlrabi, small, whole ripe tomatoes (these can be stuffed with cottage cheese), and a delicious, less familiar vegetable, finocchio or Italian fennel, cut in wedges. Be adventurous; use whatever succulent vegetables your market offers. And—you can enjoy these crisp vegetables without a fatty dressing. All I serve with finger salads is a shaker filled with a delightful mixture of spices, herbs, and sea salt. Sprinkle this over the vegetables and you add only flavor, not calories.

For those who are reducing, these crisp vegetable hors d'oeuvres keep the stomach busy and filled. You can eat them to your heart's content. For extra-special parties, serve several of these big plates of crisp vegetables with a bowl full of my special lean dressing in the middle of each tray, for "dunking" (see my suggestions in chapter 23, "Sunlit Food").

Smart hostesses are also offering their guests a healthy alternative to the usual cocktail—a glass of fresh vegetable or fruit juice. It's a delicious choice for the nondrinker. I first learned about drinking fresh fruits and vegetables in Carlsbad (Karlory Vary), Czechoslovakia, many years ago. There was a famous sanatorium there where two brilliant doctors (Mayr and Zukor) decided to give their patients fresh foods in liquid form, by extracting the "blood" of the plant. The results have made history.

Fortunes have been made in the United States and Europe by companies putting out canned juices; and this is all to the good. But nothing can compare with the deliciousness of fresh, fresh juices. These vital juices contain vitamins, minerals, chlorophyll, enzymes, and many as yet undiscovered food factors in the most appetizing form.

It will pay you to invest in the best juicer you can buy. It can become a veritable health mine for you and your family. There are several types on the market. Make certain that all parts that come in contact with the juice are made of stainless steel. This is important if you want to keep the appetizing color of the juices. Also, be sure that the machine you buy does not vibrate and is easy to clean.

Unfortunately, the poisonous sprays used on our fruits and vegetables to keep pests away still cling to them when they reach the kitchen. The safest and simplest method to remove all traces of sprays is this:

> Buy a large earthenware crock and fill it with a 1 percent hydrochloric acid solution. This is made by mixing 1 ounce of chemically pure hydrochloric acid with 3 quarts of water. Because pure hydrochloric acid may cause severe burns, ask your druggist to mix this for you. The solution can be used for a week. Place all suspicious fruits or vegetables in this solution, leave in for 5 minutes, and rinse well. Also, health-food stores now carry a special *harmless* detergent for washing vegetables.

Fruit for Dessert

The ideal dessert is fresh fruit, and with all the tempting varieties from all parts of the world piled in our markets, there is a new and delicious fruit treat available for every day in the week. Some fruits we stew with a little honey. Some we serve, on special occasions, as open-faced pies or tarts on a delicious lean whole-grain or wheat-germ crust.

For some of my favorite desserts, see chapter 26. If you are looking for pastries, puddings, and gooey desserts, close this book and take a walk. Go to your nearest pastry shop, take a good look at everything in the window, and say, "You will be a few seconds in my mouth, two hours in my stomach, and a lifetime on my hips. You are not for me!"

Let's Dine Out

I want to show you that the world is yours—that you can eat wherever you want, whenever you want, and you can eat healthily. We are going to dine out here, there, and everywhere. But before we start, I want to tell you something: don't be afraid of the waiters, not even of the maître d'. Order what you want to have, the way you want to have it. Don't be frightened into ordering too much or too rich food. Be your own person; your body will thank you for it.

---

*Five Points to Remember
When You Dine Out*

1. Eat something fresh, preferably to start the meal.
2. Eat lots of first-class protein, not less than 20 grams with each meal.
3. Eat some carbohydrates, but let them be natural. If you are overweight, skip bread, rice, and potatoes.
4. Avoid hard fats and use vegetable oils, or margarine made with vegetable oils.
5. Eat fresh or stewed fruit for an ideal dessert.

Keep these five points in mind, and soon you will order good food *automatically*. And here's another tip for your first few weeks of intelligent eating. Instead of munching bread and butter and sipping icewater while you wait for your main course, ask the waiter please to bring your salad early. Millions of pounds of fat could be prevented by just this simple habit of satisfying the first hunger with a big, fresh salad.

Let's take a healthy gourmet tour.

Chicago—the Pump Room

While in Chicago, we'll go to the Pump Room of the Ambassador East Hotel, internationally known for its good food and interesting people. Our menu?

Pump Room special salad
Butterfly steak
Fresh pineapple
Demitasse

It was Irene Castle—that beautiful, vital lady—and Pat Dougherty, the society editor who had lost forty pounds by eating intelligently, who introduced me to the Pump Room's famous butterfly steak. This is a small sirloin split in two with the bone in the middle; it is shaped like a butterfly. It takes only a few moments to broil such a steak; when our steaks arrived, piping hot, all three of us, in unison, automatically cut off the outside fat.

With the steaks we had the Pump Room special salad made of that very tender Kentucky-limestone lettuce, mixed with bits of hearts of artichoke; and when the maître d' asked what kind of dressing we preferred, we three, again almost in unison, asked for a light dressing—which meant olive oil well mixed with the greens, some wine vinegar, a pinch of vegetable salt, and salad herbs. This salad bowl was unbelievably delicious; we devoured it all with our butterfly steaks. The perfect dessert, after this, was a slice of juicy, ripe pineapple, and with it we enjoyed a small cup of black coffee. (Who could possibly want sugar and cream?)

New York—"21"

You do not see many overweighters at the Pump Room. The people who go there are really smart. This is true of most famous restaurants where people go not only for good food but also for interesting people—Jack and Charlie's "21" Club, for example, which is one of my favorite restaurants in New York.

By all means, let us go to "21." I was first taken there long ago by Adele Astaire, and throughout the years Jack and Charlie have maintained their high standard of excellent food. Let's go after the theater; in New York we are so busy that many times we haven't time for dinner at the usual hour. We will see many celebrities. Last time I was there, Helen Hayes and my friend Anita Loos were at the tables on either side of mine. My companion and I started with honeydew melon, sprinkled with lime juice. We followed with the famous "21" hamburger—sizzling hot, deliciously brown, served on a piece of rye-bread toast. With the hamburger we munched celery and olives, and since it was late we ended our meal with a cup of Swiss coffee.

New York—Mercurio

I have lived so much in Italy and know the Italian cuisine so well that it hurts my feelings to hear, as I so often do, that "all Italian food is fattening." There are many so-called Italian restaurants in America; they serve too much pasta, and some of them specialize in a rather awful dish called Italian spaghetti and meat balls, which is unheard of in Italy. But, believe me, smart Italians, like smart Americans, know the secret of good eating.

Let me take you to a truly fine Italian restaurant—Mercurio in New York.

Here is our menu:
- Large salad bowl
- Saltimbocca
- Cooked greens
- Fruit dessert
- Café espresso

On my last visit, in honor of my dinner guest, the famous designer Mme Fontana, the maître d' himself brought out the biggest salad bowl I have ever seen and placed in it dark-green lettuce leaves, escarole, dandelions, and ripe tomatoes. With loving care he marinated the whole with golden olive oil; then he poured on some wine vinegar and, last, a pinch of fragrant herbs.

Saltimbocca is made with thin slices of veal, each covered with a slice of lean ham, about the same size. Add a pinch of herbs, preferably fresh sage. Roll up and secure with toothpicks. Then sauté in butter or olive oil until golden brown. Add a little bit of wine, cover, and cook a few minutes until tender. How appetizing it smells and looks! With this delicious fare we have our cooked mustard greens (Italians know so well how to prepare them). After such a meal it would not occur to me to offer a guest a rich dessert. We end with fresh fruit cup, and, of course, café espresso.

Buenos Aires—the Alvear Palace Hotel

You will be amazed at the superabundance of meat, milk, eggs, and cheese in Buenos Aires. In this city you can dine like a king without paying a king's ransom.

We will go to the Alvear Palace Hotel. I lived there when I was lecturing in Buenos Aires, and I ate most of my meals in the Grill Room, with government officials and with friends. One meets many North Americans there, and many celebrities.

Meats are prepared wonderfully well here and—can you believe it?—it is not unusual for an Argentine to eat a two-pound steak for lunch. However, we'll settle for half of that. With our big steak let us order a big salad made of leaf lettuce, unpeeled cucumber, chopped-up radishes, and green peppers. We will also have artichoke hearts, which are plentiful in the Argentine. These are topped with a bit of butter and taste unbelievably delicious. Once again, there is no room for a big dessert. We end our meal with a slice of juicy pineapple, sprinkled with a bit of kirsch, a demitasse, and a salute to the cuisine of the Argentine!

London—Restaurant Caprice

Now we are in London, and again, we shall have good food. We will go to the Restaurant Caprice, which was brought to my attention by the slim, Austrian-born painter Anna Meyerson. Anna knows good food; the meal she ordered for us is one I will long remember:

Belgian endive
Steak Diane
Green asparagus amandine
Wild strawberries with yogurt
Demitasse

We were treated like royalty. The headwaiter himself cooked the special steak right at our table. He put just a little oil in a heavy skillet and in less than five minutes the steak Diane was tender and delicious. With this we had the green asparagus, sprinkled with a teaspoon of toasted almonds. The wild strawberries were the last of the season and tasted especially delicious. We ate them with yogurt and honey—who could possibly prefer heavy cream?—and ended the meal with a steaming demitasse.

Paris—Maxim's

Yes, I know. French cuisine is heaven to eat but can be hell on the waistline! But here is good news: slowly and cautiously the wonderful chefs of France are changing their ways. They are not getting less wonderful—perish the thought. But they are being influenced by the Centre Gayelord Hauser, which has offices at 4 faubourg Saint-Honoré in the heart of Paris.

The new center was formed by a group of influential Parisians, headed by Philippe de Rothschild, a member of the famous Rothschild dynasty. Through their efforts, intelligent eating in all its branches is being taught to thousands. French chefs are listening and learning that they can cook leaner foods without sacrificing a soupçon of flavor or deliciousness. I have high hopes for this new awakening. Those miraculous chefs of France are among her best goodwill ambassadors; I believe that Paris may yet rule the world of intelligent eating.

Let me tell you about my happiest day at France's beloved Maxim's. The entrance was garlanded with great festoons of fresh vegetables in a riot of colors. People passing exclaimed, *"Ça, c'est fou!"* But it was no crazier than I am. In fact, it was a party given in my honor.

This was a novelty for the conservative French people; more than five hundred turned out to see *"Qu'est-ce que c'est que ça."* On one side of the famous restaurant was a Hauser bar, where fresh vegetable juices were served in champagne glasses. On the other side was a champagne bar, where the driest (which is the leanest) champagne was served. Most of the Frenchmen had first a glass of freshly made vegetable juice and then a glass of champagne; and the Paris newspaper *Figaro* the next day called me a wise man. Why? Because I featured not only my vegetable juice (which they liked) but also their French champagne, which after all is, as *Figaro* said, one of the most delicious fruit juices in the world!

After this cocktail party, I dined at Maxim's with Mme de Saint Hardouin, the French lady ambassador, who entertained me so royally at the French Embassy in Istanbul. Our menu was a celery-shrimp cocktail, followed by delicious *poulet* (tender chicken) surrounded by many small white roasted onions and served with tender *haricots verts* (green beans). For dessert, Mme de St. Hardouin, who knows exactly what I like, ordered a *coupe de fruits* made with small wild strawberries, fresh peaches, and bits of toasted almonds, to which was added just a touch of kirsch for its delicate flavor.

Venice—Taverna della Fenice

It was festival night in Venice. The hotels were packed with people from all over the world. I had arrived by plane from my vacation in Taormina to be a judge at one of those fantastic celebrity parties given by Earl Blackwell. There were many attractive and interesting people to meet—dukes and princesses everywhere—but the lady who interested me most was Gloria Swanson, also one of the judges. She was tiny and slim in her maharani costume, full of life and radiant with the spirit of tomorrow.

Gloria and I dined at the Taverna della Fenice in one of the small, intimate squares—one of the world's fine restaurants, where good food has been served for more than a hundred years. We sat in a comfortable corner where we could relax and talk. Here is what we ordered from the big menu:

> Italian salad bowl
> Grilled scampi (shrimp)
> Peach flambé
> Café espresso

While we waited for dinner, Gloria told me the why and wherefore of her great interest in food. I was amazed at her knowledge; she is a real crusader and knows from personal experience what good food can do for you. She eats little and is a connoisseur; so much so that, wherever she is, she has organically grown vegetables and fruits flown to her from California. One of her favorite meals is a salad bowl that is a complete meal; occasionally she makes this for her friends.

Dining with Friends

If someday you find before you nothing but a greasy patty shell loaded with gooey chicken à la king and a tired salad already smothered with pink dressing, cross your fingers, eat two or three bites, and keep yourself busy as the Duchess of Windsor does under such circumstances—pretending that she's busy eating, taking sips of water, and chatting with the other guests—and never accept another invitation to eat at that house! Of course, if you particularly like your hostess, you might do some missionary work: return the invitation, and give a practical demonstration of good, lean food, attractively served, in *your* home.

THREE

YOUR GOOD HEALTH

Body Works

Your Body Architecture

Visualize your skeleton—206 bones, arranged in a complex yet beautifully symmetrical pattern by the Master Builder. The bones are living entities, not the dead, dry, rattling things you imagine. They are pinkish white on the outside, filled with living yellow or red bone marrow (the red marrow produces red corpuscles). The bone surface seems hard at first glance, but if you look carefully you will see minute openings through which are intertwined the arteries, veins, nerves, and connective tissues that keep your bones alive and healthy.

Your bones are made of living cells, which determine their tenacity and elasticity, and mineral component (calcium phosphate and calcium carbonate), which gives bones their hardness and rigidity. You know how light your bones are; but have you any idea of their strength? It has been calculated that bone, weight for weight, is almost as efficient as steel.

STRAIGHTEN YOUR SPINE

Visualize your spine. When you do, you automatically "brace up," do you not? It is not by accident that we speak of moral strength as "backbone," of weakness as "spinelessness," that we call an honest person "upright" or "straight." It is your spine that makes you superior to the lower animals, or invertebrates. It is your erect backbone, plus your well-developed hand (particularly the thumb), that makes you superior to the higher animals.

Visualize a flexible column a little over two feet long, consisting of thirty-three separate vertebrae—cylindrical bones all containing a central canal and strung on the spinal cord, almost like beads of a necklace. Almost, but not quite—since the support that holds the vertebrae together is not the spinal cord running through them but the ligaments that run along their outside and the very close fit they have upon each other due to the presence, between each vertebra and the next, of a spongy, elastic circle of cartilage called a *spinal disc*. The fact that the vertebrae are so separated gives the spine its remarkable flexibility and helps it absorb shocks, such as the impact of the body weight hitting the ground with each step in walking.

Let us begin at your tail. The lowest four vertebrae are fused into one bone, the coccyx, or vestigial tail, whose office is to close the floor of the pelvis. By the time you are twenty-five years old, the next five vertebrae also have been fused, to become the sacrum or "sacred bone"—so called because at one time this was thought to be the seat of the soul. Next come the five lumbar vertebrae, which support the abdominal organs; next, the twelve dorsal vertebrae, to which the ribs are attached; and at the top are the seven cervical vertebrae, which I have saved for the last because they particularly concern us.

Let's Turn Your Head

Turn your head to the left. And to the right. Nod it up and down. Now rotate your head slowly. How is it that you are able to do this? Because of those seven cervical vertebrae, particularly the last two—the topmost, or atlas vertebra, named after the mythological giant who supported the globe (in this case, your skull) and, just under it, the axis vertebra, so called because your head turns on it as the earth turns on its axis.

Here is the crossroads between your body and your mind. Here, in these bones, muscles, and nerve cells, is where, in time of danger, you instinctively thrust forward to initiate action or draw back to defend yourself. Here, in the simple gesture of nodding your head or shaking it, is where you register your opinions, reactions, and decisions. Is it any wonder that human beings, who so often are tense, confused, and flooded with conflicting desires (in other words, whose yes-no signals get jammed at the crossroads), so often suffer from stiff neck?

Now we have reached your skull. Its top part (cranium) is the container for that vast and powerful organ, your brain. It is egg-shaped and is one of the toughest bone structures you have. Though it gives the impression of surface smoothness, it is a complex jigsaw puzzle of eight different bones, fitted together with incredible precision. The lower part of the skull is the part organized for the purpose of eating—mostly cheekbones and jaws. It is interesting that the teeth are not considered a part of the skeleton, but, like the fingernails, are derived from body cells related to those that produce skin.

Your Torso, Arms, and Legs

Attached to the spine is the bone framework of the chest—twelve pairs of ribs and the breastbone, which form a protective cage for the heart and lungs and give the latter "houseroom" to expand and contract during breathing.

The bone structure of arms and legs is basically the same—a single long bone (upper arm, thigh) and a pair of bones (forearm, leg) to which are attached the hand or foot. Both extremities are fastened to the spinal column by special bones of their own—the shoulder blades (scapulae) for the arms and the pelvis for the legs. You can easily visualize your joints and the "ball-and-socket" principle on which they are constructed, giving you freedom of movement and activity.

But stop a moment to pay homage to your two forearm bones, the radius and ulna, whose rotation around each other allows for the extra action capacity of your hand. There is evidence that, in the course of evolution, the exploring function of the ape's hand was one of the major factors in the development of the higher centers of the brain, those of the cerebral cortex. This started something, evolutionary scientists tell us. It led to the development of the human animal, man, and eventually of civilization and culture—all of which are the result of coordination of the hand with the brain, of using the hand for intelligent purposes.

Your Muscular Body

With the mental picture of your skeleton in mind, follow with me the handiwork of the Master Sculptor who has fashioned on this framework (helpless in itself) the glistening forms of reddish muscular clay that give it shapeliness and make it capable of movement. Two materials have been used—muscle fibers and connective tissue.

Muscles, generally speaking, are of two kinds—voluntary and involuntary. The voluntary muscles perform as your conscious mind directs them, ache when you are bruised, rest when you rest. These have been attached to your body armature in broad or narrow bands or crisscross like basketwork. They are the instruments of your power, strength, skill, mobility, and self-defense.

Stop reading for a moment and clench your hands, feet, and jaws; wrinkle your forehead and tense your belly and buttocks. Then let yourself relax. You have just brought into play virtually your entire equipment of voluntary muscles, and these muscles, incidentally, constitute 42 percent of your body weight.

THE INDEPENDENT MUSCLES

Unless you happen to be a yogi, you cannot give your involuntary muscles the same workout. Hidden deep in the recesses of your body structure, these muscles are entirely controlled by your involuntary nervous system. You can neither set them in motion nor stop them, though they are responsible for all your internal bodily activity except chemical action. They relax and regulate themselves, independent of your will. Their steady contraction and release is slow, rhythmic, and perpetual, pushing food through your digestive tract, milking body fluids and glandular secretions along to their appointed destinations, moving your blood stream, and collecting and disposing of waste material. You are usually unaware of their action unless something gets blocked—the ureter by a kidney stone, for example—in which case you feel rhythmic pain as the muscle strains to dislodge the obstruction. The most noticeable involuntary muscle contractions are those that cause your normal breathing, the "hunger pangs" of an empty stomach, and cramps in conjunction with menstruation.

A Natural Corset

Your muscles would be useless without their "cement" of connective tissue. A muscle is actually a bundle of muscle fibers bound together in sheaths of connective tissue. Muscles, in turn, are fastened to your bones by more connective tissue in the form of tendons and bursae (little bags filled with semifluid material that serve as pulleys at some of your joints). Bones are joined to other bones by connective tissue in the form of ligaments. Connective-tissue fibers, knitted into open webbing, form the groundwork for the construction of your skin and membranes. Spread out into great flat sheets, connective tissue wraps your viscera, heart, and lungs in a strong windingcloth; it forms a large part of the wall of the digestive tract and lines the entire body cavity with a firm, elastic underpinning. When I speak of the "natural corset" that my stomach-lift exercise (chapter 9) helps you to develop, I am talking about connective tissue.

Your Digestive Laboratory

Your digestive system is an amazing, completely automatic laboratory, in operation twenty-four hours a day. What you eat is still being digested by your small intestine eight or nine hours after being swallowed and may remain in the large intestine at least ten (or as long as forty) hours after that.

Your body needs energy for operation, and building blocks for repair of structures involved in its operation. To supply this energy and these building blocks, you must eat. But food, as is, won't nourish you. It must first be changed into the smaller building blocks (glucose, amino acids, fatty acids, and glycerin) that can pass through the narrow portals of the intestinal wall. These changes take place in the digestive tract, which has the following functions: to take in food; to break down the more complex foodstuffs into small particles by (1) mechanical and (2) chemical processes; to assimilate these particles, store them, and finally eliminate from the body undigested waste material. The digestive system consists of (1) the alimentary canal, through which food passes while it is being processed, and (2) the accessory glands (liver and pancreas) that aid this digestion.

Your alimentary canal, a hollow tube which begins with the mouth and ends with the rectum, is anywhere from twenty-five to thirty feet long—five times as long as you are. While you are "digesting" this remarkable fact, here comes another: the inner lining of your small intestine, because of the way it is made, presents an absorptive surface of well over one hundred square feet. (You probably know night clubs whose dance floors are not much bigger.)

Actually, your alimentary canal is composed of four tubes, one inside the other. The innermost tube, called the mucosa, supplies many of the glands that produce the digestive juices (there are 35,000,000 of these glands in the stomach alone) and also contains the blood vessels into which the food is finally absorbed. The next tube, proceeding outward, is the submucosa, composed of connective tissue and mainly protective and supporting. Outside of this is the muscular coat, with smooth muscle fibers running both circularly and longitudinally. This allows the two basic types of motion: one to grind up and mix food with the digestive juices, and the other the long, sweeping, wormlike peristaltic waves that move food down along the tract. The outermost layer, called the serosa, is smooth, glistening connective tissue, continuous with the lining of the body cavity.

Chew It Well

Now watch. Food goes into your mouth, which bites it off and grinds it into pieces small enough to swallow. Digestion starts here, in the action of saliva, which contains an enzyme called ptyalin. (There are twenty or more digestive enzymes, agents that promote chemical reactions without themselves being changed.) Ptyalin converts starch part way into sugar; that is why, when you chew up a piece of bread, it begins to taste sweet; it is also one reason why you are urged to chew food well.

The tongue pushes the food into the pharynx (back of the throat). While you are swallowing, the soft palate rises to close the nasal passages, and the lidlike epiglottis drops to close off the entrance to the lungs, so you won't choke. Now the food is propelled by muscular contractions down the ten-inch-long esophagus and into the stomach. If you have overeaten and feel "stuffed," I'll tell you why: the stomach has had all it can hold, the valve at its entrance has closed, and food is massed in the esophagus.

The Stomach

Now the food has reached the stomach, which lies under your left rib margin, not in the center of the abdomen, as often is supposed. Empty, the stomach is more or less tube-shaped and rather small: distended by food, it is pear-shaped and has a capacity of one to one-and-a-half quarts. Its functions are storage, mechanical mixing, and chemical digestion. It operates like a churn, producing three wavelike motions a minute. Tea, coffee, and broth pass through the stomach almost as soon as they are swallowed. Milk takes somewhat longer; it gets mixed with rennet, which curdles it for digestibility. Thin cereal may pass through in two to three hours; a heavy dinner may linger six hours. The digestion of protein goes on apace in the stomach; that explains why bulky vegetables and fats "stay with you longer" than most proteins; they do, literally, stay longer in the stomach. Stomach activity reaches its peak about two hours after you have eaten; in about four hours' time you begin to feel the "hunger contractions" that tell you it is getting empty again.

Twenty-Foot Trip

From the stomach, food passes into the small intestine, which is more than twenty feet of mechanical and chemical action. If you have had a hearty meal, the small intestine is in for five or six hours' ceaseless activity—squeezing shut to break food into smaller and smaller bits, churning it, moving it by peristalsis along the tract. The innermost lining of this intestine has rough, ridge-like folds covered with millions of tiny hairlike protuberances called *villi;* this provides the huge surface area I mentioned, necessary for the body to absorb all the food it needs, either directly into the blood stream or (especially in the case of fats) into the small canals called lymphatics which then empty into the blood stream.

Now take a side glance at your liver and pancreas, which went into action the instant food began passing through the pylorus, or gate, between the stomach and the duodenum (the first nine inches of the small intestine). The secretions of the stomach are acid; of the intestine, alkaline. To achieve this acid-to-alkaline change, the liver pours in bile. The pancreas also helps, and the intestine itself secretes alkaline fluid.

The food, as it has been traveling along hour after hour, has been churned and mixed into a sudsy froth; by the end of its twenty-foot journey, almost all that is usable has been absorbed into your body. It has been transformed into the four essentials of life: glucose, amino acids, fatty acids, and glycerin. The fatty acids and glycerin have been picked up by the hairlike villi and passed into the lymphatic system; glucose and the amino acids have been passed through the intestinal wall, picked up by the blood, and carried to the liver. Each of your body cells knows what it needs—to build skin and hair cells, repair muscles, kidneys, etc.—and picks it up in exactly the right combinations from the blood stream. The miracle has happened: your food has become *you*.

What is left? Waste products—dead bacteria, shed cells, mucus, and indigestible cellulose such as vegetable fibers, peel, and seeds. Still in very fluid form, this passes into the large intestine (between five and six feet long) where it is compressed into feces, thus saving the body water that would otherwise escape (as in diarrhea) and lead to body dehydration. The large intestine takes its time over this—ten to forty hours. The digestive tract absorbs nearly everything that can be utilized. And any food it doesn't need, it stores—as you know—as body fat.

Your Circulatory System

Perhaps the best way to appreciate the wonders of your circulatory system is to think of your body lying flat and of yourself looking down on it as you might look at a familiar country on an outspread color map, studying its rivers and streams.

Your Rivers of Life

You will see three rivers—one bright red, one dark red (almost black), one white—sometimes running parallel, sometimes intertwined, all traversing the entire country of your body, each intent on its own commerce, yet all three emptying at certain places into one another.

Your bright-red arterial stream forcefully spurts along, flowing out from the heart by the great aorta, coursing through smaller and smaller arteries, dwindling at last, just under all your body surfaces, into tiny networks of tributaries called the capillaries. Carrying foodstuffs, oxygen to burn them, hormones, and repair material, it also maintains your body's even temperature. Its capillaries flow into the venous stream, which, through veins that coalesce to become even larger and larger, ebbs back toward the heart. Heavy with waste products, its hemoglobin is black with the carbon dioxide (smoke) from burned foodstuffs. And the third—the lymphatic stream, white though it is, transports an even denser cargo of debris than the venous river. Think of it as your body's drainage canal.

Your Heart Is a Pump

Now for a breath-taking experience. Look into your heart—a hollow muscular organ, just a bit larger than your clenched fist, lying behind the lower part of your breastbone, a little toward the left. You will see four chambers—two auricles above, two ventricles below. The auricle and ventricle on the left side are filled with bright-red arterial blood; the right auricle and ventricle are dark with venous blood. Both your auricles and the right ventricle are thin-walled chambers, but the muscular walls of the left ventricle are about three times thicker than those of the right and develop pressure six times greater—and soon you will understand why.

Your auricles receive blood, force it through very efficient valves into the ventricles, which contract their walls to send it out again—bright blood from the left, which goes to the body for maintenance; dark blood from the right, which goes to the lungs for purification. Both ventricles contract together, and when they do, it sends a throbbing wave through your every artery and capillary. This occurs sixty to seventy times every minute of your life if you are in good health, and you know it as your pulse beat.

Your Life Blood

Pure, sparkling, oxygen-laden blood, entering the left auricle from the lungs, flows into the left ventricle and is pumped by those extra-powerful muscles through the arteries to the capillaries of your head, toes, fingertips, and everywhere in between. Reaching the venous stream, the arterial river empties into the venous capillaries and turns back heartward. At the upper part of your chest, the white lymphatic stream, fed from tissues all over your body, dumps its entire contents. It has been laving your tissue spaces in a sort of bath of nutrient, and into your venous river, already heavy with waste material, it empties its dishwater. Dreary and black now, the venous river reaches the right auricle of the heart, passes into the right ventricle, which pumps it back into the lungs, from which—presto!—bright and sparkling again from oxygen, it goes back to the left auricle and instantly begins all over.

It takes less than two minutes for your blood streams to traverse your entire body. What you have just witnessed happens thirty times every hour, every hour of your life.

There are about ten pints of blood and plasma in your body, and this represents about 10 percent of your body weight. Blood consists of liquid plasma and cells, or corpuscles—the red ones that transport oxygen and the white corpuscles that combat infection. Lymph is blood plasma minus red corpuscles; that is why it is white. Your heart pumps five quarts of blood a minute through the circulatory system at rest, and as many as twenty-five quarts during exercise or exertion.

TUBES WITHIN TUBES

The tubes that carry your blood and lymph are similar in structure to your other body tubes—the alimentary canal, for instance, with which you already have become familiar. That is, they consist of tubes within tubes—in this case, three: an inner tube of tissuelike cellular membrane, a middle tube of involuntary muscle fiber, and a strong protecting outer coat of connective tissue. Like your other body tubes, they are controlled by the switchboard of your central nervous system, and when this operates smoothly, all goes well with your blood circulation. Let the different telephone exchanges disagree, however, and send contradictory orders from brain to heart about the amount of blood needed in different organs, muscles, and glands, and your whole body feels the effect of the quarrel.

Your Respiratory System

Air (oxygen) is taken into your nasal cavities, where it is warmed by contact with the warm vascular structures of the nasopharynx and cleaned by the hairs at the entrance to the nose and by the very tiny hairs deeper inside. Mucus cells in the nose help humidify the air to make it more acceptable and less irritating to the more delicate structures inside the chest. Passing through the nasal passages, the air enters the pharynx, a fibromuscular structure about five inches long, through which, as we have seen, your food also passes. Now air and food passages separate, food continuing down the esophagus at the back of the throat and air entering the larynx or voice box at the front of the neck (from the outside, this is seen as your Adam's apple).

Next, air proceeds into the trachea or windpipe, an elastic tube about five inches long, about as big around as your index finger. Behind the important Angle of Louis, the bump on your breastbone, the windpipe branches into the two main bronchi and thence into the much smaller bronchioles, which divide into small ducts that lead into the lungs proper—large, spongy half-cones occupying the chest and consisting entirely of alveoli or air sacs, so called because they are hollow—*alveolus* means "a little hollow" in Latin. The walls of the alveoli are a busy network of capillaries through which your blood cells continually hurry in single file, giving off carbon dioxide and then taking up the oxygen you have just inhaled.

As you breathe in, your diaphragm, a large flat muscle separating your chest from your abdomen, contracts, moving itself somewhat downward and thereby increasing the capacity of the chest. Also, your ribs rise from a sloping to a more horizontal position, increasing the front-to-back diameter of your chest. It is this creation of a partial vacuum in the chest, followed by the inrush of air, which fills the alveoli of your lungs. For exhalation, your diaphragm relaxes and is pushed upward by your abdominal viscera; the ribs return to their former position. And thus your breath (now containing carbon dioxide) is squeezed out of the alveoli, into the conducting tubes, and out into the world again.

Your Cells Must Breathe Too

All right. You have drawn breath and released it. Now watch the way your circulatory and respiratory systems combine in your best interests. Every living cell in your body—organs, glands, tissues, bones—must do what you are doing: it must breathe and keep on breathing. That is, it must maintain constant interchange of health-giving oxygen and death-dealing carbon dioxide. In those moist, membranous air-filled sponges—your lungs—is accomplished this transfer of the two gases into and out of the solution in the blood stream. Your lungs have breathed the breath of life on every drop of bright-red blood in your arterial stream. Moreover, the suction of your breathing is felt by all the branches of your venous system, whose muscular walls need the extra power of this suction to return their dark blood from the peripheral tissues to your heart. And think especially of this: so perfectly do the speeding and slowing of your respiration, the shallowness and depth of it, respond to your various *emotional* states that they transmit your every mood and temper to the remotest recesses of every one of your bodily structures.

Take a Big Breath

There is nothing that can give you a greater instant lift than filling your lungs with clean air. Yes, plain fresh air is one of the most important elements in your life. Air contains the vital properties that cleanse the body. The thoroughness with which those thirty trillions of cells of your body are pepped up and energized depends on the way in which you breathe. Just as air is the most important element of nature, so breathing is the most important function of your whole body.

The Hindus, more than any other people, took their breathing seriously (perhaps because they had so little food). Their yogis were the first to develop breathing into a vital part of their daily living. The respected Vivekananda taught his millions of followers that all the good things in life—inner peace, poise, good health, and longevity—depend on right breathing. Yogis are also taught that fresh air contains *prana,* which contains the vital spirit. Whether this is so, we Westerners are hardly in a position to tell. What we do know—and scientists have been able to prove this—is that deep rhythmic breathing, charging the body with as much fresh air as possible, is the quickest way to pep up, vivify, and energize a tired body. There are many schools of "breath culture," but I believe diaphragmatic breathing is the best and most successful method. My pupils call it "belly breathing," because that is where deep breathing starts.

Whenever your spirits sag, when your thinking becomes foggy, or whenever you feel tired, tank up with more oxygen. Step outside, or at least open a window, and inhale as much fresh air as possible through the nose. (As you do this, your stomach pulls inward and your chest expands.) After you have inhaled all you can of fresh air—through the nose, remember—exhale the air slowly through the mouth, making a slight whistling sound. The longer you can make the exhalation last, the better. I believe the million-dollar secret of the yogis, who have perfect breath control, is their long exhalation. Do this inhalation through the nose and longer exhalation through the mouth about five times. Do it quietly, in a relaxed manner. You will be amazed how mental cobwebs and fatigue disappear almost instantly. Professor Tiralla, in Vienna, discovered that even the tension that causes high blood pressure is reduced by slow, rhythmic, deep breathing.

If you smoke, or if you live in a city with bad pollution problems, you should make special pains to get air into those oxygen-starved lungs. Take yourself to the country and breathe deeply.

Your Nervous System

To visualize your nervous system, we will use the classic analogy of the telephone exchange. This vast and busy mechanism not only consists of visible brain cells, tissues, and nerve fibers but also is the invisible stuff your awareness, knowledge, memory, emotions, and experience are made of. So I want to present it to you, first, not as a bodily structure but as an over-all concept.

Your nervous system has two parts—the voluntary (or cerebrospinal) system and the involuntary (or autonomic) system. The voluntary system controls your conscious activities; it serves your voluntary muscles (biceps, triceps, muscles of the eye and jaw, etc.); it needs about eight hours in twenty-four for rest and recuperation in sleep. The involuntary system controls your unconscious activities; it serves your involuntary muscles (those which accomplish digestion, gland secretion, blood circulation, etc.); from the moment you are conceived until the end of your life, it never sleeps.

Voluntary nerves activate your five senses and your external physical response to the outside world; they get their signals from your conscious mind. Involuntary nerves activate your internal bodily processes and your emotional responses; they get their signals from your unconscious mind. I like to think of it this way: your voluntary nervous system says, "I see, I hear, I smell, I taste, I touch; I think, speak, decide, act." Your involuntary nervous system says, "I am."

A Living Telephone Exchange

Now let us look at this central nervous system—your personal, built-in telephone exchange. "Central" is your brain, which fills your skull and, at the base of the skull, narrows to become your spinal cord, which is about one-half inch in diameter and is threaded through the vertebrae of your backbone down as far as the small of your back (about eighteen inches). The brain and spinal cord weigh about three pounds. They are fashioned of spongy gray matter and bundles of incredibly fine white fibers—the nerves. From this switchboard Central sends out wires (peripheral nerves) to every part of your body—voluntary or fast nerve fibers, over which messages travel more than 500 feet per second, and involuntary or slow nerve fibers, which carry messages at 15 feet per second. This network of trunk lines establishes and maintains contact between you and your environment. In addition, it has local telephone exchanges that keep the different parts of your body in communication with one another. Also, it has private telephones connecting one portion of the brain with another. Most remarkable of all, perhaps, it has a two-way 'intercom" phone over which your conscious and unconscious minds talk back and forth—and how they argue, at times!

Truly, your body is one of the great wonders of the world of nature. Do you now see why it must have good nutrition to function efficiently?

Resistance to Disease

> If you have a health problem, be sure to discuss it with your family physician. He or she alone is in a position to advise you. In the next few pages, let us consider how certain food elements help take care of some specific needs. Whatever vitamins and supplements your doctor prescribes, be sure to take them faithfully, and buy the best and freshest high-vitality foods your budget permits. Make every effort to find a doctor who has studied and applied modern nutrition. Many doctors have a woeful knowledge of this area.

Infections

You can reduce your susceptibility to many infections that are commonly accepted as inevitable in life by building up your body resistance.

Your blood stream, the river of life that can bring health and nourishment to every part of your body, is a two-way river. Flowing in one direction is your arterial blood stream carrying nourishment, along with the oxygen needed for its utilization, to every cell of your body. Flowing in the other direction is your venous blood stream removing carbon dioxide and other waste matter from your body cells.

For the proper nourishment of every organ in your body and for building resistance to infection, the arterial blood stream must contain an adequate daily supply of nutrients.

According to one study presented at an annual meeting of the American Dieticians' Association, "infections are likely to have more serious consequences among persons with clinical and subclinical malnutrition, and infectious diseases have the capacity to turn borderline nutritional deficiencies into severe malnutrition."

Proteins containing all the essential amino acids are of first importance if the body is to produce its own army of antibodies and cells known as *phagocytes,* which destroy bacteria and viruses invading your life stream. Experiments have shown that when a high-protein diet replaces one low in protein, as many as a hundred times more antibodies are produced within a week. (See page 18 for high-protein foods.)

Not less than 60 to 70 grams of complete protein should be consumed daily. Higher amounts (100 to 150 grams) are recommended prior to or following surgery, when infection has taken hold, and during convalescence. In severe burns the amount climbs even higher. If possible, at least one third of the protein eaten each day should come from animal sources. One of the cheapest, most palatable, most concentrated, and most completely digested of all protein foods is powdered skim milk. Two tablespoons provide 6 grams of protein. The non-instant type (available in health-food stores) has not been exposed to as much processing as the instant variety and so retains more nutrients. The addition of half a cup of dry skim milk to such dishes as cream soups, milk drinks, junkets, and custards will give you an unbelievable amount of protein value to fight foreign invaders. For example, cook hot cereal with milk instead of water, and sprinkle in powdered milk for superfortification. You might also mix it into scrambled eggs, ground meat, sandwich fillings (such as egg salad), cottage cheese, mayonnaise, or any casserole dish.

Of all the vitamins, A and C are the two most important for building up resistance and combating infections. It is a well-known fact that epidemics are rampant during famines and wars when the diets are deficient in proteins and vitamins A and C. Drs. King and Menton have reported that resistance to diphtheria is increased by taking large amounts of vitamin C, and Kaiser reports that streptococci are less likely to be found in the tonsils of patients who have been given large amounts of this vitamin. Vitamin A is of value in combating infections of the lungs and bronchi; it maintains the health of all mucous membranes, including the lining of the respiratory tract. As Dr. Walter Eddy has pointed out, "Vitamin A is necessary for resistance to germ invasions."

Mucus is a natural secretion that protects underlying tissues from bacterial penetration and also has a cleansing effect on the underlying cells. Bacteria cannot survive where normal amounts of healthy mucus stand guard.

Vitamin A is found in all yellow and green vegetables and fruits and in liver, cream, and butter. It may not be possible to eat these foods in quantity during illness, in which case vitamin A requirements can be supplied by taking fish-liver-oil capsules immediately after meals, or by preparing a juice of blended raw green vegetables (most palatable when mixed with tomato or carrot juice).

For a list of other sources of vitamin A, see page 34. Make sure that your daily diet contains adequate supplies of this life-giving nutrient; it is "A" must for a healthy life stream.

Vitamin C (ascorbic acid), equally important to healthy resistance, is found in all fresh fruits and vegetables, especially in rose hips and orange juice. Its precise function is not understood, but it is known to be an important factor in the formation of collagen—a protein that holds cells together and a vital substance in the process of wound healing. Clinical experiments have shown that when body temperature increases (as in fever), blood levels of vitamin C decrease. Some studies show that for the phagocytes (bacteria-destroying white blood cells) to be effective, they must contain a certain concentration of ascorbic acid. Just how vitamin C affects viral infections (like the common cold) has not yet been deduced. Two or three glasses of fresh citrus juice daily will give you an adequate supply of the potent vitamin C so necessary to a smooth-flowing life stream. On page 46 you will find a list of other sources of vitamin C.

For those who cannot take that quantity of fresh juice daily, I recommend the substitution, when necessary, of a 100-milligram tablet of ascorbic acid or, still better, rose-hip tablets, nature's richest source of vitamin C.

Five hundred milligrams of ascorbic acid (vitamin C) can be taken every hour to good advantage at the beginning of any infection, including the common cold. Take it with a glass of milk or calcium tablets. However, if the infection is severe, consult a nutrition-minded physician.

In combating any infection, the entire diet must be made adequate not only in protein and the vitamins A and C but in all nutrients.

FOCAL INFECTIONS

Focal infections are bacterial infections that occur in various localized areas, such as teeth or tonsils; they can occasionally trigger other infections, even in remote parts of the body. Certainly a sound diet will help you in your fight against them, as well as in your need for a superabundance of certain special factors; but why prolong the fight when a good doctor can help you track down the seat of your difficulty, and in many cases offer measures that lead more quickly to its elimination?

The location of focal infection is often difficult to track down. Teeth, for instance, in which the nerves have died can easily become infected—they have nothing with which to fight back. If you are fatigued and "all dragged out" from toxins pouring into your blood due to infections at the roots of devitalized teeth —get them pulled out.

Focal infections long were blamed for arthritis. In some cases, the elimination of the focus is accompanied by a dramatic subsiding of the arthritic symptoms. In many other cases, the focus may be eliminated but the arthritis remains. What does that mean? Is the theory of focal infection, as the cause, wrong? Perhaps yes—in an individual case—perhaps no, even for the particular case in question. There may be other foci present in the body. A focal infection of long standing not infrequently migrates to remote parts of the body to set up new foci.

Focal infections are sometimes responsible for neuritis, which can be most painful. The foci also may be located in the blood vessels themselves. This condition occurs most often in the veins of the extremities, producing phlebitis. Sinusitis, or "sinus trouble," represents a discomforting and sometimes very painful infection, stubborn in responding to treatment.

Quite apart from any direct kind of treatment, the most valuable measures in combating focal infections are those that build up the general health—diet, rest, sunshine, and fresh air. The High-Vitality Diet in chapter 4 should be followed. Moreover, you should give special attention to vitamin C. Eat as much as you can of foods that are rich in it. Eat your green vegetables raw in salads, or short-cooked, to preserve as much vitamin C as possible. Your physician may recommend fortifying your diet with vitamin C tablets. It is an established fact that in the presence of bacterial infections the vitamin C content of the body fluids is grealy decreased. Moreover, both vitamins B_1 and C are excreted in perspiration, and you must make up for this loss, particularly in hot weather.

Summarizing the treatment of infections caused by disturbances of the blood circulation, we find that the first step is to locate and remove focal infections. With these sources of infection removed, the blood stream, freed of pollution, can re-establish a balanced circulation in all organs of the body, especially when all of the vital nutrients are taken not just for a week or two but for all the rest of your long life.

Diabetes

In talking about diet and disease, diabetes almost immediately comes to mind. Diabetes mellitus is a metabolic disorder characterized by a lack of insulin, a substance secreted by the pancreas that effects the transfer of glucose from outside the cell to within. It is a complex disease and all diabetics should be under a physician's care. Each person's tolerance for carbohydrates is governed by the state of his insulin sufficiency, and the patient must be guided accordingly. As practically all foods, apart from meat and fats, contain varying amounts of carbohydrates, proper diets can be furnished only by direct medical supervision.

There are, however, several general comments that I would like to make about the diet in diabetes. Frequently it is reduced to such a preponderance of protein and fat that little room remains for foods that are rich in many of the vitamins and minerals. I would advise the patient to discuss with his physician the use of as many vegetables as possible. The low-carbohydrate vegetables generally can be eaten, and most of them provide important sources of vitamins; try, with your physician, to select the vegetables that give you as many and as much of the various vitamins and minerals as possible. Then, if the diet is not adequate in vitamins and minerals, ask your physician to recommend a proper vitamin and mineral supplement for you to use.

The incidence of vascular disease is significantly higher in diabetics. In our discussion of hardening of the arteries, I make clear the role played by dietary fat in atherosclerosis. We find also that choline and inositol have been shown as effective in preventing hardening of the arteries. Discuss this matter with your physician. His purpose is to help you, and he will welcome your intelligent interest in your own care and what he is doing for you.

The great task in our program is to *prevent* diabetes. The overeating of refined sugars, for years and years, may well overwork and depress the insulin-producing cells until they finally break down. Obesity combined with inactivity seems to enhance the susceptibility to diabetes. If diabetes has ever occurred in your family, don't weigh one pound more than you should, and keep active. And make sure you're getting a superabundance of the B vitamins. These are extremely important. In Europe, vitamin B is sometimes called the poor man's insulin.

Hypoglycemia—Low Blood Sugar

Although low blood sugar is regarded as the opposite of diabetes, many specialists believe that it is actually a different stage of the same disease.

In his book, *Dr. Atkins' Diet Revolution*, Dr. Robert C. Atkins writes: "I've done 8,000 glucose tolerance tests on overweight people . . . out of the 75% who showed a problem response, 25% revealed varying degrees of diabetes, and 75% showed varying indications of low blood sugar . . . 80% of the diabetic responders showed manifestations of *both* diabetes and low blood sugar. These two seemingly opposite conditions can and do coexist—and quite commonly." Dr. Atkins adds: "Addictive people seem to have one thing in common: an underlying hypoglycemia [low blood sugar]. We certainly see hypoglycemia in sugar addicts, in alcoholics, in coffee and cola addicts. People who have studied hard-drug addicts report to me that hypoglycemia is common among them."

Those who suffer from hypoglycemia have a problem metabolizing refined carbohydrates, such as white sugar and white flour. An excessive intake of these foods stimulates overproduction of insulin in the pancreas. Insulin floods the blood stream, causing the blood sugar to fall. The brain has no storehouse for sugar and relies on a steady supply via the blood stream. When that supply is inadequate, brain function slows down and the victim becomes extremely tired.

There are many other symptoms of low blood sugar besides constant fatigue. The most common are: headaches, depression, insomnia, leg cramps, vertigo, forgetfulness, staggering, unusual heart action, irritability, blurred vision, gout, lack of concentration, gastrointestinal disorders, suicidal tendencies, cold sweats, allergies, anxiety, itching, uncoordination, arthritis, drowsiness, nightmares, excessive daydreaming (especially among children), and nervous breakdown. In severe cases, the sufferer may go into a coma or have convulsions. Surely, anyone suspected of being mentally ill, every alcoholic and drug addict, and anyone arrested for criminal or disruptive behavior should be examined for low blood sugar. In fact, I suggest you make the five-hour glucose-tolerance test a part of your annual physical checkup.

Hypoglycemia can be controlled by diet. Small, frequent, high-protein meals (five or six each day) are most helpful.

Dr. John W. Tintera made the following suggestions for the treatment of hypoglycemia in the July 1, 1955, issue of the *New York State Journal of Medicine*:

Foods Permitted

1. Meats, fish, shellfish
2. Eggs, milk, cheese, butter, and other dairy products
3. Nuts and seeds (normally I would recommend the unsalted ones, but, since this type of diet often results in sodium depletion, especially during hot weather, Dr. Tintera has suggested unrestricted use of salt)
4. Peanut butter, sugar-free (I suggest the many fine nut butters at your health-food store)
5. Decaffeinated coffee and weak tea (herb teas are preferable)
6. Soybeans and soybean products (here is a rich, inexpensive source of good protein)
7. Low-carbohydrate bread in moderation
8. Dill pickles, olives, and cider vinegar
9. All fresh fruits and vegetables not on the "Avoid" list

Foods to Avoid

1. All sugars and sweets (see following chart)
2. Dried fruits (dates, raisins, etc.)
3. Soft drinks and other sweet beverages
4. Coffee and strong tea
5. Alcoholic beverages and other stimulants
6. Breads, pies, cakes, cookies, pastries, candies, etc.
7. Cereals, both hot and cold, except possibly oatmeal
8. All high-carbohydrate foods—such as macaroni, corn, rice, peas, beans, spaghetti, potatoes

For People Who Bluntly Tell Me They Eat No Sugar, Let Them Look at This List and Blush

FOOD	AVERAGE PORTION	TEASPOONS OF WHITE SUGAR
FRUITS AND JUICES		
Canned pears	3 halves	3½
Canned apricots	4 halves	3
Canned fruit juice	½ cup	2
Canned peaches	2 halves	3½
Fruit compote	½ cup	2
Canned fruit salad	½ cup	3½

DAIRY PRODUCTS

Ice-cream cone	1	5
Ice-cream soda	1	5
Ice-cream sundae	1	7
Malt chocolate shake	1	6

BEVERAGES

Cola	8 ounces	4
Root beer	8 ounces	4
Seven-Up	8 ounces	3½
Sweet soda pop	8 ounces	5
Ginger ale	8 ounces	5

CAKES, COOKIES AND PASTRIES

Pound cake	1 average piece	5
Sponge cake	1 average piece	2
Angel food cake	1 average piece	7
Cheese cake	1 average piece	2
Cup cake	1 average piece	5
Fruit cake	1 average piece	5
Brownies	1 average piece	3
Fig newton	1 average piece	5
Macaroons	1 average piece	6
Oatmeal cookies	1 average piece	2
Chocolate eclair	1 average piece	8
Cream puff	1 average piece	5
Doughnut	1 average piece	3
Danish roll	1	4½

MISCELLANEOUS

Custard	1 cup	4
Jello	½ cup	5
Apple pie	1 average slice	7
Blueberry pie	1 average slice	10
Cherry pie	1 average slice	10
Lemon pie	1 average slice	7
Chocolate mousse	½ cup	4
Rice pudding	½ cup	5
Sherbet	½ cup	8

It is most important to begin the day with a hearty, high-protein breakfast. Lunch and dinner should also be high-protein and relatively high-fat, and between-meal snacks should be milk, cheese, nuts, meat, hard-boiled eggs, or other proteins. Since the blood sugar level begins to sag two or three hours after meals, office workers can prevent that midmorning and midafternoon letdown by keeping high-protein wafers or tablets (available at health-food stores) in their desk.

Suggested Menu

On Getting Up:	Small glass of unsweetened fruit or tomato juice
Breakfast:	½ grapefruit, eggs, fish, hamburger, cheese, or ½ cup nuts
2 Hours after Breakfast:	Your choice of fresh fruit or vegetable juice
Lunch:	Your choice of meat, fish, eggs, or poultry; fresh salad; fresh fruit for dessert
3 Hours after Lunch:	Protein snack, your choice of nuts, seeds, hard-boiled egg, soya beans
1 Hour before Dinner:	Fruit or vegetable juice
Dinner:	Salad; meat, fish, or poultry; green cooked vegetable; fresh fruit; decaffeinated coffee
2 Hours after Dinner:	High-protein snacks, seeds, nuts; just remember to avoid sugar and other carbohydrates like the plague!

Cancer

The diagnosis of cancer in its earliest stages is of the utmost importance. Much can be done then that is not possible once the growth has gotten out of control. The cancer cell is a runaway cell, one that has lost all restraint. It goes on, at an accelerated rate, producing new cells, proliferating new tissue, until it crowds out the surrounding tissues, impairing and ultimately obliterating them.

In the past few years we have learned a great deal about the characteristics of cancer, much about means of its identity and diagnosis, and something about its treatment in the early stages. Its causes, however, remain elusive. There are theories galore. They run the gamut, from diet to the endocrine glands, highly involved aspects of physiologic chemistry, and even the very genes that pass on to us our total heredity. Guesses and hopes are abundant, but facts are still scarce.

Early diagnosis and treatment is so important that a possible cancer should not be neglected for one single moment after suspicion arises.

> In cancer, as with any other disease, general well-being is important. If you have eaten well, if your body is in good shape, and if you have a positive attitude toward life, you will be better equipped to fight off any disease, even cancer.

Kidney Disease

The kidneys have an incredible reserve capacity, so that even if only one sixth of the one million nephrons (the filtering units) in each kidney are functioning, wastes are sufficiently eliminated from the body. But like every other organ, the kidneys are susceptible to destructive diseases. Infection (pyelonephrosis), inflammation (nephritis), and degeneration (nephrosis) can disturb kidney functions and cause irreversible damage.

There is a definite relationship between good kidney functioning and good heart functioning. The normal blood pressure of the kidneys is necessarily higher than that of other parts of the body in order to force blood plasma into the kidney tubules, in the urinary processes. An abnormally high bodily blood pressure, superimposed, over a period of years, on the already high but normal pressure in the kidneys, can readily bring about deterioration of these delicate tissues. There are also many other causes of kidney troubles, and much damage is caused by the presence of kidney stones, or gravel. In experimental animals, kidney stones can be induced through severe deficiency of vitamin A, and when vitamin A again is supplied in rich quantities, the stones slowly dissolve and pass away. A lack of vitamin A may be involved in the formation of the stones, but the affliction is one that should be treated by your physician.

The accumulation of minerals in the formation of kidney stones is often accelerated in vegetarian diets when too large amounts of fruits and vegetables and too little meat, eggs, and milk are eaten, thus making the urine too alkaline.

Infections of the kidney can bring about destruction of the tissues, so that the walls of the kidney tubules become somewhat like a sieve, or strainer. In that event, blood proteins, which normally cannot pass into the urine, go through the damaged tubules and are lost. In normal health, these proteins attract into the blood stream the waste materials from all body tissues.

When blood proteins are lost in the urine, or the diet is so deficient in protein that normal amounts of blood protein cannot be produced, liquids tend to accumulate in the body, especially in the feet, ankles, and legs. When kidneys are damaged to such an extent that too much blood protein is lost and wastes cannot be collected, the result can be fatal uremic poisoning through failure to excrete uric acid.

Urinary Troubles

Having to urinate during the night may be indicative of no more than a naturally small bladder, but if the urges are overly frequent, particularly in older men, a checkup is in order, and all the more so if the need is of relatively recent origin. Infection of the urogenital tract, incipient diabetes, and enlarged prostate, among other disorders, may be the cause. Prompt attention is most important, for urinary trouble caught in its early stages is easier to treat, and a very great deal of trouble can be avoided.

In the dietary management, vitamins A and C should be kept high; proteins should be adequate (at least 1 gram per kilogram, or 2.2 pounds, of body weight); and the diet should consist largely of whole-grain breads and cereals, meats, and eggs to keep the urine acid. During treatment for such irritation or infection, the use of citrus fruits and juices, and all fruits and vegetables, should be largely avoided, since they make the urine alkaline, a condition that allows the multiplication of bacteria. When all infections have been removed, the High-Vitality Diet in chapter 4 should be followed to prevent such troubles for the rest of your long life.

Gallstones

The well-known liver and gall-bladder specialist Dr. Roger Glenard of Vichy, France, has been asked thousands of times what causes some people to have constant gall-bladder difficulties. His answer has become a famous saying, "Three F's contribute to gall-bladder troubles: Female, Fat, and Forty." It seems that women are especially prone to such troubles, often those of calm temperament, rather than the tense, nervous type.

Interestingly, psychiatrists have also pointed out that persons with "inner tensions" but outer calmness are susceptible to gall-bladder troubles.

In any case, gallstones derive from a chemical imbalance in the bile. This imbalance may result in a concentration of the cholesterol that should normally have been excreted (in fact, gall-bladder difficulties first made the general public conscious of cholesterol), or it may result in deposits of calcium, or accumulations of some other solids of which the bile is composed. Under healthy conditions, the muscular wall of the gall bladder contracts sufficiently to empty completely all bile from the bladder. When the bile is not emptied, the accumulated solid, being a heavy substance, settles in the stagnant bile to form gallstones. As these stones become larger, they cannot pass through the bile duct even though the diet may have improved and the emptying of the bladder become normal. One ensuing symptom, true of all gall-bladder diseases whether caused by gallstones or by infection, is that extreme pain is experienced when fat is ingested.

B vitamins (specifically, B_6) are essential in the breakdown of fats; without B_6, for example, linoleic acid (an unsaturated fatty acid) cannot be used in the body, and the blood cholesterol cannot be maintained at a normal level. An adequate intake of B vitamins in the diet would therefore probably reduce the likelihood of gallstones caused by a build-up of cholesterol. If you believe you may have gallstones, by all means seek the advice of your physician to be rid of them.

Those suffering with cirrhosis (fatty degeneration) of the liver are found to be especially prone to gallstones. There is an obvious connection here, in that cirrhosis of the liver is also recognized to be the result of deficiencies of B vitamins, choline in particular.

To help avoid gallstone troubles for the rest of your life, make sure that your daily menu includes more than ample amounts of all the essential B vitamins.

Anemia

Marginal anemia, a much too common complaint among people of all ages, especially women, is caused largely by an inadequate diet. Lacking iron, copper, proteins, and the ever-important B vitamins, the body cannot produce enough healthy red blood cells to maintain a healthy blood stream.

Proteins are very important. (See chapter 2.) As the red corpuscles contain more protein than iron, all the essential amino acids must be supplied for the proper building of blood. Experiments have shown that diets high in iron but low in protein will not be effective in promoting blood-cell production. Dr. G. H. Whipple first reported many years ago in the *American Journal of Physiology* that liver is one of the best hemoglobin-regenerating foods because it contains both iron and protein. Women in general eat less protein food than men do; moreover, they lose blood at regular monthly intervals, and therefore are more prone to anemia than men are. This anemic condition is readily corrected when the diet contains ample amounts of complete protein, supplied by milk, eggs, meat (especially liver), wheat germ, and brewers' yeast.

All the B vitamins (thiamine, niacin, pyridoxine, para-aminobenzoic acid, folic acid, etc.) are essential to the formation of healthy red blood cells. In particular, a lack of folic acid and vitamin B_{12} appears to be the causative factor in pernicious anemia, which is a most serious complaint.

Pernicious anemia (not to be confused with the commonplace marginal types) is closely connected with decreased functioning of the liver. The American scientist George R. Minot, who discovered this connection, found that the blood vessels become saturated with immature blood cells from the bone marrow, but that the total hemoglobin is greatly reduced.

Formerly considered incurable, pernicious anemia became amenable to treatment following the epoch-making work of Dr. Minot and his colleagues. Liver therapy, and later highly potent extracts of liver, saved untold lives. Pernicious anemia was brought so beautifully under control that there were times when it was difficult to find sufferers. Now with the isolation of the active principle, vitamin B_{12}, and its synthesis, the treatment of pernicious anemia promises to become mere routine; and a fraction of a milligram of vitamin B_{12} suffices to control the symptoms of the disease.

Make a blood test a routine part of your regular medical checkup. Keep your blood stream, the river of life, flowing strongly and smoothly. Begin today to revitalize it. It needs iron and copper; the best sources of iron and copper are wheat germ, liver, and molasses. Plan to eat liver once or twice a week. Include wheat germ and unsulphured molasses in your daily meals.

Varicose Veins

Although the beating or pumping action of the heart forces the blood throughout the body, its effect diminishes as the blood passes into the thousands of miles of capillaries. The return of the blood to the heart is brought about by contractions of muscles; the back flow of the blood toward the arteries is prevented by valves in the veins. If, however, the muscles fail to contract normally, the blood cannot be pushed on in its return to the heart. Then blood stays in the veins; it clots and remains there. Other blood may be pushed into the clogged veins and, if not forced out, will likewise remain to form clots. Such clogged veins, filled with stagnant blood, are spoken of as varicose veins. In time, new blood vessels are formed around the plugged veins, but the varicosities themselves remain to become unsightly, perhaps painful, and in extreme cases ulcerous.

There are two methods for removing unsightly varicosities. One is by surgery, which eliminates the difficulty permanently; it is a comparatively simple operation but requires hospitalization. The other is the injection method, which has become popular in Europe and in America. Discuss these methods with your doctor if you are troubled with varicosities; do not spend the rest of your life trying to hide them.

More pertinent to our purpose is the prevention of varicose veins. Certainly a vitality diet, rich in body-firming proteins and vitamin C, will provide help of the first order. And so will relaxation. As we get older, the distance from the lower extremities to the heart remains geometrically the same, but in terms of heart burden it lengthens considerably. Do your heart, and your veins, a favor. Rest in the horizontal position, or better still with your feet above your head, on the yoga slant board (see chapter 9). Let the blood in your veins run downhill for a change, with the aid of gravity, instead of always against it. Added to the pressure available for returning the blood to your heart, this helps flush the veins, keep them clear, and prevent conditions of varicosity. Vitamin E may also be helpful, for, according to Dr. Evan Shute of Canada, "It is a dilator of blood vessels. It opens up new pathways in the damaged circulation, therefore, and bypasses blocks produced by clots and hardened arteries."

The bicycle exercise—thirty seconds of lying on your back with your legs in the air pretending to pedal a bicycle—is recommended by physical-fitness experts and is very helpful in preventing varicose veins.

Mental Disturbances

I am never happier than when I find that the science of nutrition is becoming more and more helpful in preventing mental deterioration and disease. Mental disease does not just happen; it is the end product of a long series of causative factors. Happily, some of these causes are simply nutritional; *these can be eradicated.*

It has long been known that a severe lack of the B vitamin niacin can result in a type of dementia. Furthermore, when human volunteers have been kept on diets lacking almost any one of the B vitamins, mental confusion, depression, and anxiety states developed. When Dr. Sydenstricker, in his studies, kept human volunteers on a diet adequate in all respects except for the B vitamin biotin, the resultant mental depression became so severe that his subjects developed suicidal tendencies and the experiments had to be stopped. Such findings indicate that the lack of the B vitamins may well be a causative factor in inducing certain forms of mental disturbance.

Groups of scientists, particularly in Sweden, have studied the brains of persons who died of mental diseases and have compared them with the brains of normal individuals who met accidental death. They found that four substances essential to the healthy nucleus of brain cells were lacking in the mentally disturbed: adenine, thymine, cytosine, and guanine. These four nutrients are found in multicellular meats such as liver, calf or lamb brains, sweetbreads, kidneys, and in brewers' yeast. Such excellent meats should be eaten frequently, and brewers' yeast should be added to the daily diet.

NERVOUSNESS

Eat and stop fidgeting. Nervousness can be a result of unwise diet. That high-strung, jittery feeling, that jingle-jangle of nerves, could readily stem from a lack of B vitamins, particularly thiamine; if your diet is high in carbohydrates, then the effect of thiamine deficiency is all the greater.

If your diet is very deficient in calcium, to the extent that the level of calcium in your blood becomes low, your nerves will become irritated. Fortified milk is the best source of calcium. It is easily prepared. Just beat one cup of powdered skim milk into a quart of fluid milk. A hand egg beater will do the job, but of course an electric blender is easier. You may consume generous quantities of calcium; but unless you do so in perfect ratio to phosphorus (and you would have to be a mathematician and check every bit of the food that you eat), it will not be absorbed from the intestines unless vitamin D is also present. If you are indoors most of the time and do not eat eggs every day, you may be getting ample calcium and still not be absorbing it effectively. In such cases it is wise to fortify your diet with a vitamin D concentrate. Many nutritionists now also recommend small bone-flour tablets containing the right amounts of calcium and phosphorus, plus the sunshine vitamin D.

Scientific experiments with human volunteers have shown that diets lacking in any one of several B vitamins can lead to nervous tension. A serious lack of thiamine (vitamin B_1), niacin, or pyridoxine (vitamin B_6), separately or all together, may lead to nervous tension.

A balanced, vital diet is essential to general good health and a sense of well-being. It follows, therefore, that it is essential to a calm and stable nervous system.

In older people, a sense of tension and fatigue can frequently be caused by failure to take a snack between meals, particularly if the oldster is normally a light eater. The sugar in the blood may have been used up to a sufficient extent to produce "physiological hunger" that is often shown by a feeling of fatigue and uneasiness. It can be corrected very simply indeed—by a glass of milk or fruit juice, vegetable juice, cheese and crackers, or almost any light snack.

Learn as much as you can about your own mental quirks. If necessary, go to a psychotherapist and let him help you uncover those trouble-making aspects of your personality that you cannot find and correct yourself.

FORGETFULNESS

Psychologists tell us absent-mindedness is a sign of something, but not necessarily a sign of old age. It can be a symptom of dietary deficiency.

One of the Philadelphia hospitals conducted tests for memory, clarity, speed of thinking, and general intelligence among a group of elderly patients living on a standard hospital diet. The tests were made before and after a number of the B vitamins were separately given them, and repeated again when the entire B family was amply supplied by natural foods. There was no change in native intelligence, but the patients showed improvement in memory and ability to think clearly after the separate B vitamins were given. Marked improvement followed, however, when *all* of the B vitamins were amply supplied. If you have difficulty in remembering or find your thinking growing foggy and confused, try adding such food nutrients as brewers' yeast and wheat germ to your diet; it may help.

Recent experimental work has shown that one of the amino acids, known as glutamic acid, is a principal component of an enzyme in the brain. When glutamic acid is amply supplied in the diet, the intelligence has been found to be actually increased, the ability to learn is accelerated, thinking is clearer, and memory becomes more keen and accurate. While glutamic acid is found in all complete proteins, it is interesting to note that milk is rich in it. Fresh and powdered milk are excellent sources of this invaluable nutrient. Glutamic acid is now available in tablet form.

Allergies, Hay Fever, and Asthma

The blood resents foreigners! It goes to work to produce an army of antibodies to entrap and render harmless the foreign substances—generally, but not always, proteins. If the same species of foreigner almost daily invades the blood, antibodies are continually produced and remain in the circulatory blood; the body is then said to be in an immune state, as far as that particular species of foreigner is concerned. If the invasion is spasmodic, say at intervals of ten days and upward, during the intervening period the antibodies attach themselves to certain cells of the body, remain there, and do not circulate in the blood stream; the body is then said to be in an allergic state.

During the allergic state, should the same species of foreigner invade the blood stream, there are no circulating antibodies to intercept it; and when it reaches the antibodies attached to the cells, an irritation is produced—so-called anaphylactic shock—which is manifested by one or more of the symptoms of allergy, according to what cells of the body the antibodies have become attached to. Nonproteins also can cause allergylike reactions; allergy to drugs is a typical example. But even in such cases, certain body proteins become involved in the reaction. That is the mechanism of allergy, as it is known today. Its cause is the invasion of the body by foreign substances.

How do they get there? Air-borne allergens—pollens, dusts, and the like—are drawn into the lungs with the air we breathe, and thus are absorbed into the blood stream. Another condition is absorption from the intestinal tract, which, it is suspected, is more likely to take place following the eating of offending foods in more than ordinarily large quantities, possibly causing the digestive apparatus to become overburdened.

What can be done about an allergy? First, it is desirable to know what substance or substances produce allergic responses. A physician specializing in allergies can frequently make the discovery. Once the offending material is known, it is best, if possible, to avoid completely the offending substance. Or you can make your own effort at immunization. If it works, you are so much ahead; if not, little if any harm is done.

First, if you suffer from a food allergy, you must know what food causes the allergy. Then try eating daily almost infinitesimal quantities of that food. Slowly and cautiously, over long intervals of at least several weeks, very gradually increase the amount. You may reach a normal amount with no more trouble. This method is a long way from being infallible, but I have seen it work. If you are allergic to any meats cooked rare, the chances are you will be able to tolerate them if they are well done. If you are allergic to ordinary milk, try powdered skim milk. Soybean milk is suggested as a milk substitute by some physicians, but remember that it does not contain the essential vitamins found in whole milk.

The wheat-sensitive person must take care to avoid all foods containing wheat and not just the obvious cakes, pastries, and crackers. Creamed soups, sauces, and gravies are often thickened with flour. Meat loaf, hamburger, and prepared meats like sausage may contain wheat fillers. Cereal and malted beverages must also be avoided. A gluten-free diet is therefore especially restrictive, as you can see, and great care must be taken to obtain nutrients normally provided in wheat from other sources. The American Dietetic Association (620 N. Michigan Avenue, Chicago, Illinois 60611) provides recipe booklets for gluten-free cooking.

The egg-sensitive person must also investigate commercially prepared foods for the not so obvious egg content. Some baking powder, for instance, contains dried egg white. So do many foaming beverages.

In all cases, if you are concerned with your diet because of allergies, remember that a diet continuously rich in all the vitamins is probably the best possible precaution in maintaining general good health.

Dr. Arthur F. Coca, Honorary President of the American Association of Immunologists, says, "If a person is not suffering sunburn or an infection such as the common cold, any variation from his normal pulse rate in usual activity is probably due to an allergic reaction." Following the systematic pulse-dietary method described in Dr. Coca's helpful book *The Pulse Test* (Arc Books), you can be your own detective—tracking down allergy-inciting foods. Rather than using drugs to control the symptoms of allergy, this fact-finding investigation helps you eliminate the cause.

Psychosomatic Difficulties

Psycho refers to the mind and *soma* to the body; *psychosomatic* therefore refers to the relationship and reaction of mind and body, one to the other. In recent years, much has been written about psychosomatic difficulties. We have all become increasingly aware that worries, emotional upsets, and anxieties can have such a tremendous effect on general health that they can be causative factors in producing severe illnesses.

Such abnormalities as asthma, hay fever, and other allergies, hypoglycemia, migraine headaches, digestive disturbances, diarrhea, and high blood pressure may be caused by several things. All, however, *can* be induced by psychosomatic disturbances.

The person suffering psychosomatic illness all too often has allowed himself to develop multiple deficiencies of the B vitamins to such an extent that he is readily upset emotionally. If an allergy has also developed, and a restricted diet supplying even less of the B vitamins is followed, the whole psychosomatic condition becomes worse. Several heaping teaspoons of brewers' yeast, half a cup of wheat germ, and from a pint to a quart of fortified milk should be included in the daily diet.

Arthritis

Arthritis is an inflammatory, often chronic, process involving the joints; its cause is not known. However, in experimental laboratories, arthritis has been produced in animals by depriving them of vitamin C over a period of weeks and then injecting bacteria into them. The bacteria were carried throughout the body and lodged in the small joints first; there the body tried desperately to stop the infection by depositing calcium all around it. Pain and swelling developed and arthritic stiffness followed. On the other hand, where animals had been on a balanced diet with optimum amounts of vitamin C, the injected bacteria did not enter the blood stream but caused an abscess to form at the point of injection. When the abscess broke, the dangerous bacteria were drained away and there was no arthritis. The lesson to be learned from this is: do not tolerate any infection anywhere in the body. Consult your doctor immediately.

To insure against conditions that might lead to arthritis, use maximum amounts of vitamin C daily. Get plenty of protective proteins, especially lean meats, cheese, and yogurt. Use only wholegrain breads and cereals, and eat generous amounts of fruits and vegetables. Calcium should never be restricted as it was in old-fashioned incomplete diets. Iron and vitamins are also essential.

I cannot accept defeatism in regard to even so serious a problem as arthritis. As with so many other ailments, we can at the very least stop its progress. I have known many cases in which arthritic patients have overcome many of their difficulties by means of nutrition and exercise.

I would like to pass on to you another encouraging report from a physician who almost made the century mark. Dr. William Brady, in his book *An Eighty-Year-Old Doctor's Secrets of Positive Health* (Prentice-Hall), noted the confusion in terms used to denote disturbances of the various joints. Dr. Brady settled on the term *rheumatiz* to describe serious arthritic conditions. This degeneration of joint tissues, he said, is due to nutritional deficiency throughout the years, chiefly a lack of vitamins B and D and of iodine. For an optimum supply of vitamins B and D, he recommended fish-liver oil, whole-wheat kernels, at least 1½ pints of milk a day, and B-complex and other food supplements, plus iodine from seaweed.

Sex and Menopause Problems

Vitamins A and E have long been identified with sexual and reproductive functions, and more recent knowledge has included many of the B vitamins in the same category. Deficiencies of B vitamins affect the production of sperm and ovum, the mating urge, and the entire sexual cycle, embryonic development, lactation, and the maternal instinct (all functions which fall under the control of the endocrine glands). Dr. R. Hertz links failures of these functions to the direct part played by the B vitamins in the maintenance of general health, which is another way of saying general nutrition. As it is the quality of the diet that determines nutrition, diet must supply the B vitamins.

The liver is truly a great workshop of the body. A list of its functions is almost unbelievable. But the one that is of special interest to us here is that of maintaining the balance between the hormones that stimulate the sex glands. The adrenals secrete both androgenic and estrogenic hormones (substances that stimulate male and female characteristics, respectively), in one and the same individual. The liver maintains the balance between the two by inactivating excesses of either hormone.

It has been shown that, in laboratory animals, deficiencies of B vitamins, notably thiamine and riboflavin, cause the liver to fail in the inactivation of estrogens but not of androgens. On this basis the Drs. Biskind have reported successful use of B vitamin therapy in cases of premenstrual tension, excessive menstrual flow, morbid discharges, and cystic breasts.

Dr. Roger Williams and his colleagues point to cases of greatly enlarged breasts among many male prisoners of war in the Orient, which were always accompanied by a serious condition of malnutrition.

Some women find menopause as free from difficulty as was the experience of puberty. They are aware only that the ovaries become less active and cease to bring about the conditions necessary to conception. And few indeed are the women over forty who wish to continue bearing children.

Other women, a majority perhaps, experience difficulties all the way from "merely annoying" to serious nervous and bodily upsets. Frequently it is sheer fear of the unknown, fear that can be set at rest through talks with a physician or psychologist. Equally as frequently, it may be a glandular imbalance, which indicates hormone treatment by a physician.

It is my belief that the truly healthy woman—healthy in mind and body—finds her menopause quite uncomplicated. Deficiencies bring about a variety of disruptions in the mechanisms of the body, many of which contribute to nervous upset and accentuate the fears of menopause. While a well-balanced diet is always of the utmost importance, it becomes even more necessary under the stresses of menopause. The inclusion of foods extra-rich in B vitamins, calcium, and iron is most advisable. Brewers' yeast, wheat germ, yogurt, and molasses can all be used with profit. Some gynecologists recommend vitamin E to relieve menopause symptoms.

According to Dr. N. R. Kavinoky, from 10 to 25 milligrams of vitamin E give relief from hot flashes, backache, and excessive menstrual flow. And a dosage of 100 milligrams of vitamin E daily also minimizes high blood pressure and muscle pains.

Before leaving the subject, let me remark about some general attitudes that prevail and may cause needless concern.

For the healthy woman, sexual desire does not end with the end of the reproductive functions. It can continue indefinitely, and with adjustment to the menopause she can embark upon a new life that is satisfactory and harmonious.

All too often, both men and women mistakenly believe that a woman's capacity for sexual feeling disappears after the menopause. They quite fail to realize that her sexual feelings come from many sources which are in no way affected by decreased ovarian activity. Freed from the fear of unwanted pregnancy, a woman's sexual enjoyment may be greatly increased after menopause.

Loving and being loved is the fundamental human experience, essential to the formation of character and a positive attitude toward life. Sex is both spiritual and physical; from a mutual exchange of affection emerge tenderness and security, which bring health and harmony and enhance the total personality. Longevity statistics indicate conclusively that older people who are happily married have the best chance of achieving a healthy long life.

If false sex education has given you latent hangovers of guilt, or if the destructive influence of possessive parents has created a problem, have no hesitation in discussing such problems fully and openly with a doctor or psychiatrist, and be guided accordingly. Know that thousands upon thousands of other humans have had such troubles and have overcome them. Know also that sex is a natural and normal function, that it can be one of life's greatest blessings for both men and women.

Take Care of Your Glands

The endocrine glands (i.e., those glands whose secretions pass directly into the blood or lymph) have been a subject of widely publicized research because their malfunction can produce profound and sometimes bizarre changes in the body. They have been proved to be subject to the state of our nutrition. A vital diet, well balanced in all of its nutritive factors, with special emphasis on vitamins, is basic to their health and proper function. Although the nutritional and medical sciences have not yet been able to give us a complete picture of all the interrelationships between diet and glandular function, certain specific ones have been clearly defined.

THE THYROID GLAND

This gland lies in the foreground of the throat, astride the windpipe, and has been called the "watchman" between the physical and mental body. The thyroid secretes a hormone, thyroxine, which is constantly poured into the blood stream and carried to all parts of the body.

A weak or lazy thyroid can make the sex glands lazy, and an overactive thyroid overstimulates the sex glands. The great Don Juans you read about are the overactive thyroid type, and the indifferent lovers usually have a lazy thyroid.

One of the functions of the thyroid is that of controlling the body's metabolism. An underactive thyroid lowers (to 15 to 30 percent or more below normal) the basal rate (the rate of energy production that supports the "inner" activities of the body). It does this through thyroxine, which it secretes into the blood. A deficiency of thyroxine reduces the need for calories; but if one eats at the required level, one will not become fat, contrary to popular supposition. Drs. MacKay and Sherrell have brought this out. I quote from them as follows: "Although it is well known that patients with myxedema [extreme hypothyroidism] are not obese as a rule, the idea persists in the clinical literature that hypothyroidism may be a *cause* for obesity." Dr. W. A. Plummer has given clinical evidence that much of the supposed obesity of myxedema is, in fact, water retention in the body. *One does not have to become fat as a direct result of hypothyroidism, but it is much easier to do so.* Mental sluggishness, difficulty in remembering, and the constant desire to sleep are also typical problems of thyroid starvation. The hypothyroid sufferer should seek the counsel of his physician for treatment of this specific condition.

When the thyroid gland is overactive, the metabolic rate is increased (15 to 20 percent above normal). In animals, overactive thyroid causes loss of weight, interrupted sexual cycle, liver damage, disorders of the heart and vascular system, nervousness, fatigue, and a fall in liver glycogen. These symptoms can be relieved through the use of B vitamins, which function as part of the metabolic enzymes and are found in brewers' yeast and liver. Thiamine administration is accompanied by beneficial effects in some cases of exophthalmic goiter. Thus the *symptoms* of hyperthyroidism really are symptoms of vitamin deficiency, the deficiency being caused by the elevated metabolic rate. Nutrients are burned so rapidly that additional fuel is drawn from body tissues. Dr. Roger Williams and his colleagues point out that there is a real possibility that the thyroid and other glands have a marked influence on vitamin metabolism, particularly in regard to absorption and excretion.

Goiter, an enlargement of the thyroid gland, is caused by a lack of iodine. This enlargement is an attempt by the body to compensate for the shortage of iodine by making more thyroxine-producing tissue. As a result, the production of thyroxine is usually normal and there are no drastic physical changes other than a slight fullness and perhaps a mild pressure in the neck. The goiter is a danger sign, pointing to possible trouble ahead. If it is at all suspected, call your physician.

Toxic goiter or exophthalmic goiter occurs where the thyroid is already weakened because of lack of iodine and the body fails to inactivate excess thyroxine. Patients with this disease lose weight, are extremely nervous, suffer from heat excessively, and have a fast heartbeat; often their eyes become prominent and somewhat protruding. This type of goiter must be supervised by a physician, who will probably prescribe large amounts of iodine, with other nutrients (copper, magnesium, calcium, etc.). Here, more than in any other disease, diet is important. Because the body is in effect racing its engine, all vitamins and minerals must be given in extra-large doses.

The thyroid has so many important functions in keeping us slim, trim, and alert, in keeping the hair, nails, and complexion healthy, that it could also be termed the "beauty master" of the body. Not only can wrong diet disturb the balance of this sensitive gland, but the resultant depression, fear, worry, and constant strain can further weaken it.

Adequate iodine is of foremost importance for normal, healthy functioning of the thyroid. Without it, we grow old before our time, are always tired, and wonder whatever became of our usual pep. Without essential iodine, we may find ourselves becoming soft and flabby of flesh; mentally lazy, and unable to take much interest in anything; lapsing into the blues; and never feeling warm enough, especially in the hands and feet.

Dr. Russell Wilder of the Mayo Clinic found that when human volunteers do not get sufficient vitamin B_1, the thyroid gland becomes less active and the basal metabolism drops far below normal. The condition was not corrected by giving thyroid extract; it was corrected by giving vitamin B_1 without any thyroid. Probably thousands of people who now take thyroid extract would be helped far more by following a diet rich in all the B vitamins.

Here, then, are the essential foods for a well-balanced, smoothly functioning thyroid. First-class proteins: meat, eggs, cheese, and fortified milk. Abundant iodine: shrimps, oysters, salmon, radishes, tomatoes, watercress, sea greens, and iodized vegetable salt. All the B vitamins, which are richly contained in brewers' yeast, yogurt, wheat germ, and dark molasses. And for the rest of your long life, season all foods with iodized salt, preferably iodized vegetable salt.

THE PITUITARY GLAND

Weighing only six-tenths of a gram, it is located just back of the nose and beneath the brain; but small as it is, the pituitary has been termed the "director" of the entire "glandular symphony." This tiny gland manufactures ten or more hormones that are tremendously important in their effect on every other gland in the body. A deficiency in proteins, fat, or the B vitamins will adversely affect the production of these hormones. One of the pituitary's hormones directs the growth of bones and tissue; through its sex hormone it directs sex stimulation and the activities of the ovaries. It controls the thyroid gland, the adrenal glands, and the insulin-producing gland (the pancreas).

One condition of malfunction of the pituitary gland appears to be manifested as a fatty deposit around the chest and abdomen, in a girdle-like fashion. Men take on female characteristics and women become somewhat masculine. The external genitalia of the male appear to become smaller—so-called fatty degeneration. That this girdle-like fat is not necessarily true obesity has been shown by Drs. Freyberg, Barker, Newburgh, and Coller.

When the pituitary gland does not function properly, it adversely affects the ovaries and brings about premature menopause. It is interesting to note that whereas underfunction of the pituitary produces an earlier menopause, the underfunctioning of the thyroid causes a later-than-normal menopause.

The Adrenals

There are two of these glands, weighing only half an ounce, and located one atop each kidney like little caps. The adrenals produce the hormone *adrenaline*, which is poured into the blood stream in time of danger or strong emotional upheaval, to brace us for action or to sustain us against shock. A deficiency of adrenaline causes slowed-down reactions. The adrenal glands appear to have power to affect certain toxins and have been termed "the glands of survival." While much remains to be learned about these glands, it has been found that nicotine, lead, and other chemicals can cause them great damage, and that an unbalanced diet is definitely injurious. It is also suspected that malfunctioning of these glands plays a part in graying of the hair. For example, in animals with a pantothenic acid (a B vitamin) deficiency, a section of the adrenal glands develops changes that cause the hair to turn gray. If the glands are removed from such animals, either the graying of the hair is prevented or the color is restored. If after the glands have been removed, deoxycorticosterone is administered, the hair turns gray! Deoxycorticosterone is only one of many similar hormones secreted by the adrenal cortex. A panthothenic acid deficiency has definitely been shown to affect the adrenals adversely. Many authorities believe that a certain abnormal "steroid" produced by the adrenal cortex may also play a role in cancer and mental diseases. This shows a distinct relationship between diet and an endocrine gland, though there is no reason to suspect that such a relationship is unique to a single gland.

The cortex of the adrenal glands has recently become a focal point of considerable scientific interest. Cortisone, one of the hormones it secretes, has been shown to be of extraordinary clinical value in the treatment of rheumatoid arthritis, rheumatic fever, bronchial asthma, inflammatory diseases of the skin and eye, and Addison's disease, which is manifested by, among other symptoms, a bronze coloration of the skin and is due to changes in the adrenal cortex. The adrenal cortex produces glucocorticoids, hormones involved in turning protein into glucose and the release of insulin. Hypoglycemia often results from insufficient production of these hormones.

Here we may mention that the pituitary gland secretes a hormone (known as the adrenocorticotrophic hormone or ACTH) that affects the adrenals and is also of considerable therapeutic use in cases of deficiency. When the pituitary gland is removed (as in the treatment of cancer, for instance), the adrenal glands atrophy.

The Pancreas

As is well known, this gland manufactures the hormone we call insulin, whose chief purpose is to help the body utilize and store sugar, or glycogen. When the pancreas becomes damaged and no longer secretes insulin, sugar is lost in the urine, and we have diabetes. (Hormonal disturbances can also affect insulin production.) This vital gland, which is several inches long, lies across the middle of the abdominal cavity. In addition to the production of insulin, it pours enzymes into the upper intestine for the digestion of proteins, fats, sugars, and starches.

While the exact cause, or causes, of diabetes is not entirely known, there is reason to believe that the overeating of sugars overworks the pancreas, and after years of such abuse it finally slows down the production of insulin. (See discussion of diabetes earlier in this chapter.)

Some researchers believe that pancreatitis, or inflammation of the pancreas, with its accompanying sharp and instant pain, is an indirect result of vitamin A deficiency. Insufficiency of vitamin A creates a proliferation of mucous-membrane cells, which die quickly and block narrow ducts, including the pancreatic duct. Some healthy, cleansing mucus is necessary for bacteria fighting, but too much becomes immovable, obstructing debris.

The Sex Glands

A basically well-balanced diet is the first step toward improvement of the general health, hence that of all glands. When nutritional deficiencies have been overcome, improved health and vigor will be reflected in greater virility and normal libido. Remember that first-class proteins, as well as vitamins A, C, E, and all the B vitamins (especially pantothenic acid, para-aminobenzoic acid, and folic acid) are imperative.

When a woman's ovaries do not function properly, a type of fat is deposited on the breasts and upper thighs, usually at middle age. While glandular therapy can be of great help in such cases, a common-sense reducing diet is necessary to get rid of the fat.

In men, fear and worry may be the worst troublemakers in preventing normal sexual functioning, especially in later years. And such fears and worries may be brought on by a lack of B vitamins as much as by a man's own erroneous beliefs concerning sex. How often, and how wrongly, a man views an active sex life as the symbol of youth. Medical records show that libido, the ability to have intercourse, and the production of living semen are sometimes sustained up to a very great age.

Sexual emotion depends upon the amount of internal secretions delivered to the blood by the gonads. These in turn must depend upon the amount of nutrients available to maintain the health of the ovaries and testicles. People who have lived on inadequate or starvation diets (as did those in concentration camps) invariably report that sex interest quickly and completely disappeared.

Animals maintained on diets low in protein, or inadequate in any of the essential amino acids, show so little sex interest that mating soon ceases. On a high-protein diet, restoration of sexual potency and the resumption of mating quickly take place. The importance of a diet adequate in all nutrients in maintaining sexual potency cannot be overemphasized. A lack of the amino acid arginine causes sterility in male animals. In experiments with young men, it was shown that inadequate arginine, over a period of only one week, resulted in a marked decrease in sperm production.

The studies of Reynolds and Macomber showed that calcium deficiency had the same effect as that of protein starvation, while too little vitamin A can cause in animals a marked reduction in fertility, disturbed sexual behavior, and, in severe cases, complete loss of libido.

I believe that, with our ever-increasing understanding of the glands and their vital secretions, we are about to enter the "Hormone Age," and I predict that the day is not distant when diets rich in hormone-producing vitamins, to protect our life-giving and life-sustaining glands against depletion and disease, will be the general rule rather than the exception.

Megavitamin Therapy—the New Science

A Los Angeles psychiatrist, Dr. Harvey M. Ross, is one of two hundred physicians and psychiatrists using massive doses of vitamins to treat schizophrenia and alcoholism, and hyperactivity in children. These specialists believe that, because of biochemical imbalances, patients with mental disorders require very large doses of specific vitamins along with a high-protein diet and other supplements in order to stay well.

Dr. Ross tells the story of Mitch, an eleven-year-old boy who wet the bed and had hallucinations (his dead grandfather appeared in the room as a purple ball). He fought with his sisters (he imagined they were talking about him), set fires in his room, and disrupted his classes at school. Such behavior is typical of the hyperactive and schizophrenic child. Also typical was his obesity and his low blood sugar. At times he ate sixty candy bars a day, most of them stolen from neighborhood stores.

To correct the hypoglycemia, Dr. Ross immediately placed Mitch on a high-protein, low-carbohydrate diet consisting of small, frequent meals and high-protein snacks. After each meal, Mitch took 500 mg. of vitamin B_3 (niacin), 500 mg. of vitamin C, 100 mg. of vitamin B_6, 100 mg. of pantothenic acid (another B vitamin), 200 I.U. of vitamin E, and a multiple-B tablet. After one week, Dr. Ross increased the B_3 dosage to 1,000 mg. This larger dosage made the boy nauseous, so Dr. Ross switched him to niacinamide, which is another form of vitamin B_3. The nausea subsided. After a month, the vitamin C dosage was increased to 1,000 mg. Later, Dr. Ross supplemented the boy's diet with L-glutamine, an amino acid. After three months on megavitamin therapy, Mitch's mental health improved considerably.

"Mitch and his vitamins are going to be together for a long time," Dr. Ross said. "If his symptoms do not reappear, he will continue his present treatment for several years. Then I will reduce the doses slowly to see if he can function normally with less vitamins, or with none at all."

Dr. Abram Hoffer is one of the pioneers in megavitamin therapy, along with Dr. Ross, Dr. Humphrey Osmond, Dr. Allan Cott, Dr. David Hawkins, Dr. Russel Smith, Dr. Carl Pfeiffer, and Dr. Linus Pauling.

When asked about his treatment for schizophrenia, Dr. Hoffer replied that each case is different. "Many times, though," he said, "a daily intake of 3 to 5 grams [3,000 to 5,000 mg.] of vitamin C, up to about 20 grams of niacin, the right diet, and good vitamin and mineral supplementation will, within a few weeks or months, bring most acute schizophrenics around to what we call normalcy. Other cases may involve—until the megavitamin therapy is well under way—the addition of some of the commonly accepted tranquilizers and anti-depressants, plus even electroconvulsive [shock] therapy, if the disorder is far advanced."

In order to stabilize the biochemical malfunctions, the massive doses are apparently necessary; some doses can be reduced while others must be taken for a lifetime, just as a diabetic has to take insulin.

Megavitamin therapy, or orthomolecular psychiatry, as the professionals call it, is a young science that promises hope for millions. I believe it is much more sensible than the many drugs that often cause serious damage. If you are interested in megavitamin therapy, ask your doctor to contact the Huxley Institute for Biosocial Research in New York City for the name and address of the nearest physician or psychiatrist who uses this therapy. For physicians who want to know more about megavitamin therapy, I recommend *Orthomolecular Psychiatry: Treatment of Schizophrenia* edited by Dr. David Hawkins and Dr. Linus Pauling, W. H. Freeman & Co., San Francisco, 1973.

Fight Fatigue with Exercise and Relaxation

Fatigue is a deadly enemy in our busy lives, one that we must wipe out right from the start. Many years ago I discovered that people who eat enough of the good protein foods, good breads, and only natural sugars never complain of being tired. The tired ones were those who ate white breads, overrefined cereals, and lots of white sugar and cola drinks.

For men and women who cannot afford tension and whose lives demand a full, steady flow of energy all day, every day, my program is basic. There are just two secrets for living and working at a sustained pace, without strain, without overdoing, without knowing the meaning of fatigue. The million-dollar secrets are: a high-vitality diet and the art of relaxation.

The Million-Dollar Secret of Relaxation

A balanced, superbly nutritious high-vitality diet can gradually establish for you a state of healthily balanced nerves to cope with life's ups and downs. But it is also necessary for you to learn how not to *waste* energy. You must learn the art of banishing tension.

Relax. Remove the hectic tensions from your face, and it will become tranquil, more harmonious and attractive. Relax your body, and it will serve you better.

When you first learn the art of relaxation, it is best to be alone. For complete comfort, you might buy some small pillows. These should be placed under the neck, the elbows, and the knees.

I believe one of the secrets of Winston Churchill's long success was his ability to relax completely. He retired every afternoon to his private room to relax, to let go, to forget the stresses and strains of his hectic career. One wonders how many of our present world leaders bother to learn how to relax.

You may not have the problems of a world leader, but learning the art of relaxation will help you cope with the tensions in your everyday life. Lie comfortably on a couch or bed. Let your imagination help you. Make believe you are floating on a cloud, or that you are a rag doll with entirely loose and floppy joints. Be the branch of a bush blowing in the wind, or seaweed in the ocean going back and forth with the waves. If it helps, put on gentle, relaxing music—or try one of those records of "white" sound, the sound of the ocean, for instance. Think of anything that helps you to let go, so that your muscles become loose and free.

I find it best to start with the feet. First, turn each foot a few times to loosen it up; then think of your feet as being very loose, as dangling like two tassels. Now relax the calves and thighs. You might flex them a couple of times, or shake each leg a bit—then let your legs lie heavy, heavy as lead. Think of your legs, and your feet, as utterly relaxed—no tension, no tightness, anywhere.

Now take a few breaths, as deep as possible. Breathe gently and make your exhalations longer than your inhalations. Feel your body sink into the bed. Banish every thought of tension and tautness. Next tense your arms; stretch them as long as you can. Tense your fingers, spread them apart, make them as rigid as you can. Now make tight and hard fists, as though you were boxing.

Relax the muscles of your hands and arms, and let them drop heavily by your sides. Your hands and arms should now be as relaxed as sleeping kittens. Now comes the neck, the part of the body that shows so much tension, and is so susceptible to it. Roll your head from side to side a few times, as though you were saying no. You will probably find several kinks in your neck. Make believe your head is unbearably heavy, and then let it sink deep into the pillow—assume that the neck has no power to move it.

The eyes are next, and it is very important that you learn how to relax them. This can be accomplished in many ways. First of all, squeeze the eyes a few times by just closing them tightly. Now open and close them a few more times, but lightly, delicately, loosely. If you are still tense and nervous, the eyelids will quiver. So keep on letting go, breathe calmly until the eyes don't quiver and flutter. With the eyes closed, make believe that the muscles that control the eyeballs are loose, very loose, and completely relaxed—let go of all tightness and tension here too.

This head-to-toe relaxation will do you good any time of the day, but it is ideal when done just before going to sleep. It has helped many insomniacs to overcome their tensions and sleeplessness. The whole relaxing procedure takes between five and ten minutes. Don't feel silly about doing it. Try it. Do it at least once a day. But if you are weary, and really anxious to conquer the strains and tensions of life, do it two or three times a day, until you have learned to prevent tightness and tension. Even then, though, do it each night before going to sleep. For when you sleep in a relaxed and peaceful attitude, you will wake up refreshed, with added strength and energy for the new day.

THE GREAT ESCAPE

Here is a simple way, and a quick one, for relaxing and relieving yourself of nervous tension during the day. It is my favorite method when I am on television (which is perhaps the most killing of all work) or when I am on a lecture tour. It only takes a few moments and is most helpful. Open your nearest window, sit on an upright chair or at your desk, and sit straight. Close your eyes and keep them closed. Now, breathe as deeply and as slowly as you can. Remember to breathe in through the nose and to exhale through the mouth, slowly, slowly, and as long as you comfortably can. Hum on the sound of "Om" as you exhale, but not so loudly that those within hearing range will think you are going berserk. While you hum and breathe slowly and peacefully, allow yourself to escape for a few moments. Use your imagination, and think of your favorite pastime—fishing in a brook—lying under a blossoming apple tree—floating in the Mediterranean; think of anything and everything that brings you happy, peaceful, and calm memories.

This letting go, this breathing deeply and slowly, plus a few happy thoughts, can refresh you miraculously.

The Magic Yoga Slant

The ageless Lady Mendl was famous for standing on her head when she was eighty. The Great Om, a yogi from India, had promised her a long and youthful life if she stood on her head for three minutes each day. There were other famous headstanders in the twenties, too, such as Ina Claire, Anne Morgan, Blanche Yurka, Greta Garbo, and Leopold Stokowski. I learned to do the headstand under the tutelage of Miss Garbo, and there is no question of its efficacy; nothing relieves the constant downward pull of the face and abdominal muscles so quickly as this upside-down position. But I also discovered that some of my students who practiced the headstand hurt their necks and backs. I was glad when another yogi introduced the *magic yoga slant,* which is so easy to do; anyone, regardless of age, can lie in this comfortable position. Many of my students, especially in California, have installed what they call the *beauty slant,* a wooden or plastic board with the foot end raised 12 to 15 inches. (It should never be higher, or the position becomes uncomfortable.) At this elevated angle, you can obtain all the benefits of the headstand without the possibility of injury. It is actually the laziest and most effective way of stopping the downward pull of gravity. Lady Mendl was full of praise for this yoga slant and used it constantly in place of her headstand until her ninety-fourth birthday.

All you need to make one for yourself is a solid board, one and a half feet wide and six feet long (a little longer if you are very tall). You simply raise the foot end of the board to a low chair or attach two legs to the foot end, not higher than 12 to 15 inches.

For more comfort, you can pad the board with a thin sheet of foam rubber and cover it with canvas or plastic. On expensive and sophisticated beauty farms, the yoga slant boards are in every room as well as clustered around the swimming pool. The lovely and ageless Ann Delafield, who was director of the Elizabeth Arden beauty farm, says that this yoga slant brings the spine and inner organs into proper alignment and lifts falling faces and chin lines from within, via your own red blood stream. Ann Delafield insisted that all beauty-farm guests take the beauty slant at least twice a day, for fifteen minutes during the afternoon and fifteen minutes before retiring. Poor circulation may cause some discomfort initially. Begin slowly, adding a minute more to slant time each day until you can recline comfortably for the full fifteen minutes.

Serious yoga experts believe that this position forces the blood into the vital centers of the body. In the yoga slant position, the spine straightens out and the back flattens itself. Muscles that ordinarily are somewhat tense, even in easy standing or sitting, are relaxed and at ease. The feet and legs, freed from their customary burden and the force of gravity, have a chance to release accumulated congestions into the blood stream and tissues, and thereby reduce the possibility of swollen limbs and strained blood vessels. Sagging abdominal muscles get a lift, and the blood flows more freely to the muscles of the chin, throat, and cheeks, helping to maintain their firmness. The complexion, hair, and scalp benefit from this increased blood circulation. In this position the brain also is rested and cleared. In fact, Dr. Donald Laird, of Colgate University, has said that the brain functions 14 percent better when the head is lower than the feet.

Take the yoga slant for fifteen minutes, twice a day. Take it whenever you can—on arising, before retiring, or, best of all, when you come home tired from work.

Midriff Flattener—the Stomach Lift

Lying completely relaxed in the yoga slant position, draw in your stomach as you count one. (Continue breathing naturally while doing this exercise.) Draw your stomach in and up, farther, on the count of two. On the count of three, you draw it in close to your spine, which is pressed flat against the board. Try to hold this position to the count of ten. Then relax. Repeat the exercise as often as you wish.

I call this exercise the stomach lift. In the years when people were flocking to Munich to learn it at Dr. Bauer's famous clinic, it was called the *Bauchgymnastik* or "belly gymnastic."

Do the stomach lift for the rest of your long life, and save your waistline permanently. You will be saved from sagging shoulders, middle-age spread, "jelly belly," face and throat wrinkles, bulges, and rigidity. Why? Because you will have a strong, permanent "muscle corset" supporting the center of all the vital processes of your body.

Dr. Erich A. Mueller, after ten years of research, came up with a related discovery that should be exciting to many busy people —especially men who dislike exercise. He found that one intense muscular contraction, the maximum possible, held for only seconds, and performed just once a day, will rapidly strengthen the muscle. His research showed that the one maximum contraction, performed once a day, makes the muscle 6 percent stronger in one week, 66 percent stronger in eleven weeks. These quick muscle-tensing exercises have become very popular in England, Germany, and Italy.

Good health depends upon abdominal firmness; this region is the center of absorption, assimilation, and elimination. Energy and emotional health also depend on it. Behind the stomach lies what is known as the "abdominal brain," a sympathetic nerve apparatus connected with all the other abdominal organs.

Master the stomach lift and, when you walk, you will keep your stomach flat without effort. Take long steps when you walk, feel the good, rewarding "pull" in the muscles of your legs and buttocks, feel your shoulders go back, your neck straighten to carry your head proudly. Imagine that you are a movie heroine walking down a long corridor toward the dramatic climax of the story, or a model on the runway at a fashion show. Or a dignitary crossing the platform of a huge amphitheater to receive the decoration of the Legion of Honor.

Muscular Joy

Rediscover Your Favorite Sport

If you have a favorite sport, one that you have allowed to slip out of your life in recent years, go back to it. Do not be discouraged if your skill has become a bit rusty and your muscles protest at first. No one ever forgets how to swim, dance, ski, bicycle, ice-skate, play tennis, or swing a golf club. Your body remembers; only give it a chance, and start slowly!

And give it the energy of your high-vitality diet to draw on. You will soon feel again the exhilaration you used to enjoy. Even if you are not, and perhaps never have been, a champion, what of it? The muscular joy of using your body will keep you happy at your sport.

Swimming is, as you know, one of the most joyous exercises. If you are at all skilled in the water, I urge you to locate a pool or beach and begin to swim regularly, all year round. But I do mean swim. Just dunking yourself in the water will be fun, but not really enough fun for real muscular joy. Swim your one, two, or three steady laps across or around the pool. Speed is not important.

Swim, ride, walk, dance—enjoy whatever you like, but *enjoy* it.

Seven Exercises / Seven Minutes

For the apartment dweller and the other millions of people who do not have much opportunity to pursue their favorite sports, just seven minutes a day spent doing simple rhythmic exercises can do wonders.

Here is some cheerful news about exercise: it does not have to be a long, complicated, strenuous routine. All the men and women who have told me how they successfully made exercise a part of their daily lives have confirmed my own experience. A few well-chosen, basic, *simple* exercises make the best routine. They can be gone through in a few minutes as part of the getting up, bathing, and dressing ritual that begins your day.

I have studied countless exercise routines—American, European, and Oriental—for every country has its favorites. The best ones have been developed out of natural body movements and do not demand a contortionist's or an acrobat's abilities. Let me give you seven basic exercises. You can do them well and thoroughly in no more than seven minutes of your day, and they will keep you trim and fit all your life. Remember, we do not exercise only to keep slim, we exercise because it helps us to feel so much better.

1. *Stretch:* Rise up on your toes, arms up; with your hands, try to touch the ceiling. Drop arms. Relax. Do ten times.

2. *Bend:* Down, down, from the waist, hands reaching for the floor. Stretch, stretch, until you can touch the floor with the palms of your hands. Each time bend down as far as you can comfortably—but don't overdo. The best vitalizing exercise and cure for backache. Do ten times.

3. *Torso twist:* With arms outstretched to the sides, reach to the left, to the right; twist at the waist and reach backward to the left, then to the right. Back and forth. A wonderful, easy way to keep your waistline. Do ten times.

4. *Hip roll:* With hands on hips, rotate the lower torso first to the left, then to the right, holding the shoulders still—the way a belly dancer does. Do ten times slowly in each direction.

5. *Bicycle:* Lie on the floor on your back, legs up; pedal slowly and rhythmically. The more you breathe, the better it feels. Do for two minutes, then relax. This helps to counteract varicose veins.

6. *Stomach lift:* Pull your abdominal muscles in, hard, harder. Hold tight for about thirty seconds, or until muscles quiver, then relax. Do at least once a day, but regularly (or do this, as I have suggested, on the yoga slant).

7. *Shoulder shrug:* Important for neck, face, and scalp. Lift the shoulders to the ears and hold for ten seconds. Relax. Repeat ten times.

Now shake yourself all over, take a few deep breaths, and off to your shower or tub. You have done your muscle work for the day. Any other exercise, sport, or physical work you do will be so much gravy. Try to make these easy, lazy twists and stretches a daily fun habit.

Every one of these seven exercises has its particular as well as its general value for your health and good looks. The stomach lift explains itself; you can reduce several inches in just a few weeks. But you must do it regularly. The bicycling and hip roll take care of circulation in the legs and middle. The stretches, bends, and twists do wonders in loosening spinal and torso tensions. Those large muscles across your back and ribs contract by reflex, without your conscious effort; in your sedentary life, they are in tension most of the time. The same is true of the shoulder shrug, which loosens tension in the neck, face, and scalp and creates revitalizing circulation to the brain; it also strengthens and firms the muscles that hold the chest high.

Rock Away Your TV Bottom

Since we became a nation of sitters, a new nuisance has arisen called TV Bottom. To counteract the effect of constant sitting in front of television, here is an easy and effective exercise to strengthen those large and flabby buttock muscles and help to reduce an oversize derrière.

While watching TV, sit on the floor, pull up your knees, take hold of your ankles on the outside, and rock-rock-rock like a little rocking horse; swing back and forth. You will feel the buttock muscles getting a terrific squeezing, your whole circulation is pepped up, and, what's important, you will discover that rocking is fun! You might even feel energized enough to get up, turn off the set, and go for a walk.

Walk Your Way to a Longer Life

Most people will do almost anything to avoid walking, but there are exceptions—and they are exceptional people. Greta Garbo for years walked on the beaches and hills of Hollywood; it kept her going during her strenuous film-making days. Lynn Fontanne, one of the most enduringly beautiful women, was known for her walks over the rolling hills of her Wisconsin farm. Marlene Dietrich, famous for her young legs, is a walker; even in New York she still takes long walks in the park. Ingrid Bergman is another woman who walks, whether she is in Hollywood, Rome, or Paris, often with her children. I could go on endlessly with this list.

Perhaps you think I'm going overboard about walking, but I'm not. Walking preserves health and lengthens life. A New York physician said bluntly that half the patients in his waiting room could cure themselves of what ailed them if they would spend an hour walking every day. Walking cures tensions, insomnia, chronic fatigue, and a host of minor physical and mental complaints that drag down the spirit and body and take the joy out of living. Walking—free striding, free-swinging, rhythmic, brisk but unharried walking—is the perfect aid to digestion, elimination, circulation, relaxation of body, mind, and spirit.

The next time you feel low, go out for a walk. Put on your most comfortable shoes. (See also page 205.) Walk with your head up, take long steps, let your arms swing freely and easily, and deepen your breathing. Keep a good rhythm—not necessarily fast, but steady. See how your mood changes, how the dark color of your thoughts becomes gradually brighter. Your low spirits will not accompany you very far on a good walk. Psychologists remind us again and again that the mind cannot remain depressed when the body is in motion.

Walking does all this for you; and furthermore, it is a very special pleasure. Why do you suppose so many intelligent, gifted people, who could choose any recreation they like, enjoy walking? Because it is sheer muscular joy.

Sleep

Deep, sound sleep is a gift from heaven, and if you have it, give thanks, for nothing is as rejuvenating as a good night's rest. I hope that you are not in the habit of taking barbiturates. Figures show that more than 6 million people in the United States are unwise enough to shorten their lives by taking these so-called sleeping pills. Do not worry about sleeping; the more you worry, the more sleepless you become. It is a vicious circle that you create for yourself.

Many food factors contribute to the relaxation that is necessary for sound sleep. The four most important, however, appear to be calcium, magnesium, vitamin D, and vitamin B_6.

Vitamin B_6 seems to have a sedative effect on the nerves. It has even been used in the treatment of St. Vitus's dance and palsy, with excellent results. In any case, it does seem to be essential to a healthy nervous system. Although some lesser-known vitamins of the B family have not as yet been definitely identified with specific deficiency diseases, they do seem to play a role in many deficiency conditions. For example, many of the nervous symptoms that remain after treatment with thiamine, riboflavin, and niacin respond rapidly to the administration of B_6. But B_6 is not found in many common foods. It is removed during the refining of grains, and is not added to "enriched" flour. To get adequate amounts of vitamin B_6 you must eat such foods as wheat germ, brewers' yeast, molasses, and liver—not occasionally, but often.

Magnesium deficiency often causes restlessness and the inability to relax enough to fall asleep. Magnesium oxide supplements, taken a half hour before retiring, have replaced the sleeping pill for many insomniacs. Magnesium deficiency is caused by eating too many refined foods and not enough green vegetables and whole grains.

A lack of calcium can also be responsible for much sleeplessness. Every person, regardless of age, should get one gram of calcium daily. This can be obtained most easily from a quart of milk. It may be skim milk, buttermilk, or yogurt; the choice depends on your weight and on your own preference. Since calcium dissolves in acid, "soured" milks such as buttermilk and yogurt, which contain lactic acid, supply calcium in a form more quickly and completely absorbed into the blood. Those milk drinks that have been advertised as conducive to sound sleep depend primarily on the calcium in the milk you make them with; it helps the nerves to relax and thus promotes sleep.

Although calcium is abundant in dairy products, it is found in very few other foods. Green leafy vegetables, for example, have calcium; but it is in an insoluble form that cannot pass into the blood. But a tablespoon of dark molasses supplies as much calcium as does half a glass of milk. A cup of hot milk with 2 teaspoons of the darkest molasses to be found is still one of my favorite "sleep cocktails." All dishes prepared with meat on the bone should include a little lemon, vinegar, tomato juice, yogurt, or cooking wine to help dissolve calcium from the bone and make it available. Many primitive peoples, such as Eskimos, get their entire calcium supply from eating bones.

Here in the United States some baby foods are now fortified with very fine bone flour. Let's hope that bone flour fortification soon will also be applied to foods for adults. Dr. Sherman repeatedly stated that the need for calcium in adults does not decrease and the intake should be kept high.

Calcium cannot be efficiently absorbed and utilized without vitamin D. And vitamin D is found in only a few foods—vitamin D milk, eggs, certain fish, and that rare delicacy caviar. The best source is sunshine. If it is impossible for you to have a half-hour sunbath daily, get your vitamin D by taking fish-liver oil. (It comes in capsule form.)

Fresh skim milk fortified with dry skim milk powder also ensures a rich supply of calcium. However, where a calcium deficiency is of long standing, nutritionists recommend calcium tablets with vitamin D. When the body is brought into positive calcium balance, the ability to sleep readily and soundly should follow.

Calcium tablets must never be considered a substitute for milk. The person whose health is so below par that he suffers from insomnia also needs the protein, vitamins, and minerals that dairy products supply; deficiencies do not occur singly.

For restful sleep, base your menus on this sample:

Breakfast:	Fruit or fruit juice; egg or whole-grain cereal with wheat germ; whole-wheat toast; milk or Swiss coffee—half hot coffee, half hot milk
Midmorning:	Buttermilk, yogurt, or skim milk flavored with molasses or cinnamon; plus 2 calcium tablets
Luncheon:	Fruit or vegetable salad with cottage cheese; milk, buttermilk, or yogurt; junket or custard
Midafternoon:	A tablespoon of brewers' yeast stirred into tomato juice; plus 2 calcium tablets

Dinner: Vegetable juice or fruit cocktail; meat or broiled liver; 1 or 2 short-cooked vegetables; milk, buttermilk, or yogurt; fresh fruit or cheese with whole-wheat crackers

Before Retiring: Hot milk drink, yogurt, or cheese and whole-wheat crackers; plus 2 calcium tablets

---

Tranquilizing Nightcap

1 tablespoon powdered skim milk
2 teaspoons molasses or honey
1 teaspoon brewers' yeast

Stir into cup of warm milk and sip slowly.

10

Keep Your Body Young

Prevention is vastly better than cure. So much can now be done to prevent many conditions of ill-health or an aging body through good nutrition and will power. When I see anyone feeding his body unwisely, I ponder on the tragedy that may be in store for that individual, a tragedy that may be completely unnecessary. So let's talk about some common-sense secrets for long life.

Smokers Need More Vitamin C

I myself do not smoke, but this does not mean that I am unsympathetic to the problems of stopping this habit. Once started, a smoker needs an iron will to quit. Many people use cigarettes as a substitute for food and worry that if they stop smoking they will gain weight. But if you eat properly, with respect for your body, there is no reason for this worry. For a better, longer life, stop now. If you can't stop, at least keep your smoking in moderation. And certainly, if you have a circulation problem, stop entirely.

If you must smoke, remember extra vitamin C is necessary for cigarette smokers. Dr. W. J. McCormick of Canada has studied many of his patients who smoke and discovered that the smoking of *one* cigarette destroys about 25 mg. of vitamin C, or about the amount found in half a medium-size orange.

Excessive Drinking Destroys Vitamins

ALCOHOL STEALS VITAMINS. That is not a news headline. It is an everyday fact. The drink you enjoy before dinner, when the day's work is done, is a B vitamin thief. Don't misunderstand me; I am not a teetotaler or a killjoy. I just want to caution you that alcoholic beverages increase your need for vitamins. Why? Because alcohol, like carbohydrate foods such as candy and pastry, requires B vitamins for its metabolism. So the body borrows from your daily stores, and then you need more B vitamins to offset the loss.

In a remarkable little book entitled *Nutrition and Alcoholism,* Dr. Roger J. Williams relates the discovery of how alcoholism is tied up with nutrition. Experimental research and clinical trial showed that lack of vitamins was a factor in the overwhelming urge to drink, and that large amounts of B vitamins plus good nutrition eliminated the drinking problem. As long as Dr.Williams's patients abided by his nutrition-plus-vitamins plan, they could drink in moderation or leave it alone, as they preferred. When they neglected their established requirements of vitamins, the old alcoholic urge came back. As with other aspects of the nutritional picture, it was pointed out that there are wide variations in the individual requirements for B vitamins, and this in turn influences the wide variations in individual reactions to drinking.

Alcohol and sugary desserts and candy are remarkably similar: you can "get drunk" on any of them, all are B vitamin thieves, all are loaded with hidden calories that carry excess weight.

Have a relaxing drink, if you wish it. Make it wine rather than hard liquor, if possible. Wine is festive and it contains digestive enzymes, a factor in its favor. But do not make the mistake of having an extra drink because you are reducing and want to reward yourself for eating less. To help you make your own decision on this point, here is a chart that will show you that alcohol, though it does not nourish, definitely can add poundage.

BEVERAGES	CALORIES
Beer (12 ounces)	170
Brandy (1 ounce)	75
Cocktails (3 ounces)	
daiquiri	130*
manhattan	170
martini	145
old-fashioned	185*
Eggnog (1 scant cup)	200
Rum (1½-ounce jigger)	105
Tom Collins	180*
Whiskey (1½-ounce jigger)	
rye	120
bourbon	120
Irish	120
Scotch	110
Wine (3½-ounce glass)	
red	75
white	90
port	160

* More, if you like them sweet.

Prevent Brittle Bones

Bones need not become brittle and fragile with age. In general, such bones are the cumulative effect of years of eating foods deficient in the nutrients essential to good bone strength. Experiments with animals have shown that when their diet is always rich in bone-building elements, their bones retain strength even in most advanced age. Of course, a serious glandular disturbance could upset the calcium metabolism in later life, but this is not a major cause of brittleness.

The substructure of the bones requires vitamin C to produce collagen, which is responsible for its soundness. Vitamin A is required in the bone remodeling process. Experiments have shown that when growing animals are fed diets deficient in vitamin A, bones are not formed properly and structural defects occur. Calcium and phosphorus are deposited on the substructure to produce dense, hard bones; the diet must therefore also supply calcium and phosphorus. When not enough calcium is supplied for the body's other needs, such as in the blood, calcium will actually be pulled from the bones to maintain the supply in the blood and for necessary daily excretion. The resulting *demineralization* leads to very breakable bones. Chronic demineralization is one reason why many people get shorter as they grow older. Back pain, stemming from weakened, compressed lumbar vertabrae, is another common result of calcium lost from bones. Furthermore, without vitamin D, calcium is not absorbed from the intestines, and so we must have this vitamin, too. Supplementing the diet with a vitamin D concentrate is advised.

Older people, especially women, are frequently deficient in calcium. This comes about in several ways. Dairy products, milks, and cheeses are often shunned or taken in too small quantities. Many vegetables contain large quantities of calcium, but much of it may not be available to the body, for a variety of reasons. The calcium in spinach, for example, is unavailable because it is present in an insoluble form and cannot be absorbed. Also, vegetables with considerable fibrous matter may not be well chewed; with poor digestion, the calcium may never be liberated in the intestines. Yogurt, however, is an excellent source of calcium. It is easily digested and its calcium is highly available.

Elderly people should also watch their calories; overweight increases the pressure on already weak bones. But, most important, keep your diet rich in the bone-building elements: calcium and vitamins A, C, and D. If citrus juices, excellent sources of vitamin C, are not liked, many of the vegetable juices can be used to replace them. (You will probably not be deficient in phosphorus, so don't worry about that.)

Ward Off Hardening of the Arteries

When arteries become hard, they lose their elasticity. This condition is called arteriosclerosis, and there are two types. One, which is common in older people, is caused by calcium deposits on the insides of the arteries. This is the so-called pipe-stem arteriosclerosis. The other is the result of an accumulation of cholesterol within the walls of the arteries (atherosclerosis), which leads to hardening and thickening. This second type can be influenced directly by diet. Too much cholesterol, too little lecithin can both contribute to early occurrences.

When the arteries have become hard in this way, not only do they lose their elasticity, but they become smaller in diameter, ultimately being reduced to inadequate channels. Since the amount of blood in the circulatory system remains the same, the strain on the heart increases as the diameter of the plugged arteries decreases and the blood pressure rises. Fatalities occur when the coronary arteries become so diminished that blood supply to the heart muscle is inadequate for its function. As we know that smoking greatly reduces circulatory functions, the strongest recommendation as regards a smoker with arteriosclerosis is to stop smoking at once.

Dr. William Kannel of the Department of Preventive and Social Medicine at the Harvard Medical School warns that the chances of an American male having a heart attack before age sixty are about one in five. Dr. Kannel, who is also the director of the Framingham Study of the National Heart and Lung Institute, told the American College of Physicians that, as of 1974, "there is a 14 percent increase in the coronary events under age forty-five."

Prevention is truly the life-saving word in regard to coronary arterery disease, for many of its victims do not get another chance. Eight percent of the fatalities occur during the initial attack.

I myself have seen intelligent people put a halt to this process of hardening by following a diet low in animal fat, increasing their vitamin intake, and drinking freely of fresh green- and yellow-vegetable juices. I am delighted to report that the experimental work of Dr. Lester Morrison and others has been instrumental in finding the cause and developing the prevention and control of atherosclerosis.

In 1947 Dr. J. R. Moreton published his first study of arteriosclerosis. This work pointed to a fatty degeneration of the elastic tissues, which occurred when the fat content of the blood was high. It was also shown by Dr. J. W. Gofman that an overgrowth of the outer layer of the arteries occurs, and that it takes place when certain constituents of fats are circulated in the blood, as a result of fat in the diet. Then Drs. Moreton and Necheler demonstrated that when excessive quantities of cholesterol were fed to various animals, atherosclerosis always followed promptly. And so a disease, a killing disease, was being tracked to its lair.

Now comes the dramatic news. Once the habitat of the "killer" was discovered, we learned how to set about getting him. And that way lay through diet—B vitamins! Drs. Steiner, Morrison, Rossi, Herrman, and others showed that nutritional hardening of the arteries could be prevented and even cured by the use of vitamins that *mobilize* fat, and its associated substances, and also accelerate its assimilation in the body. These three most important vitamins of the B family are choline, inositol, and pyridoxine (vitamin B_6).

We have known for a long time that diseases such as diabetes mellitus, nephritis, myxedema (a species of dropsy), and a skin disorder called xanthomatosis (which appears as very small patches of connective tissue that has undergone fatty degeneration) are all associated with high blood fat and are frequently accompanied by hardening of the arteries. Dr. Morrison recently offered evidence that the converse also is true—that in diseases accompanied by low blood fat, such as exophthalmic goiter, arteriosclerosis rarely occurs. Work in the laboratory brings forth more and more evidence. It shows that arteries hardened by excessive fatty matter in the blood display approximately the same composition of fatty matter as that circulating in the blood.

One reason the United States leads in circulatory and heart troubles (the number-one killer) is that it leads the world in excessive fat consumption, especially of the hardened and hydrogenated kinds.

Of course, there are other causes of the constant increase in vascular diseases. Man really asked for trouble when he started to denude and refine the staff of life—our grains and bread. The throwing away of the wheat and other cereal germs, the richest source of vitamins B and E, parallels the increase in heart difficulties. Vitamins B and E probably lead all other vitamins in nourishing the heart. Chemical additives may also play a role in the atherosclerosis epidemic. Dr. George V. Mann, of Vanderbilt University, found that when surfactants (additives used in mayonnaise, ice cream, chocolate, and commercially baked goods) were added to the diet of laboratory animals, blood cholesterol levels rose significantly.

It has been shown that atherosclerosis (arteriosclerosis caused by the faulty metabolism of fatty substances) can be prevented and cured through the administration of the B vitamins choline and inositol, either with or without pyridoxine. Little courage is now called for to classify it as a dietary deficiency disease. I am going to ask you now to solemnly promise yourself that from this day forth you will take special pains to see that your diet contains generous amounts of choline and inositol—in fact, all the B vitamins, plus vitamin E, which, according to the Drs. Shute in Canada, has helped thousands of their patients, when taken regularly in large enough amounts.

Yogurt may be the new anticholesterol drug! Dr. Mann's laboratory experiments led him to the Masai tribe of East Africa. He decided to study this particular nomadic tribe because of their resistance to heart disease despite their high-cholesterol diet (twice the amount recommended by the American Heart Association). The tribesmen also consume about a gallon of yogurt a day each. During the study the tribesmen *doubled* their yogurt intake and the cholesterol level actually dropped. According to a report in *The New York Times* (June 23, 1974), Dr. Mann said: "Yogurt made by adding a commercial American yogurt culture to whole milk or to skim milk has been found to lower cholesterol..."

Take the precaution of eating natural foods wisely, for that is good common sense. But, in being vigilant, do not jump to extremes. Many individuals have consumed normal amounts of fat and lived a long and vital life, with never a touch of arteriosclerosis—perhaps they always ate wisely! If you have the slightest suspicion that to any degree you may be tending toward hardening of the arteries, have an examination made of the state of fatty material in your blood. But be sure to have a reliable examination made.

Once your doctor has confirmed that your blood contains too much cholesterol, you should be guided in your diet by the following:

1. Go easy on high-cholesterol foods; especially avoid hard animal fats and rich cream.
2. Use liquid vegetable oils in place of hard fats for salads and for cooking.
3. Increase your protein intake to 100 grams daily.
4. Cut down on carbohydrates and use only the unrefined variety.
5. Reduce fat to not more than 20 to 25 grams daily and use cold-pressed vegetable oils.
6. To compensate for the vitamin A loss due to omitting animal fat, use other vitamin A and E foods generously.
7. Be sure that the diet supplies ample quantities of vitamin B_6, choline, inositol, and lecithin. When choline and inositol are taken together, they heighten each other's effect; as means of therapy, 3 grams of choline and 1.5 grams of inositol should be taken daily. When therapeutic measures are called for, it is advisable to take these vitamins in the pure form, immediately after meals; you can obtain them in capsule form.

Even if your physician gives you a clean bill of health as regards atherosclerosis, you should still take precautions. Everyone can profit from a diet that supplies generous quantities of choline, inositol, and pyridoxine (vitamin B_6). See chapter 3 for complete lists of foods rich in these substances. Remember that brewers' yeast is an especially good source for these and all the B-complex vitamins. And, I shouldn't have to add, stop smoking.

Your Heart and Your Diet

The muscles of the heart are continuously at work every moment that you live. The energy demanded by the heart is very great, both in amount and in the rate at which it is required. From your diet you must get the food factors—the vitamins—necessary for energy exchanges in the body.

For instance, anything that disturbs the fundamental metabolism of the body, as deficiency of most B vitamins does, must in some degree affect the heart. Unless we select our diets with care, heart disease will remain a scourge.

So many everyday foods do not supply you with a generous amount of B vitamins. Here is where you can turn to the wonder foods for help. One cup of yogurt, two tablespoons of brewers' yeast, one half cup of wheat germ, and one half cup of dried skim milk, together give seven times the vitamin B_1, twice the vitamin B_2, and 130 percent of the niacin necessary (on the basis of the dietary allowances of the National Research Council) for a moderately active person.

Not only do you get vitamins B_1, B_2, and niacin but you also get choline, inositol, vitamin B_6, panthothenic acid, and other B vitamins too. Natural foods that are particularly rich in any of the B vitamins generally contain virtually the entire B family. That is why I picked certain foods and called them wonder foods. (See chapter 2.) We know now that many of the B vitamins work together rather than, as was once thought, in a sharply specific manner. Not all of the accompanying symptoms of the classic niacin deficiency disease, pellagra, are helped by the administration of niacin alone; riboflavin and pantothenic acid are also needed. That is why brewers' yeast achieved such outstanding success in the treatment of pellagra. Moreover, rarely is there a deficiency of only one B vitamin. If you wish, you may take capsules that give you thiamine (vitamin B_1), riboflavin (vitamin B_2), and niacin, even those that add a little pyridoxine (vitamin B_6) and pantothenic acid. But my advice is to eat also the B-vitamin rich foods such as brewers' yeast and wheat germ. Had this practice been followed, many of us would have obtained choline and inositol in more adequate amounts, and it is more than a probability that there would be less arteriosclerosis. But in our enthusiasm for "pure" vitamins and our tendency to ignore natural products, and because clear-cut deficiency conditions were not identified with the "lesser" B vitamins, we paid them little attention. I am prepared, always, to believe in natural foods, to which man has been adapted for countless generations; if I do no more for my students than passing this secret along to them, I will be well satisfied.

(For a discussion of the role of vitamin E and the heart, see chapter 3.)

Now let us go back to the subject of the prevention of heart troubles. Intelligent eating is one of the essentials, and unless we take to intelligent eating, I predict that heart troubles will increase. We have discussed hardening of the arteries and shown quite clearly that it can result from a poor diet. Hardened arteries lead to high blood pressure, kidney disease, and heart trouble. A sound, well-balanced diet is fundamental to the well-being of your heart, and intelligent eating is the cornerstone of a longer life.

Your heart muscles, like every other muscle in the body, are composed principally of protein. Once it was believed, by physician and layman alike, that with heart trouble one should reduce the proteins in the diet. The opposite is now known to be true. Even in conditions of heart failure, when considerable fluids collect in the tissues, a high-protein and low-salt diet is prescribed.

But once heart trouble has set in, the advice of your physician is essential to a proper diagnosis and plan of treatment best suited to the particular, individual condition. Since I have stressed so much the importance of vitamins, especially vitamin B, you will be interested in what Dr. William Brady has to say:

The real heart tonic I recommend can do no harm and may do considerable good not only for the heart and circulation but for the digestion and nerves as well. It is not medicine at all. It is my same old remedy, simply food; food which every child or adult needs to maintain good digestion and good circulation but which few children or adults get in adequate proportions because of our ultrarefined diet. It is vitamin B complex, an optimal, daily ration of it.

Type A Behavior

Hurriedness is a typical American disease. We have always known that the high-pressure executive who watches the clock and the stock market and eats too fast is a likely candidate for a heart attack. Recently two California doctors, Meyer Friedmen and Ray Rosenman, have described this type of man in their very informative book *Type A Behavior and Your Heart* (Knopf). In my long experience, however, I have found that Type B men, the slower, more easygoing type, also get heart attacks. I believe this is because they do not eat high-vitality meals with more protein, more vitamins and minerals, and fewer carbohydrates.

I am very much impressed with the ideas of Canada's stress-and-strain man, Dr. Seely. He says that we cannot live without some stress and strain, but it is our reaction to stress that can harm us. His sage advice is to counteract every stressful emotion with a positive one. I suggest you counteract stress with a positive philosophy, good old-fashioned prayer, and faith in your Maker.

Lecithin Combats Cholesterol Build-up

In 1951, at the age of fifty-one, Dr. J. Rinse, a consulting chemist, had a heart attack. He was puzzled by the violently painful attack of angina pectoris because he did not fit the usual heart-attack profile: he did not smoke, he was not overweight, he was not under undue stress, he exercised moderately, and there was no history of heart disease in his family.

In 1957 he had a second heart attack. His physician prescribed the usual drugs and gave Dr. Rinse only ten years to live and that only if all physical exercise was avoided. Dr. Rinse began an exhaustive search through medical literature to determine what causes a heart attack and whether or not it could be prevented. He read that lecithin might be an important deterrent, and so added it to his supplement intake. Within a few days he noted improvement. After three months all symptoms of angina had disappeared. In July 1973 Dr. Rinse wrote in *American Laboratory:* "Starting with an hypothesis that deficiencies in my food could be causative factors, dietary changes were explored, resulting in the complete alleviation of angina and related heart disease."

Dr. Rinse compares the human body to a chemical plant, "that is, a chemical energy plant, producing various kinds of energies—

for moving and thinking, for electric energy, and for heat . . . The human body needs secondary materials such as minerals, metals, vitamins and enzymes. These are needed to run the numerous chemical reactions of metabolism, for the production of energy, and in particular for the digestion of proteins, fats and carbohydrates, which are the primary raw materials for the body. Therefore, food must contain everything in adequate quantities and should be varied as much as possible."

What about cholesterol? Again Dr. Rinse thoroughly studied the literature as only a chemically minded person does when faced with a dilemma. "Although statistically the chance for atherosclerosis [hardening of the arteries] is higher if the cholesterol content of blood is high, many persons are healthy with a high cholesterol content," Dr. Rinse reports. "Therefore, it is doubtful whether the efforts to lower cholesterol content by all means are justified. Such efforts include avoidance of food containing cholesterol—such as eggs and butter, or using drugs that affect the production of cholesterol in the liver. It has been demonstrated that the liver produces more cholesterol if food contains less. Reducing its production by the liver by means of drugs can be dangerous and has caused serious side effects like cataracts and hair loss . . . It seems," he continues, "that one cannot change cholesterol production in the body without penalty. On the other hand, if lecithin is added to the diet, the unwanted deposits of cholesterol derivatives do not form, because the lecithin-cholesterol compound is soluble. Both materials occur in eggs, and therefore an atherosclerotic patient should not deprive himself of eating eggs. We have seen that polyunsaturated oil also should be present. Any excess of cholesterol in the bloodstream is removed from the body through the intestines." Dr. Rinse believes that the consumption of polyunsaturated oils without the use of lecithin is not effective. He says: "Only in the presence of sufficient lecithin can polyunsaturated fatty acid help in dissolving cholesterol."

At the time of the *American Laboratory* article—sixteen years after Dr. Rinse's last heart attack—none of the agonizing symptoms had returned. Thousands of people, many through word of mouth, have benefited from Dr. Rinse's regime.

"The following combination of vitamins and minerals has proved to be beneficial for the cure and prevention of atherosclerotic complications such as high blood pressure, angina pectoris, cataracts, obstructions in the arteries of the neck, legs, arms, and kidneys," Dr. Rinse reports.

---

1. Make a mixture of 1 tablespoon each of soybean lecithin,* debittered yeast, raw wheat germ, and bone meal. (It is recommended to prepare a larger quantity for storage. For debittered yeast, buy brewers' yeast.)
2. Mix in a bowl:
   2 tablespoons of the above mixture
   1 tablespoon dark-brown sugar (if you can take the mixture without the sugar, I suggest that you do)
   1 tablespoon safflower oil or other linoleate oil (soybean oil, for example)
3. Add milk to dissolve sugar and yeast.
   Add yogurt to increase consistency.
   Add cold cereal for calories as needed, or mix with hot cereal such as oatmeal or porridge. Raisins and other fruits can be added as desired.

* For severe cases of atherosclerosis the quantity of lecithin should be doubled.

This mixture can be taken at various meals, but most logically it should come with your usual breakfast. Most of the ingredients could be baked into a loaf of bread; many of them could also be used with a salad, meat loaf, etc. After one year on this regime, Dr. Rinse was able to resume heavy outdoor work (such as cutting down trees) and running.

Dr. Rinse also recommends that you take daily:

500 mg. vitamin C
100 I.U. vitamin E
1 multiple vitamin and mineral tablet

Any other normal food may be used, including eggs and butter, but high-melting fats (regular margarine) must be avoided. Soft (linoleate-containing) margarines are helpful, but butter is preferred, because it contains medium-chain triglycerides.

In summarizing his conclusions, Dr. Rinse says, "Atherosclerosis is a deficiency disease which can be counteracted successfully by the use of food supplements, in particular lecithin and unsaturated oils."

Vitamin P and Your Capillaries

If you want firm gums, strong, supple, and pliant connective tissue, and reasonable freedom from bruising, you should have a generous supply of vitamin C in your diet. Vitamin C is essential to the formation of collagen, the substance that cements the cells together into firm tissues. A lack of vitamin C causes the capillaries to become fragile and bruises to form with only slight injury. All conditions of bruising, however, are not caused by vitamin C deficiency. That was discovered very early in the development of vitamin C. When first the relationship between vitamin C and fragile capillaries was discovered, the hopes of medical men were raised that a cure for the dreaded disease of hemophilia had been found. (This disease recognizes no rank or station. It is hereditary, being transmitted only through the female line, and has afflicted many of the royal families of Europe.) However, those hopes soon were dashed. When the Hungarian scientist Szent-Györgyi isolated a factor from peppers that made the capillaries less permeable (less able to be passed through), again hopes were raised, and again dashed.

The cause and cure of hemophilia remain elusive to science, but the discovery of Szent-Györgyi was not useless. It promises results that were little suspected at the time, when the need for them did not exist—Szent-Györgyi's discovery may quite possibly lessen certain effects of atomic bomb explosions! The factor which Szent-Györgyi discovered is now known as vitamin P, not because it was first isolated from peppers, but for its effect in decreasing the permeability of the capillaries; it was originally called the antipermeability vitamin.

Capillary fragility and capillary permeability are entirely different. Fragile capillaries are easily ruptured; highly permeable capillaries pass considerably more fluid in a given time than is normal. Vitamin P is given together with vitamin C in the treatment of scurvy, for it seems to prevent the destruction of vitamin C by oxygen in the body.

Vitamin P belongs to a family of plant substances called the *flavonoids* or *bioflavonoids*. They occur in the peel of citrus fruits and in black currants; one active principle, called rutin, occurs in buckwheat. The flavonoids have come in for considerable research recently and can now be obtained in concentrated form.

Problems with Digestion and Elimination?

The best insurance of freedom from digestive disturbances is the eating of a sound, well-balanced diet composed of natural, unrefined foods—living foods that have not been destroyed by processing.

The diet must give you proteins that contain the essential amino acids, along with vitamins, especially the B vitamins, needed by the enzymes that digest the food. B vitamins maintain the tone of the digestive tract, the stomach and intestines. You need sound teeth to chew thoroughly the food you eat, and for your teeth's sake you need vitamin C and calcium.

You need hydrochloric acid in your stomach to act with the enzymes in order to digest the proteins completely. People who are addicted to the baking soda "relief," or the constant "alkalizers," are making the mistake of helping to produce the very trouble they hope to avoid. Gas pains, more frequently than not, are caused simply by air that has been swallowed. Air swallowing is a pernicious habit. Gum chewing is conducive to air swallowing. Many of us swallow copious quantities of air when we drink beverages; you chronic gas sufferers, try drinking through a straw, and you will be amazed at your freedom from gas.

The crime of crimes is to eat while you are doing something else or while you are under any kind of tension. The stomach works hard on the food you put into it—it has to churn it about and turn it over and over. Nerve tension makes the stomach relatively rigid—spastic. If you want it to work efficiently for you, relax. Serious organic disease often stems from chronic "tension" indigestion.

Do not discuss annoying subjects at the table. Do not fight with the children. The less attention you pay to them, the better they will eat. At mealtimes members of your family can get to know each other as interesting people and can be helpful to one another through quiet reasonable conversation. Banish worry and contention from your dining room.

About those business lunches—let lunchtime be a period of social intercourse with your business associates. Relaxed and at ease, you can get to know each other better and establish a friendlier relationship than by spending the same precious few minutes talking about disturbing business matters. You will live longer and more comfortably for it.

Eat at your leisure, relaxed and in a contented frame of mind. Eat serenely and slowly. Food bolters deserve ingestion, and fast eating is one crime that almost invariably is promptly punished. Chew your food, divide it very finely, give the stomach juices opportunity to penetrate. When you eat, do not include great volumes of air. Drink slowly; do not gulp.

Metchnikoff, the Russian bacteriologist, was the first to tell the world that within the gastrointestinal canal there are millions of bacteria, some friendly and some unfriendly. Under the microscope these bacteria look rather like flowers, and that's why we speak of the intestinal flora. It was also Metchnikoff who first discovered that through bad eating habits most people encourage the unfriendly flora and thereby suffer from digestive difficulties, excessive gas, and constipation.

Biochemists were able to prove that certain foods are especially helpful to feed the friendly flora. For successful intestinal gardening, all milk products are recommended; but speedier results are obtained from foods containing the lactobacilli acidophilus and bulgaricus. These are found in fermented acidophilus milk and yogurt, and also in certain kinds of cottage cheese. For those who are unable to use these milk products, whey powder or whey tablets, derived from fermented milk and in cheesemaking, are highly recommended for feeding the friendly bacteria.

Lazy Elimination

"A man whose bowels move regularly and normally will live very long," said Herodicus of Selymbria. That observation, made before the Christian era began, holds true to this day. Physicians have long noted that health and longevity are connected with the condition of the alimentary tract. Centenarians, who usually enjoy excellent digestion, often attribute a great deal of their longevity to the healthy functioning of the entire intestinal tract.

"Obey that impulse" is one of the best prescriptions for constipation. Pressure in the rectum is the body's signal to defecate. It makes a forthright request, even gives you fair warning; if you do not heed it, the body metes out its punishment—constipation. What happens when you don't heed the urge is precisely this: the rectum, when full, exerts pressure on the nerve endings, causing a feeling of the need to defecate. If you put it off, the pressure remains, but the nerve endings become overstimulated; fatigue sets in, and they no longer react. You lose the signal. You forget it, and constipation results.

Constipation, sufficiently prolonged, can become chronic and can lead to physical injury to the rectum, ultimately producing hemorrhoids. One of the functions of the colon is to retain water and allow it to be absorbed back into the body. When food wastes remain too long in the colon, they are robbed of much of their water content, and the stools become relatively dry and hard. In that form it is difficult for the normal rhythmic waves of the colon's walls to propel them along toward the exit. Moreover, when they do reach the rectum, they are discharged from the body with difficulty, and mechanical injury frequently results. The entire process is accompanied by a considerable degree of discomfort to the victim, both mental and physical.

Good habits can do much to improve evacuations. Regularity in habits induces regularity in bowel movements. Many conditions of chronic constipation have been relieved through "training." If one creates the conditions conducive to evacuation, regularly, every day, at the same time, preferably on arising in the morning, sooner or later the bowels will respond and continue to do so with most satisfying regularity. Sit comfortably, relax, do not strain, and give the bowels a real chance.

When you first get up in the morning, drink a glass of lukewarm water to which a half teaspoonful of vegetable salt has been added. This drink, on striking the empty stomach, arouses the reflexes and sets peristaltic waves in motion throughout the intestinal canal. If the bowels then are given an opportunity, evacuation generally follows. Moreover, the addition of the salt prevents the water from being absorbed before it reaches the colon, where it is useful in maintaining the food wastes in a moist and plastic condition. Patience is required at the start to train the bowels to regularity, but the result is satisfying; you will be rewarded over and over again, for the rest of your long life.

Too many people become addicts of laxatives early in life, partly because of clever advertising and partly because of bad habits and laziness. Children are fed laxatives by intestine-minded mothers from the earliest age. Small wonder, then, that the natural function of bowel movement, which works like a clock *without artificial interference* and is well able to take care of its small disturbances, becomes degenerated in more and more adults.

A daily bowel movement, or even two, is a sign of good intestinal health, and don't let anybody tell you differently. If the diet supplies appreciable quantities of bulkage, derived from vegetables and whole-grain breads and cereals, there will be more waste reaching the colon, and the movements may be more frequent.

A diet lacking in bulk leaves little for the colon to work on, and the stools become dry, hard, difficult to pass; constipation results. This type of constipation can be quite discomforting. It is the typical constipation of the white-flour, refined-sugar, meat and potato eater. The introduction of vegetables, fruits, whole grains, and a daily salad should suffice to rid you of this condition.

The B vitamins are essential for the maintenance of the normal tone of the intestinal tract. The simple inclusion of the wonder foods in the diet will give you a sufficiency of them. But the colon requires a reasonable quantity of bulkage, too. The salad bowl, colored vegetables, and fruits answer that purpose, in addition to giving you a rich supply of vitamins and minerals.

Sufficient protein is essential to maintain good muscle tone. Forceful contractions of the muscles that form the intestinal wall push wastes along the digestive tract. Production of digestive enzymes also depends on adequate protein intake. There is no substitute for vital eating; hardly a function of the body can be considered fully without reference to it. A man can be only as good as his digestive tract, for he can use only what he takes out of it—and he can take out of it only what he puts into it! Again, we return to the very wellspring of life—the diet.

There are circumstances that can induce temporary constipation, even in the most regular. Then the question arises as to what to do. First, do not jump to the conclusion that you need a laxative. Give nature a chance; she may correct herself. Stewed fruit, especially prunes, is usually helpful. Mineral oil and products containing it are undesirable. This oil is wholly indigestible, and it robs the intestines of the oil-soluble vitamins A, D, E, and K.

Your Natural Corset

For better elimination, I suggest you strengthen your inner and outer stomach and intestinal muscles with the laziest and best exercise in the world—the stomach lift (see chapter 9). Doing this muscle-tension exercise for two minutes each day can strengthen and flatten a protruding abdomen; and as the muscles regain their elasticity, lazy elimination becomes a thing of the past.

An overall run-down condition, flaccid muscles, and general lack of tone in the intestinal tract are frequently accompanied by constipation. But as the diet is improved, with emphasis on the B vitamins and protein, the general health will in turn be improved and constipation eliminated.

Nothing is so conducive to an easy bowel movement as the squatting position. Many wise people have adopted the use of bathroom stools about ten inches high on which to rest the feet during eliminations. This lifts the knees, bringing the thighs close to the abdominal muscles, and approximates the natural squatting position.

Natural Laxatives

Food yeast (or *brewers' yeast*) is a natural laxative because it is so rich in B vitamins and protein. By all means add a teaspoon of good-tasting dry yeast to fruit juice, tomato juice, milk, and other beverages. Use it daily and be generous with it.

Dark molasses is one of the finest laxatives of all times, as our grandmothers knew. Their favorite spring tonic was old-fashioned molasses and sulphur. We no longer need to take this evil-tasting combination; the sulphur we get in young radishes, celery, and green peppers, and the molasses, the darkest you can buy, can be mixed with all sorts of foods and used in place of empty white sugar.

Honey is another natural laxative. It is so mild that pediatricians recommend it for babies. An interesting combination is honey and molasses, half and half; it provides both vitamins and iron. Thousands of my students enthusiastically use this honey-lass combination for all sweetening purposes.

Yogurt, besides being a delicious food, is also helpful in cases of faulty elimination. The bacteria in this cultured milk utilize the sugar in milk and convert it into beneficial lactic acid. Milk sugar also helps to make soft, bulky stools, which are passed with great facility. The friendly bacteria of yogurt also synthesize the B vitamins so important to good elimination.

Wheat germ is by far the most valuable of all cereals for its vitamin and protein content and is also a natural laxative par excellence. When you use the fresh and vital kind, available at your health-food store, such "live" wheat germ, sprinkled freely on your morning cereal or into fruit juice, makes a fine self-starter for lazy bowels. Fresh wheat germ is "unpreserved" and should be kept tightly covered in a cool dark place (or in your refrigerator) to prevent rancidity.

Quick salt-water flush. This efficient flush has been recommended by Dr. E. V. McCollum of Johns Hopkins, and also by Dr. Victor Heiser, author of *An American Doctor's Odyssey*. Simply add two rounded teaspoons of salt to a quart of very warm water and drink the whole quart on an empty stomach the first thing in the morning. In about thirty minutes a copious flushing will result. Be sure not to eat breakfast until after you have flushed. For a more pleasant-tasting quick flush, many of my students put three level teaspoons of vegetable salt into a quart of very warm water and drink the entire quart. Such a flushing, taken occasionally, is harmless, and thousands swear by it. It should not be taken habitually, however, because the water-soluble vitamins are also flushed away.

Natural herbs. Following a highly nutritious diet should automatically banish constipation. The ideal way is to get along without any special help. But for those who for some reason are not eating intelligently, and therefore suffer from occasional constipation, instead of synthetic laxatives, pink pills, or oils, I recommend a combination of dried, natural herbs which I discovered in Switzerland. It is as natural a formula as I could find and is made up of seventeen crushed herbs. Thousands of pounds of these herbs were formerly imported from Switzerland; but since this formula became such a phenomenal success, it is now made here. So, if you must use a laxative occasionally, try this Swiss formula. It is obtainable at all health and diet shops and drugstores.

Swiss vinegar-milk tonic. For upset stomach or for lack of digestive juices, thousands of Swiss swear by their *Essigmilch* drink. Cider vinegar or wine vinegar can be used. (In Switzerland they add herbs.) Simply put one tablespoon of vinegar into four tablespoons of buttermilk or skim milk and drink it down.

Laxative home brew. A delightful and very effective laxative tea can be made by brewing a level teaspoon of Swiss Kriss herbs in a large cup of water. Let water come to a boil and add the herbs. Turn off the heat; let stand for three minutes, and strain. Add a teaspoon of honey and a few drops of lemon. (Do not boil, or the tea becomes *too* laxative.) When feeling bloated after eating too much, a cup of this mild laxative tea brings amazing relief.

The Niehans Cellular Therapy

A great deal of publicity has been given to the Niehans treatment. This cellular therapy is quite popular throughout Europe, although today it is relatively unknown to the average person in the United States.

After reading all the French and German reports on this treatment, I had the pleasure of meeting Dr. Paul Niehans in Paris. He was an amazing-looking man, full of enthusiasm—especially for his treatment. It consists basically of *Frische Zellen,* fresh living cells taken from unborn animals, usually lambs or calves. These tissues are ground up and added to a saline solution to make a serum. The secret lies in the fact that the tissues take only twenty minutes to go from the unborn animal to injection in the human patient.

Perhaps the best-known person among those to benefit from this treatment was Pope Pius XII, on whom it worked wonders. Other people who have taken this treatment are Winston Churchill, Bernard Baruch, Somerset Maugham, Charlie Chaplin, Bob Cummings, the ever-young Gloria Swanson—and over 40,000 other important people.

At the clinic La Prairie in Switzerland, Dr. Niehans's work is still carried on and visitors include many physicians who come to learn more about his therapy. Although Dr. Niehans worked in this field for thirty years, American doctors say more research is needed before cellular therapy will be used in America. One of the problems relating to the treatment is the fact that live tissues are not always immediately available; and, because of the painstaking care in the preparation of these *Frische Zellen,* the treatment necessarily is still expensive. One of the latest accomplishments of cellular therapy research is the injection of young cells of pancreas tissue for diabetics. This offers great hope that many diabetics may be freed from the inconvenience of daily insulin injections. Certain specific pancreatic cells that Dr. Niehans succeeded in separating may achieve lasting results. For more specific and detailed information, I recommend that you read Dr. Niehans's book *Introduction to Cellular Therapy.*

There are many doctors in Europe who claim to have improved on the Niehans method. Dr. Alfred Pfister, of the Revitalization Center Lemana, Clarens, Switzerland, calls his treatment Cellvital Therapy. In a beautiful Swiss setting, not far from Lausanne, one can rest and receive Pfister's diet and cellular therapy under strict medical supervision.

FOUR

YOUR GOOD LOOKS

11

Eat and Grow Beautiful

Your Eyes

Every body requirement—every vitamin, every mineral, every amino acid—probably plays some part in the health of your eyes. Your best possible vision depends on your blood stream carrying to your eyes a consistent, steady supply of vitamin A, vitamin B_2 (riboflavin), vitamin C, and vitamin D.

Dr. Russell Wilder of the famous Mayo Clinic predicted a world of the future where expectant mothers will eat such a superior diet that no one will need to wear glasses. He also said that if we apply our *present* knowledge of nutrition, we can delay the development of presbyopia, the kind of farsightedness that often comes in middle life. So decide, from today on, to feed your eyes for the rest of your long life.

Vitamin A is manufactured in the liver from carotene, the yellow coloring matter found in carrots, apricots, and other yellow foods, and in all green foods such as parsley, spinach, and mustard greens; one generous serving will give you your eyes' daily requirement. (You can also get vitamin A in liver, eggs, butter, and cheese.) Milk and liver will supply riboflavin; citrus fruit juice will furnish vitamin C; eggs, milk, fish-liver oil, and sunshine will provide vitamin D.

Do you know why vitamin A is important for your vision? It is an interesting story.

Vitamin A

At the back of your eyes, lining your eyeball like the thin inner skin that lines an eggshell, is the retina, the film of the eye-camera. It is composed of the very special cells of vision. In each eye there are about 137 million of these seeing cells. They are developed from the same tissue that goes to make brain and nerve cells, but they are specialized to respond to light. They are even further specialized among themselves. Some, which are cone-shaped, do all our seeing in bright light, and they also see colors. Others, which are rod-shaped, are for seeing in dim light.

Each kind of cell reacts to light with its own kind of sensitive chemical substance. The cone-shaped cells have special substances that react only to bright light and to light of different wave lengths for the different colors. There is still a great deal the scientists are trying to solve about the differences among the cone cells.

The rod cells have a substance for dim light called visual purple; the cells themselves make this substance out of a special protein plus vitamin A. When the visual purple becomes bleached out by very bright light, its return to normal (the regeneration of visual purple) depends on the amount of vitamin A available.

One result of a lack of vitamin A, the most apparent one, is the inability to see in dim light—what is called night blindness. By measuring the ability to recover visual acuity in low light, vitamin A deficiency can be determined.

The fighter and bomber pilots who flew night runs in World War II were given heavy doses of vitamin A. Long before that, in my first book on beauty and nutrition, *Manger Pour Être Belle*, I told of the experience of thousands of Belgians in World War I who suffered from a mysterious eye affliction, apparently incurable—until spring came and they began to eat fresh green vegetables and butter and cheese and to drink their good rich milk. And then, miraculously, their eyesight recovered! The explanation was that the enemy had confiscated all their fresh foods, and their apparently incurable eye ailment was nothing else but a serious lack of vitamin A. Vitamin A is also vital for the maintenance of mucous membranes. When the moist epithelial layer of the eye is affected by deficiency, the conjunctiva becomes dry and thick, tear ducts fail to function, and the cornea clouds over. Infection and even blindness can result.

But the story of vitamin A and the eyes is a great deal older than our two world wars. Four hundred years before Christ, the wise Greek physician Hippocrates recommended raw liver to his patients who had difficulty in seeing at night. Today we know that liver is a rich source of vitamin A.

Vitamin B

When there is a lack of vitamin B_2, or riboflavin, the eyes become bloodshot, itchy, burning; they water frequently, and they are sensitive to light, the condition called photophobia. Accompanying frontal headaches are also common. Laboratory animals that were deprived of riboflavin over a long period of time have developed cataracts. When these symptoms appear, the recommendation is not only to take the riboflavin but to increase the whole B group in the diet, just as it occurs in natural foods such as food yeast, wheat germ, and liver.

In my classes I have told the story of a famous motion-picture star who suffered for years with burning, bloodshot eyes. She blamed the studio lights, and since she was past her fortieth birthday she also blamed her age. She undertook to follow the nutrition program I recommended, with the same vigor and persistence that made her one of America's most distinguished artists. The results surprised even me. After three months her eyes were clear and beautiful as they had not been for years. The diet that worked this magic was nothing mysterious—simply a diet rich in vitamin A and the entire B complex: vegetable broths, food yeast, liver, milk, all the natural foods that restore health and beauty to hard-working eyes.

Vitamin C

Some exciting studies have been made with vitamin C in connection with the serious condition of cataract, the clouding of the eye's crystalline lens. Some years ago Dr. Donald T. Atkinson of San Antonio, Texas, found that when he persuaded many of his patients who habitually lived on salt pork, corn meal, and coffee to add fresh greens, oranges, and tomatoes to their diet, as well as eggs and other good proteins, the condition improved or the growth of the cataract was arrested.

We do not know just how vitamin C is connected with this serious ailment of the eyes, and anyone suffering with cataract urgently needs the help of an ophthalmologist. But we do know that the eye, and especially its lens, normally contains more vitamin C than any other part of the body except some of the endocrine glands. And we know that in cataract the vitamin C is conspicuously missing from these tissues.

We also know that vitamin C is crucial to the health of the capillary walls in the body generally, and that a lack of it goes hand in hand with aging of the connective tissues. And if healthy eyes keep up such a high level of vitamin C, there must be a reason!

So let us give them this vitamin in maximum, not minimum, amounts. The body does not store it, and you need to replenish the supply every day. With plenty of vitamin C in your diet, so easily supplied with citrus fruits, green peppers, tomatoes, and the richest of all foods in vitamin C, rose hips (in tablet form), you are feeding your eyes what they themselves take in great quantity from the body's supply.

Vitamin D

Vitamin D is the sunshine vitamin that the body must have to absorb calcium and make good bones and teeth. Now here is a curious fact that came out of two separate experimental studies: a lack of vitamin D and calcium produced nearsightedness in puppies, and the addition of vitamin D to the diet of nearsighted children improved their vision or at least prevented it from getting worse.

Here again the scientist cannot explain exactly how this worked. We do know that a proper balance of calcium in the blood is essential, and that if this balance is disturbed, cramping spasms of muscles, big and small, can occur. Quite possibly, especially in young growing puppies and children, a disturbance in the calcium and vitamin D balance could result in excessive tension of muscles and ligaments, so that the eye fails to accommodate for near vision.

And finally there is good evidence that amblyopia, a general dimming of vision without any apparent defect to account for it, can be a result of general nutritional deficiency. Dr. A. J. Cameron, surgeon at the Royal Eye Hospital in London, found this to be so during the postwar years of austerity diet in England. We can go a step further: in countries of generally poor nutrition—for example, India, and in the Soviet Union during the war years—cataracts appear at a much earlier age than the average in well-fed countries.

There is still one more point in this feeding of the eyes. It is not enough to take the food into your body. It must also be distributed, and this means good circulation of the blood via exercise.

Gymnastics for the Eyes

Good food, remember, creates a good blood stream, but only exercise can bring that blood stream where it is needed. Attached to your eyeballs are six fine, silk-like little muscles that can be exercised and strengthened like all other muscles of the body. Simple eye drills, which take only a few minutes a day, can greatly improve the looks and function of the eyes. Here are two simple eye drills to keep your eyes young:

1. Turn your head from side to side as if saying an emphatic no. Do this ten times.
2. Hold your index finger or a pencil about ten inches away from your eyes. Look at its tip, then into the distance. Do this ten times.

Do these two simple eye drills every day; do them especially when you are using your eyes intensely for close work or for reading, and your eyes will serve you better.

How to Relax Tired Eyes

Palming is still the best way to relax tired eyes. This simple method was discovered by Dr. William H. Bates of New York

City. It is the same exercise I recommend for relaxing tensions.

Sit in front of a calendar or a picture. Look at it. Now, gently, close your eyes and cover them with your cupped palms. *Be sure not to press on the eyelids.* Rest your arms. Relax. Let go. Breathe slowly and deeply thirty, forty, fifty times. As you relax, your covered eyes will only see restful gray-black, and as you gradually let go of all tension, your eyes will see a deep, dark black. Then open your eyes. Look at the calendar or picture again. You will see it more and more clearly the more you relax. Your eyes and your whole face lose their tension whenever you palm. Do it often.

Another wonderful and lazy way to relax tired eyes is, every once in a while, to look into the distance, just as far as possible. (Remove your glasses, if you are wearing them.) Do this especially when you are on your vacation, for looking at green scenery in the distance is especially beneficial.

Eyeglasses

My students in many lands have made relaxation and these simple eye drills part of their daily living, and many have had remarkable success in keeping their eyes young. Some have succeeded in keeping their eyesight sharp and keen. I have actually met hundreds of men and women who believe that good nutrition, exercise, and the eye relaxation originated by Dr. William Bates have kept their eyes young.

I definitely do not belong to the school that says, "Throw away your glasses." Unless you are willing to work on your eyes constantly and daily, I suggest that you consult the best eye doctor in your city and let him decide, after a thorough examination, whether or not you need glasses. There are few things so damaging to a person's looks as a straining, squinting effort to see. Not only is it detrimental to the eyes, the tissues around the eyes become a mass of fine, squinting lines. Along with the muscles of the eyes, your whole face and even the muscles of your neck and shoulders become tense in the struggle to see. The decision should rest entirely with you and your eye doctor. And if you need glasses, wear them boldly and confidently. Or try contact lenses, which have been greatly improved in the last few years.

New Ways to Hear Better

Most of us are born with more acute hearing than we ever need. Nature starts us out in life with the kind of hearing that primitive man needed to keep alert and alive. Many people keep this acute hearing throughout life; but if in later years the hearing of high tones shades off a bit, there is nothing to worry about. It is a wonder that we retain hearing at all under the constant barrage of loud noises in our modern cities.

Naturally, a thorough checkup by the best ear specialist is the most important thing. In former years, doctors could do very little to prevent or check hearing loss. They removed wax, treated running ears, and dispensed sympathy. Today they can do so much more. Dr. Samuel J. Kopetsky published the clinical studies of 581 cases of different types of deafness and found consistently high levels of cholesterol. He recommended a better diet, low in fat and high in proteins; extra emphasis was put on brewers' yeast, which is high in choline, inositol, and methionine.

Impaired hearing can stem from many causes. It can be congenital or result from infections or accidents. If your diet ever becomes grossly deficient, and remains that way long enough, impaired hearing could follow. The various specialized tissues of the ear and the nerves that receive and transmit the stimulus of sound, like all other tissues and nerves in the body, require proteins, vitamins, and minerals for their integrity. For the rest of your long life be sure to eat for a sound body—each and every part of it.

If you are hard of hearing, face it with courage, patience, and a wide-open mind. Courage, because impaired hearing is one of the most difficult of all the handicaps to live with. Patience, because there is no easy cure for impaired hearing. An open mind, because impaired hearing is now gaining the widespread attention of top doctors, educators, and electronic engineers. Today, whatever your type or degree of hearing loss may be, you may be sure that otologists, audiologists, speech and speech-reading experts, and hearing-aid manufacturers are working on your special problems.

A good way to keep an informed, open mind is through the

American Speech and Hearing Association, 9030 Old Georgetown Road, Washington, D.C. 20014, which has many local branches throughout the country. Through this organization you can learn how and where to get speech and lip-reading training.

Your Teeth

There will always be some controversy about the exact role played by diet in the soundness of the teeth, but I have no doubt that the food we eat, or fail to eat, profoundly affects them. There are records upon records of peoples living in primitive regions on diets of fish, game, whole grains, vegetables, and fruit who have the soundest of teeth. When our civilization touches them, and the native diet is abandoned in favor of highly milled flour, white sugar, and colas, the new generations develop unsound teeth, highly subject to infection and decay.

How to Feed Your Teeth

Besides the best external care, the health and looks of your teeth depend on good solid nutrition. The teeth, hard and inert as they seem, are alive. They build themselves and renew themselves with the materials that you give them. Their materials come, as to all other parts of the body, in the blood stream. Like plants, the teeth take their nutrition through their roots. Tiny branches carry these precious molecules of building material through the living core of the tooth, the pulp within its casing of hard enamel, and the cells take what they need for their health.

"If the repair materials supplied to the blood by our daily food is second or third rate, the teeth are rebuilt with shoddy material that deteriorates as surely as a shoddy piece of cloth in a suit deteriorates," says Dr. Fred D. Miller in his very fine book *Open Door to Health*, a book I highly recommend to parents.

One of the most widely known facts about the teeth is that they need calcium. The teeth are composed of the hardest substance in the body, calcium phosphate, which is also the hard material of the bones. But here are some curious facts that few people know:

A lack of vitamin A can lead to decay of that hard substance. And a lack of vitamin D means that no matter how rich in calcium your diet may be, the body is unable to absorb and use it, and the badly needed tooth-building material will never get to the teeth at all.

Vitamin C is essential to the production of collagen, the connective tissue that provides the framework for the dentine or bony structure of the teeth. And the bone of your jaw, in which each tooth is implanted, needs its proper supply of calcium and phosphorus like any other bone.

FLUORINE AND TOOTH DECAY

All over the United States there is great controversy about fluoridation of our drinking water for the protection of our teeth, and people become very emotional and violent on the subject. I personally believe it is always safest to follow the concepts of old Mother Nature and eat plenty of fish and seafood of every kind. These gifts of nature provide us with the right kind of fluorine to protect our teeth. Sicilians usually have excellent teeth, probably because a large part of their diet comes from the sea.

PLAQUE

No one's mouth is bacteria-free, but when bacteria mix with food particles they cling to the teeth, forming a thin invisible coating, or *plaque*. It covers the teeth and gum line and supports thriving colonies of decay-causing bacteria. Sugar provides food for these germs, and in less than twenty-four hours they can start their dirty decaying work. The plaque is easily removed with thorough brushing and flossing to remove debris trapped between teeth. When plaque is not removed, it will eventually harden and produce gum-irritating tartar. Gum disease is the greatest cause of tooth loss in adults. Some 80 percent of middle-aged people (according to the World Health Organization) suffer from gum disease.

Bone Meal and Good Teeth

Where tooth decay is rampant, many dentists now recommend the addition of fine bone meal, a rich source of calcium, phosphorus, and fluorine in food form.

Here's an interesting experiment by the Swedish dentist Dr. Alfred Aslander, of Stockholm, which he carried out with his own children.

He and his wife both had very bad teeth, and he was determined to give his own children a better start. Incidentally, he thought he might prove that although poor teeth may be inherited, an unfortunate heredity could be corrected. And he did prove just that. He prescribed finely ground bone meal to be added to the family's orange juice. The result is that this foresighted father's lucky children have grown up with beautiful, sturdy teeth that will probably last them all their lives long.

When the teeth of over a thousand children were inspected in a school in Stockholm, there were only four children with perfect teeth; and whose children do you suppose they were? They were the children of Dr. and Mrs. Aslander.

Analysis of Bone Meal
(ACTIVE INGREDIENTS)

	PERCENT		PERCENT
Sodium oxide	.46	Lead oxide	.005
Potassium oxide	.20	Zinc-oxide	.018
Calcium oxide	30.52	Chlorine	.22
Magnesium oxide	.73	Phosphoric oxide	22.52
Barium oxide	.001	Boron oxide	trace
Copper oxide	.0005	Fluorine	.043
Iron oxide	.004	Iodine	.00002
Manganese oxide	.0014	Sulfur	.25

All the large packing houses now make very fine bone meal from veal and young beef bones. Many dentists prescribe such bone-meal tablets, with vitamin D for better absorption, for their patients. They feel that these tablets, added to a good diet, provide a better and less expensive way to combat tooth decay than the fluoridation of water.

Exercise Your Teeth

And here is another almost forgotten fact. Your teeth and gums need *exercise:* exercise to strengthen the surrounding tissue and to stimulate the circulation for gums and teeth. This is essential to the health of all living tissue, and your mouth and teeth are no exception.

How does one exercise the teeth? No doubt your dentist told you, when you were still a youngster, how to massage your gums vigorously with your brush, and I hope you still do it conscientiously. Another way to stimulate the circulation of gums and teeth is simply to do what your teeth were meant to do: CHEW!

Chewing your food well not only helps your digestion (and your weight); it also brings the blood stream to gums and teeth and, incidentally, it brings the cleansing, germ-killing saliva to them as well. By chewing, I mean chewing good solid food like whole-grain bread or toast and raw vegetables such as celery and carrot sticks or any of your own favorites.

Munching a handful of firm, nutritious seeds not only exercises the teeth but also gives them real nourishment. Try them, all kinds, fresh or lightly toasted, including sunflower, pumpkin, and melon seeds, plain or salted.

Cosmetic Dentistry

If your teeth are already in trouble, then you cannot chew raw or other solid foods; and the first and most important thing for you to do is to find the best dentist in your city.

If you have lost some teeth, he can skillfully replace them for you; and if you need a whole denture, a modern dentist can adjust your bite and give you chewing comfort.

Today, especially in the United States, dentistry has developed splendid solutions to repair the damage done by neglect or inadequate dentistry performed in the past. Teeth may be sturdy and still be unbeautiful if they are crooked, badly spaced, or discolored. I urge you to look into this cosmetic dentistry, which combines beautification with skillful engineering that saves teeth for many years and improves your appearance, too.

Infected Teeth

A so-called "dead" tooth is a misnomer, because if proper root-canal therapy has been done, with the nerve removed and the canal thoroughly cleaned and filled, the tooth is actually *pulpless*, not dead. It is "dead" only if the surrounding areas of the socket, jawbone, and gums have no nerves. Pulpless teeth, if properly treated, may last for many years. However, if there is any infection at the base of a root, whether the tooth has a live nerve or is pulpless, have it attended to at once. Even if you have no pain, the infection may be there—it will show up on an X-ray photograph, which you should have made by your dentist if there is any reason to suspect trouble.

I have always considered infected teeth a serious threat. Seemingly minor infections can be carried to all parts of the body and cause trouble when we least expect it, especially with the heart and joints.

If you have decayed and infected teeth I would recommend that you go to the best dental surgeon in your vicinity (borrow the money if necessary) and have all sources of dental infection removed. Healthy teeth and jaws are a must in your Live Longer program. The modern dentist, with all the aids of medical science at his fingertips, works quickly and efficiently, causing you little or no pain.

Pyorrhea

Pyorrhea is an infectious disease of the bony sockets of the teeth. If left untreated, it can cause much destruction to the jawbone—so much that even on extraction of teeth, which generally is necessary, the fitting of artificial dentures becomes difficult. Pyorrhea requires the promptest kind of treatment by a dentist.

The occurrence of pyorrhea is an indication of considerable neglect. (It should not be confused with gingivitis, in which only the gums are involved and which can be treated much more simply.)

Among native races on completely adequate diets, such as those studied by Sir Robert McCarrison of England, and the late Dr. Weston A. Price of the United States, pyorrhea is unknown. I believe that future generations, living on adequate diets, will continue to brush their teeth not to prevent decay—they will not have tooth decay—but because they like the idea of a clean mouth. In the meantime, remember that a balanced diet rich in large amounts of calcium and vitamins A, C, and D can and will help you keep sound teeth for the rest of your long life.

Your Hair

If you have hair you "can't do a thing with," nine times out of ten it first of all needs more body, and for this it needs feeding from the inside. Contrary to what you may have heard, there is nothing known to scientists which can in any way, shape, or form feed your hair from the *outside*. Dr. Irwin Lubowe, the famous dermatologist of New York's Flower and Fifth Avenue Hospitals, has said: "If the diet is unbalanced, particularly if there is an excessive intake of carbohydrates and animal fats, the sebaceous glands are adversely affected."

There is one way to correct a multitude of hair troubles, and that is to replace empty starches and sugars, cakes, candies, soda pops, and nutritionless cereals with foods that will nourish your hair. Most important are the first-class proteins like lean meat, fish, eggs, cottage cheese. Use only whole grains, good breads, fruit juices, and honey. Cut to a minimum all animal fats with the exception of butter. But be generous with the liquid vegetable oils. You have a wide choice to fit your taste and pocketbook: sunflower oil, sesame oil, soya oil, wheat-germ oil, corn oil, olive oil, and many others. These oils make tasty salad dressings. Use them singly or mix them in a salad dressing. Cook with these oils and bake with them, and if your hair is especially dry and mousy, take a tablespoonful of oil every day. You will find that these natural oils taste sweet and fresh.

Hair is protein, and so sufficient protein is essential for healthy growth and vibrant color. An extreme example of protein deficiency is found among some children of South America, Africa, and India who do not get enough milk and are fed diets low in proteins and high in carbohydrates. They develop a protein-deficiency disease, kwashiorkor, one of the symptoms of which is loss of hair color.

EXERCISE YOUR HAIR

If your hair is excessively oily and dank, it tells the nutritionist that something has gone wrong with the little sebaceous glands in the scalp. That is why, first of all, the animal fats should be cut down and replaced by vegetable oils. Excessively oily hair also shows a lack of "exercise." Brushing is one of the million-dollar secrets of healthier and more beautiful hair. One hundred strokes isn't necessary and may even damage fragile hair. Instead, brush it just a few strokes a day against the direction it is usually worn. This is enough to wake sluggish oil glands, distribute the natural oils evenly along the hair shaft, and remove surface oil.

Obviously, there are some scalp and hair conditions that are medical problems and should be handled only by a dermatologist. If you have a problem like an infected scalp, or if your hair comes out in bunches, do not waste your money on tonics and salves but get the best professional help.

There are also some hair problems that can be caused by poor thyroid function. Some years ago, in our Great Lakes region in the Middle West, the farmers complained that they were having trouble growing wool on their sheep. This is one of the areas in the world where iodine is lacking in the soil; Switzerland is another such area. When the farmers added an iodine ration to their animals' feed, the animals responded with good healthy fleece. Unfortunately, growing hair for human beings is a much more complicated affair, but it is always wise to make use of the iodine-rich foods or at least use salt that has been iodized.

What goes on inside your head, believe it or not, can also affect your hair. Stresses and strains can definitely interfere with the circulation in the scalp and so can constant worry affect the health of your hair. Obviously this is where the art of relaxation comes in.

A famous New York dermatologist tells his patients that the surest way to have a good head of hair is to choose parents with good hair. No doubt he has a point. Heredity has a good deal to do with good hair; but I insist, and I have thousands of students to prove it, that it is not heredity we should blame for many defects. We inherit not only the traits but also the cookbooks and eating habits of our parents.

Who Has Good Hair?

Our bad eating habits are more often at fault than our inheritance. Let me give you an example. The Chinese people in general have handsome, thick, black hair as long as they stick to their native diet. They rarely suffer from baldness and their hair keeps its blue-black color until late in life. Inheritance? No doubt, but it is also true that the Chinese cuisine is very high in minerals and many B vitamins. They eat quantities of soybeans and soy sauce and a great variety of vegetables, and their diet is rich in first-class proteins such as fish and sea food. They also consume quantities of iodine-rich sea greens of all kinds. The Chinese never overcook their vegetables, they never throw away the cooking water, and their cooking fat is liquid vegetable oil, rich with the unsaturated fatty acids. You never find hardened fat in a Chinese household.

The Italian people, and especially the people of Sicily, where I spend a good deal of my time in summer, have thick, black, curly hair. I have many Sicilian women neighbors who still have beautiful black hair at the age of seventy. No doubt inheritance plays a part, but listen to this: the Sicilians practically live on the foods coming from the sea. They eat quantities of clams, mussels, and other shellfish fresh out of the ocean, and also quantities of fish, broiled, boiled, or roasted over wood fires. They also eat vegetables from the sea. One of their favorites, spaghetti del mare, a sea green that looks like spaghetti, they eat both fresh and dried. And, of course, Sicily also produces some of the finest olive oil in the world. This is their only source of fat, and, as with the Chinese, you find no hardened fat in a Sicilian kitchen.

NATURAL HAIR COLOR

The Chinese and Sicilian diets are both rich in B vitamins. I am convinced that the vitamins of the B complex are important for the health, beauty, and even the color of the hair. Scientists have been able to prove in animal experiments that there are three so-called anti-gray factors. They are called pantothenic acid, para-aminobenzoic acid, and choline. In animal experiments there have been definite successes, but with human beings the results have not been satisfactory. Some of my students have reported that with large amounts of the three anti-gray hair factors, their hair did get darker. Many others found that diet had no effect on the color of their hair, but their hair did become healthier and more vigorous.

Your Skin

Your skin is not just an inert covering like the glove you put on your hand but is the largest organ of the body. Its functioning is as vital to your health as your lungs' or your kidneys'.

As an organ the skin has two main functions. It is first of all the body's protective covering, its shield against the outer environment. And secondly it is the body's principal mechanism for maintaining that steady average temperature of 98.6 degrees Fahrenheit in which all our cells and body systems are adapted to function. If the skin fails in this task, the body becomes gravely ill. In health and in illness, the skin is one of the hardest-working of the body's organs.

Think of it, the skin covering your body weighs about seven pounds. It has an area of about nineteen square feet. It is made up of living, busily working cells, and every inch of it is supplied with delicate, responsive nerves that keep your body and mind informed about your environment, whether it is hot or cold, wet or dry, soft or hard, agreeable or disagreeable.

This outer covering of your body looks fragile, but actually it is tough and amazingly resistant. It can withstand much punishment from nature. It heals and renews itself, day in and day out. It makes spectacular recoveries from disease and accident.

Your skin is your body's protection against dirt and foreign invaders of every kind. It is a barrier to the billions of germs and viruses in the air and on every surface that we touch. It lets none of these pass into the body; at worst, they may penetrate into the outer layers or pores of the skin itself and set up local infection there, but the skin must be wounded or damaged before it will let anything get into even its own deeper layers. But remember that this same barrier keeps out creams and lotions with which you may be attempting to feed the skin itself.

How Your Skin Is Nourished

Always remember that the skin needs nourishment and that nourishment comes only from within. I have been teaching this principle for many years, and each year science adds some new confirmation of its truth. There is no part of the body that can thrive without good nutrition, and there is no part of the body that derives more glowing beauty from good nutrition than the skin.

Let me tell you how remarkably your skin is made, so that you will carry a picture of it in your mind. It is thin on some parts of the body and thicker on others, as on the palms and soles; but even where it is only one thirty-second of an inch in depth, it is made up of four separate layers.

The outer layer of cells, the epidermis, is the one you see. This layer is constantly flaking and rubbing off. But that need not worry you, for it is forever being renewed from underneath. Under it is always a fresh layer, growing from the buds of living cells below. Interlaced through these growing layers are the capillaries of the skin's own circulatory system. These tiny blood vessels are of a special design, unlike capillaries elsewhere in the body. They are shaped like hairpin loops, each one curving up and down again, carrying the nutritious blood to the cells in every layer of your skin.

And your skin is being newly made every day, *every hour,* by the growing layer of skin cells below. Those cells, which you do not see, can make a finer, healthier skin for you, but only if you give them the materials to work with. Those materials can come only through the blood, flowing up and down the tiny capillary loops, in and out among the cell layers of your skin.

NEW SKIN FOR OLD

What are these life-giving elements?

First, our old friends, the proteins, the building blocks out of which new cells are made. And these must be the whole, complete proteins, containing all the essential amino acids for the healthy new protoplasm.

Then, the full list of essential minerals, especially iron, which gives your blood its power to carry a full load of oxygen. Your skin cells need a constant supply of oxygen so that the well-oxygenated red blood, flowing through those capillaries close to the surface, can give your skin its live, glowing radiance.

Finally come the vitamins: vitamin A, to preserve smooth texture and avoid drying and roughness; all the members of the B family of vitamins, to keep the skin youthful and firm, to prevent excessive oiliness, to keep the color clear and free from ugly pigmentation; and vitamin C, for elasticity and also for resistance to infection.

None of these can be fed to the skin from the outside, out of jars. These are nature's own foundation, supplied from within to the growing layers for a healthy complexion. See how simple and familiar they are.

MORE COMPLEXION SECRETS

On my lecture tours, where do you suppose I have found the most radiant and glowing complexions? In Holland, Denmark, Sweden, and Norway, those lands where women cherish their fresh supplies of milk and cheese, of greens from their gardens and fish from the seas that lap those shores on nearly every side.

The fish and sea food, which the Scandinavians eat so plentifully, are rich in iodine, essential to the thyroid gland; when the thyroid is functioning inadequately, the skin can become coarse, thickened, and dry.

Skin specialists have been paying increasing attention to the role of vitamin A in skin health. Dr. Erno Laszlo, who was an internationally famous skin specialist, did not believe in slathering dry skin with moisturizing creams but insisted on a high intake of vitamin A. I have reports from women the world over who found vitamin A a benefaction for dry, rough, lifeless-looking skin. Since there is a possibility of overdose with this vitamin (it is fat-soluble and can therefore accumulate in the body) when it is taken in other forms than food, your physician should prescribe and supervise any special vitamin A therapy of more than 25,000 International Units a day.

Skin blemished with blackheads and whiteheads, and with that affliction of many adolescents, *acne vulgaris*, is often the result of vitamin A deficiency. In severe cases, doctors administer high doses of vitamin A, not in oil, but in water-soluble capsules. They also insist on cutting down on animal fats, chocolates, pastries, and sweets of all kinds.

B Vitamins and the Skin

It may surprise you that the B vitamins are specific skin vitamins. All the B group play a part in keeping the skin youthful. Vitamin B_2, riboflavin, when liberally added to the diet, has been known to help clear those disfiguring brown blemishes, the so-called liver spots.

Long ago I began to teach the value of food yeast as one of the most potent natural sources of the B complex vitamins. Just one or two tablespoons of this wholesome food, added every day to fruit or vegetable juices, can bring a new, alive beauty to the skin.

Skin Beauty from the Outside

I want you to think of your skin in a way that might never occur to you: from the inside, as part of the wonderful interweaving of all the parts of the body. I want you to think of your skin as dependent upon the same healthful nutrition as every other part of your body, with some special nutrients that are specifically valuable for your skin. First, you must feed it from the inside.

Second comes protection from the outside. Your skin is your body's shelter. Like the outer walls of your home, your skin is directly exposed to the physical environment. It lives in heat and cold, in wet and dry climates. It copes with sharp changes of temperature, with too little sunshine or too much, with wind, soot, industrial fumes, fog and smog, dust and smoke. Your skin lives an outer as well as an inner life.

Wind and water can wear away stone, and the sun can peel and crack a painted wall or a leather chair. The skin is living tissue, and it can defend itself against the elements far better than these inert substances. But the environment takes its toll all the same. Too much sun makes the skin lined and leathery, too much cold and wind cracks and roughens it, and too much water makes it first puffy and then wrinkled.

DRYNESS, THE SKIN'S NUMBER ONE ENEMY

Even when we protect our skin from the harshest environment, as most of us are ordinarily able to do, there is one continuous threat to its outer surface of cells. That is dryness. More women complain of dry skin than of any other skin condition.

The skin has its own protective mechanism against drying. All over its surface are millions of tiny glands, the sebaceous or oil glands. There are more oil glands in the face and scalp, fewer on the throat, and even fewer on the hands. These tiny glands spread a thin invisible coating of natural oil that helps to protect the skin against losing its moisture too rapidly.

To living tissue, moisture is even more vital than food. A man can go without food for many days and survive; he will perish of thirst long before he starves. What is true of the body as a whole is also true of each cell. It must have water in order to carry on its life processes.

Your skin is exposed to sun and wind outdoors, and even more to the warm dry air of our winter heating systems and the cool dry air of our summertime air conditioning. It is constantly losing moisture, in spite of its self-oiling system of sebaceous glands.

Protection of Natural Oils

People of the ancient world, three thousand years ago, used to oil their bodies. So did our own American Indians; they rubbed their bodies from top to toe with bear grease. The first Europeans who came to these shores were apparently not too repelled by the odor of this primitive cosmetic to observe its advantages. They wrote home that this was a good way to protect the skin against insects and dirt and to keep it from becoming chapped in cold weather. Some historians give credit to the Indians for the revival of cold cream, which had been forgotten since Roman times.

Americans definitely believe that cleanliness is next to godliness. Yet each time you scrub, you wash off not only dirt and germs but also the natural oils that protect your skin. Soap, even the gentlest, dissolves these oils away. Detergents do it even more thoroughly.

There are some dermatologists who believe we use too much soap on our bodies. They urge that we should rub and scrub the skin more to keep up its circulation and clear the pores of waste. They do not recommend daily soapings, which wash away all the natural protective oils. A natural sponge, the loofah, is excellent for cleansing. It's just abrasive enough to remove dead, dry cells, soil, and accumulated excess oil.

The true value of our fine creams, oils, and lotions is not that they nourish the skin, because the skin cannot absorb nourishment from the outside, but that they smooth the outer skin and then protect it from drying.

Skin and the Sun

Today our standard of beauty includes a healthy, golden tan. We also know that in the sun the skin manufactures vitamin D for the whole body, and that water, air, and sunshine and the healthy exercise of the body out of doors are nature's best and finest beautifying agents. Unless you want your skin to become tough, leathery, and aged, though, do not overdo the sunbathing.

English women are famous for their lovely complexions. So are many chic San Franciscans. In London and in San Francisco the moist air is an ally of women in keeping the skin beautiful. By contrast, an Arab scholar a thousand years ago observed that women who lived in the desert had withered, wrinkled faces before they were thirty.

So be wise. Take your sun, but take it in safe doses, gradually, and know when your skin has had enough. Too dark a tan is unattractive, and a sunburn is unforgivable. Sunburn, like any other kind of burn, destroys skin cells. It is an actual wound to the body. One should also not forget that skin cancer has been shown statistically to have some correspondence to chronic overexposure to the sun.

One of the sun's benefits to your skin is that it draws the blood to the surface cells, a skin exercise that takes place without your having to do a thing, like massage. But for the same reason, be careful not to sunbathe for an hour or more after eating, any more than you would engage in strenuous exercise, because the sun, like exercise, draws the blood away from your digestive organs.

When you sunbathe it is always wise to give your skin the protection of a light natural oil cover. Swiss mountaineers use a combination of oil and quinine to prevent burning in the brilliant sun of their snowcapped heights.

Today the chemists have developed many kinds of protective oils and creams that filter some of the sun's rays. They are helpful to the fair-skinned, and for those features such as the nose and forehead which may get more than their share of the sun.

In Sicily, if you want to sunbathe, your Sicilian friends will hand you a cup filled with half olive oil and half vinegar. It is an old recipe, and as good as any suntan lotion you can buy. The oil intensifies the sun's rays and helps you to tan more quickly, while the vinegar protects your skin against burning. One of the best commercially available lotions is a solution of para-aminobenzoic acid (PABA for short) in alcohol, available at any good drugstore. PABA lotion acts to absorb ultraviolet rays and has the ability to build up a reservoir of effectiveness, which means it will not lose its power if you go swimming. But the best protection against overdoing is to use your watch and time your exposure. Then you can be certain of getting just the right amount that will bring a golden glow of vitality to your skin, along with a golden tan.

Lines and Wrinkles Tell a Story

There are exactly fifty-five muscles in your face; with these muscles you express all your feelings. The muscles are "wired" with nerves and these nerves are connected with your brain and are related therefore to every part of your body. Everything you think, everything you do, everything you eat—pleasant or unpleasant, healthy or unhealthy—eventually shows up in your face. Each habit, good or bad, brings into play certain sets of the fifty-five muscles and produces folds, lines, and wrinkles. It would be impossible to make a wrinkle all at once; you must tense and pull muscles fiercely every day for years before wrinkles become noticeable, conspicuous, and permanent.

A famous plastic surgeon says that lines and wrinkles are an index to personality. Stubborn, self-willed people who are set in their ways press their lips together tightly until they have deep wrinkles on the upper lip. The earliest wrinkles appear around the eyes. These are not necessarily due to age; they may be mirth or laughing lines. Wrinkles between the eyes, especially if they are deep, indicate excessive determination; they are often found in homemakers who are overly efficient or in people who drive themselves in some other way.

It is the daily overuse of the same facial muscles that forms lines and wrinkles in the skin. Unbalanced reducing diets also can cause lines and wrinkles. By no means are *all* lines caused by age. By no means are all lines undesirable. Think of how often you see a person who has been plain become increasingly attractive with age.

Psycho-Cosmetics

Years ago the well-known surgeon Dr. Frank Slaughter announced that it is impossible to put "beautiful skins on unhappy faces." Cosmeticians the world over complain about women coming for beauty treatments tense, nervous, and so rigid that creams and lotions and treatments can do precious little good. All the external treatments offered by the most glamorous beauty salons can do very little to help a tense and cranky face. Yet just one happy emotion that makes you smile, lifts up the corners of your mouth, and brings forth an inner shine, costs nothing in time or money.

In France and Germany, the science of *psycho-cosmetics* teaches that only thirteen facial muscles are required to create a happy, uplifted look, but all fifty-five are required for a depressed and cranky appearance. The modern psycho-cosmetician then says, "Why waste all that energy to look unhappy and depressed?" Naturally, people should not become pallid Pollyannas; life brings to all of us some dark moments that may make us look sad and depressed momentarily. But never should an intelligent person permit himself to live habitually in a climate of discontent, because your habitual emotional climate is registered on your face. If your habit of mind is hopeful and outgoing, the muscles of your face pull upward; if your inner life is habitually a sunny one, your face reflects its brightness.

The psycho-cosmetic treatment begins with face control in front of the mirror. First, bend your head backward, then bend it slowly forward until your chin touches your chest. Relax the lower jaw. Start shaking your head—at first gently, then more and more firmly. While doing so, expel little humming sounds, increasing, decreasing. This relaxation of the face may last several seconds to three minutes, depending on your comfort.

Now look in the mirror. Place your hands gently on your cheeks and close your eyes, bending your head back as far as possible. Remain in this position a few seconds. Then have another look in the mirror. Now it is time to send little impulses to your facial muscles. In this, the psycho-cosmetic treatment resembles autogenic training and autosuggestion. For hand in hand with the relaxation of your features goes the brightening of your facial expression through orders you give to yourself: "Life is beautiful—I am happy—the corners of my mouth rise—I smile—no wrinkles in my forehead." Later you extend these orders to the position of your body: "I stand erect—I can cope with any situation—I am strong—my chin up—I am conscious of my powers."

Remember that optimism is the best cosmetic.

After one of my classes in London, one of my students presented me with the following charming poem:

It Shows on Your Face

> You don't have to tell how you live each day;
> You don't have to say if you work or you play;
> A tried true barometer serves in its place,
> However you live, it will show on your face.
>
> The hate, the deceit you may bear in your heart
> Will not stay inside where it first got its start,
> For the skin and the blood are a thin veil of lace.
> What you wear in your heart you wear on your face.
>
> If your life is unselfish, if for others you live,
> For not what you get, but how much you give;
> If you live close to God, in His infinite grace,
> You don't have to tell it, it shows on your face.

Three Ways to Lift Your Face

You can get rid of heavy jowls and that extra chin with this gymnastic recommended by the famous German dermatologist Dr. Hans Weyhbrecht, Stuttgart. Oil the face and throat. Sit high and straight in front of a mirror. Push your chin forward as far as it will go. Now push your lower lip forward à la Maurice Chevalier. Stay in this position and turn your head slowly to the left, then slowly to the right. This brings all the weakened muscles of the throat and jaw into play. The more you push forward with your lip and the more you tighten these muscles, the sooner you will establish a firm throat and neckline. Do it daily, twelve times left and twelve times right. This takes only about sixty seconds.

How does your mouth look in your mirror? I hope the corners go up and not down. If your mouth droops, perhaps it could be because some of your upper teeth are missing. If so, have them replaced at once. Nothing can give you such an unhappy look as missing teeth. If your teeth are in order and the corners of the mouth are down, then perhaps your spirits need lifting as well.

Disappointments, sadness, constant worry, all register, especially around the mouth. All of us have our share of disappointments, but why advertise it? In the meantime, cheer up! Remember, if you do your best each day you can also expect the best.

Now this is how you can pull up the corners of your mouth so that they will stay up: put both hands on your cheeks, and hold the cheek muscles tight. Now draw your mouth as far to the right as it will go, then as far to the left. Be sure to hold your cheek muscles tight. Just exercising and pulling the mouth left and right will do you no good. It is the muscular left and right pull, against the cheeks you are holding with both hands, which can do wonders for weakened muscles around the mouth. Do this twelve times toward the left and twelve times toward the right. Dr. Rudolf Drobil, the well-known Viennese physician, has taught this scientific face-lifting-via-exercise, insisting that unless you give your facial muscles resistance, facial gymnastics are a waste of time. Dr. Drobil, in his book *Gesichts-Gymnastik* says that before considering plastic surgery, first strengthen your facial musculature via his face gymnastics; then, if the face lift is still desired, it will be twice as lasting.

If you are too busy or just too lazy to do these three-minute facial gymnastics, do as Ann Delafield taught thousands of women at the Elizabeth Arden beauty farm: lie down on your yoga slant board and let the law of gravity pull your muscles upward and flood their cells with your own nourishing, reviving blood while you rest. You can actually feel and see the lifting up of the entire face.

I have never seen a woman whose appearance could not be

improved by wise use of makeup. The art of makeup is as old as the oldest civilizations. Cleopatra highlighted her features, and I have seen, in ancient Indian temple paintings, figures of women whose lips, eyes, and brows were all accentuated very delicately and exquisitely.

The most beautiful women I know are not beautiful because of showy clothes or *striking* makeup. They are beautiful because of the force and power that emanate from within. They have sublimated the superficial, and have accentuated the positive. And, need I add, the most beautiful women I know are intelligent about their food. To be beautiful, they must care for their bodies from within, which is the only place from which the spirit can be fed.

Your Feet

More than twenty years ago, Alan E. Murray had foot trouble. He had corns, calluses, hammer toes, and collapsed metatarsals. He had plaster casts of his feet to prove it. Murray had been a skater, but his feet deteriorated so much he had to give it up. Then he tried to obtain relief and correction. Nothing and no one helped him. So, being the kind of man he is, he set about to make a pair of shoes for himself. He believed that just as feet are deformed and distorted by shoes, so can they be corrected by them. Thus were born "space shoes," and people like Arthur Godfrey, Garbo, Lillian Gish, Joe DiMaggio, and Martha Graham, together with 25,000 others, not only wear them but swear by them.

Mr. Murray's theory is to fit the shoes to the feet, not the feet to a space that is available after every concession has been made to the outside form that convention demands. So he fits the inside of the shoe to the foot, and lets the outside come where it may, which makes walking in space shoes like walking on air.

These shoes are expensive. But for those who can afford them, I consider them a highly worthwhile investment in good looks, good health, and good temper.

Shoes do affect your posture. Just take a look at the forward tilt of high-heeled ladies. Anna Kalsø of Denmark has designed a shoe that does the reverse—the heel is lower than the toe, forcing the wearer to walk in the heel-to-toe motion he would use walking barefoot on the sand. The spine straightens and leg muscles stretch, especially those cramped ones extending across the back of the knee. Many people claim backaches disappear. Kalsø Earth Shoes are now sold throughout the United States and are priced from about $23 for open sandals to $43 for boots. Learning to walk in them naturally takes time. The salesperson will probably warn you to begin slowly and wear your Earth Shoes only an hour or two a day for at least a week before you waddle forth into the world.

One more thing: whatever you do, don't be trapped by fashion into buying extremely high-heeled shoes or those dangerous platforms with soles up to six inches thick. The number of ankle injuries that are directly traceable to these shoes should scare people off, but would you believe that one of my friends this year reported seeing a young man wearing a pair of purple platforms while washing windows five stories up!

12

Treat Yourself to Beauty

Bathe Yourself to Health and Beauty

"Water contains great healing power," said Father Kneipp, and today in Bad Wörishofen, Bavaria, this inspired priest's "water cure" attracts thousands of people from all over the world. There you may see a group of men and women wading knee-deep in the cool, fresh streams. According to Father Kneipp's theory, the fresh "alive" water brings better circulation to the feet and legs and the organs of the abdominal region. You may also see another group holding their arms, up to their shoulders, in cool running water in pinewood troughs, to create better circulation for the upper part of the body, especially the heart and lungs.

You will find the scientific counterpart of Father Kneipp's "water cure" in many of our modern hospitals where hydrotherapy (water therapy), given in tubs, tanks, pools, and specially designed showers, is a standard procedure in overcoming the effects of many diseases and disabling accidents.

Whether or not we agree that water has healing power, we all recognize that it is a marvelous medium for pepping up lazy circulation when applied to the feet, face, or entire body.

With a little ingenuity and practice you can use your bathroom for all sorts of refreshing and youthifying baths. There are two schools of the bath: tub devotees and shower addicts. Since it is easier to relax in the tub, I shall emphasize tub baths.

THE ALTERNATING BATH

My favorite bath, which thousands of my students also have enjoyed, is the *Wechselbad,* or alternating bath. I recommend this highly, especially to those whose circulation needs stimulating or those who get one cold after another.

Simply lie and relax to your heart's content in a tub of pleasantly warm water. Put a small rubber pillow under your head, if you like. Do your relaxing exercises or the stomach lift. (There is definite additional benefit from exercises done under warm water.) If your skin is dry, make doubly sure that the water is not too hot. Add a teaspoon of fine bath oil. You can soap and scrub while you are soaking. Use a good superfatted toilet soap.

After you are clean and relaxed (and this is important), let half the warm water run out. As the warm water runs away, turn on the cold water full force. Then lie back, and with both hands mix the cold water with the remaining warm water. Keep mixing, while the water gets cooler and cooler and cooler. In three minutes your whole body will tingle and glow. You will feel refreshed and *not at all cold.* Have one of those immense bath towels ready and wrap yourself in it. Rub yourself dry, and, if you have the time, wrap the towel around you, go to bed, and cover up; and relax, relax, let go of all your real or imaginary burdens.

A SITZ BATH FOR THE MEN

Hot baths are wonderfully comforting and relaxing. Take them whenever you are tense, tired, and out of sorts. But remember that it is cool to cold water that peps you up. At the famous water *Kurort* in Wörishofen in Bavaria, they call this bath the "youth bath" because the increased circulation to the vital centers helps to keep a man young. They even have special sitz bathtubs.

Here is how the tired husband can get the beneficial effects of plain cold water without a special bathtub: let the cool water run into the tub until it is about half full. The idea is to concentrate the water as much as possible around the "sitz." Sit in this water for three and no more than five minutes with knees drawn up so that only the feet and "sitz" are in the water. The cooler the water, the greater the benefits. Jump out of the tub and rub dry with a coarse bath towel. It is amazing how this sitz bath can refresh you. Thousands of people have thanked me for the benefit they received from this simple five-minute bath. For many men it has taken the place of pink pills, Benzedrine, and other stimulants. Take this two or three times a week or whenever you feel the need for a lift.

Another ancient refresher was told to me by a Scandinavian friend; it was handed down from the days of the Vikings. If you haven't the time or a bathtub for a sitz bath, simply immerse the scrotum in very cold, even ice water, for one or one and a half minutes. It is a quick and simple way of increasing local circulation.

The Herbal Bath

This is especially good for older people. Into pleasantly warm water, put a bundle of your favorite herbs from the garden, or a tablespoonful of pine, eucalyptus, or mint, which are especially relaxing. Be sure that the water is not too hot. You will find a fifteen-minute herbal soak exceptionally soothing to irritated nerves.

Roman Oil Bath

As early as the year A.D. 212 at the most luxurious of all bath establishments, the Caracalla, the Roman aristocrats had a choice of twenty-five different kinds of baths. The favorite of the ladies was the most expensive one—an oil bath given in a marble bathtub full of pleasantly warm water, precious oils, and perfume. Such baths are having a renaissance here in America, probably because women have learned that the right kind of oil, broken down into millions of fine oil globules by the warm water, moisturizes and smooths dry skin. Here is a million-dollar recipe for as luxurious and elegant an oil bath as any Roman ever had:

   1 cup of corn oil (the Romans used sesame or olive oil)
   1 tablespoon of any liquid detergent shampoo
   ½ teaspoon oil of rose geranium or your favorite perfume

Pour oil, shampoo, and perfume into a bottle. Shake vigorously each time before you use it. The shampoo breaks the oil into millions of fine globules that cling to your seven million open pores. Just 2 tablespoons of this mixture in a tub of good warm water does wonders for dry skin. And it costs only pennies.

The Sea Bath

Everyone knows that this is wonderful, that it prolongs youthfulness and life. If you live near the ocean, be glad of it and make use of it. Are you afraid of the water? Learn to swim. One of my People, the beloved Annie Laurie, a brilliant San Francisco newspaperwoman, learned to swim at seventy. "What are you afraid of?" a Honolulu fisherman challenged her. "The sea, she is your mother; lie on her and she will caress and carry you." And I am delighted that bathing suits have gotten briefer. The briefer the better, for our sun- and air-starved bodies.

The Dry Bath

In France, where it is very popular, this is called the friction bath. Its value lies in the fact that it is soothing and quieting. You can obtain a coarse bath glove made of twisted wool and horsehair in any of the better drugstores, and it will prove a good investment for one whose nerves need quieting or who wishes to have baby-smooth skin all over.

With the glove on the right hand, proceed gently to massage, with a circular motion, your feet, calves, thighs, abdomen, and as much of the upper body as you can reach. Then change the glove to the left hand and massage the rest of the body. You will be surprised to find how soothing and relaxing this bath can be. In France it is taken before retiring and is proclaimed an excellent remedy for sleeplessness. In hot weather, French people sprinkle the glove with a pleasant eau de cologne, which is not only a mild deodorizer but also helps to remove dead, dry skin from the body.

The Air Bath

"Just as fish need water, so man needs air," said Dr. Benedict Lust, a medical doctor who practiced and applied the natural sciences at his Florida sanatorium. In big cities where people live closely together and apartments are small, there is little opportunity to give the body the chance to breathe freely of good fresh air. Yet even busy city people can take air baths at night in the privacy of their bedroom. Fortunately pajamas and nightgowns are becoming thinner, briefer, and more porous. But why not go all the way and sleep "in the raw"? Try it, the next time you go to bed feeling dead-tired. You will be amazed at how much fresher you feel the next morning.

Try to keep your body surrounded with fresh, crisp air. Take air baths, in the raw, or in the airiest of sleeping garments. Sleep in a well-ventilated bedroom. Wear light, porous clothing. And live outdoors whenever possible.

THE SUNBATH

In Switzerland today, sunbathing is done seriously and scientifically, due to the influence of Dr. Auguste Rollier, a prominent surgeon who fell in love with a nurse suffering from tuberculosis. Determined to cure her, he left his hospital in Bern and took her high up in the Swiss Alps where the sun is at its best. There, with the help of sunbaths, he slowly but surely accomplished her cure. Today, up in Leysin in the Swiss Alps, thousands of people come from all over the world to find health, and the Rollier clinic is still accomplishing amazing things.

The Rollier technique of sunbathing is gentle and easy to apply. Dr. Rollier has absolutely forbidden people to take uncontrolled sunbaths. When overdone, sunbathing can be positively dangerous. First of all, that part of the body which is exposed to the sun is oiled with a cream that filters out most of the harmful rays. Second, the head is *never* exposed but always covered or shaded. And the duration of the sunbath for older or sickly people is never more than fifteen minutes.

Here is the most important part of the Rollier sunbath technique: only the legs are exposed for the first few days. The upper part of the body is covered with a towel or a shirt. When the legs have a glowing color, then and then only is the upper part of the body exposed. There again, the abdomen and chest are exposed only for fifteen minutes for the first two days. The same procedure is applied to the back and the buttocks.

When the whole body, back and front, is fairly pink and glowing, sunbaths can be extended to thirty minutes for three or four days. After that, you can work it up to one hour, but not more; Dr. Rollier has found excessive sunbathing weakening. At all times, the head should be covered to prevent the possibility of sunstroke.

The best time to take sunbaths is around ten o'clock in the morning. The least desirable time is at noon. If you can, go to the seashore and get the combined benefits of sun and water. If you cannot, do manage to let the sun caress your body, not through a windowpane, but directly. The sun, like water, has magnificent healing and rejuvenating power and it is free for the taking. If you cannot go to the beach, why not arrange a small place on your porch or in your bedroom and on sunny days take these short, stimulating, and invigorating Rollier sunbaths? Start now, and you too will become an enthusiastic "sun worshipper."

For the rest of your long life, let your bath be not merely a daily habit but a daily ritual. Join the new "Order of the Bath" and get as much as possible out of it, for health's sake as well as for beauty and cleanliness.

Unless your daily schedule requires it, do not take your bath at the same time every day. Try to plan your bath for a time when you have nothing else to do for at least an hour. Follow it, if possible, with fifteen minutes in the yoga slant position. I cannot suggest too often that you invest in a good strong board that does not sag in the middle and is comfortable enough so that you will be able to relax and do the stomach lift. Relax, relax. Do the stomach lift. One, pull in. Two, pull in more. Three, pull in and flatten still more. Keep the muscles tense for about ten counts, then let go, relax. Do this ten times and know that you are permanently flattening your abdomen, taking inches off your waist, and giving your whole body firmness, youthfulness, and dignity.

Superfluous Hair and Moles

As the years go by, superfluous hair on the face becomes a real problem for many women. A thorough physical examination is in order in all such cases, along with a check on various glandular functions, including a basal metabolism test. If endocrine deficiencies are present, they should be treated. Then, for vanity's sake, have the hair removed. In mild cases depilatory wax is best. For permanent removal the only safe method is electrolysis. This treatment should be given *only* by a trained technician. Strong hairs are difficult to destroy; often they must be removed more than once. But with patience and a skilled operator, permanent results can always be obtained, and without scarring.

A new mole or small growth should always be reported immediately to your doctor. Sometimes a mole that has been present for years will suddenly show signs of growth; this, too, should be observed by your doctor. He can remove it, not only for cosmetic reasons but for your health.

The Case for Plastic Surgery

If there is something about your face that really troubles you, a scar or an ugly feature, or if deep lines and sagging muscles make you look older than your years, consider having the condition corrected by a first-class plastic surgeon. Plastic surgery is an art and a science that has developed fabulously since the end of World War II. Today it is no longer frivolous or vain to have plastic surgery when it is desirable.

If you have a really troubling facial problem and want to consider plastic surgery, this is my advice: take the utmost pains to find the best doctor within your reach. Travel to find him, if necessary. Write to the state medical society at your state capital; you will get from them a list of three specialists in your locality. If you live near a large hospital or medical center, ask there for the names of staff surgeons or affiliated surgeons who specialize in plastic surgery. When you have the names of several, find out all you can about them. Consult the doctors themselves and ask, if possible, to see some photographs of their work.

In other words, if you are considering plastic surgery, find a first-rate doctor, an artist in his profession. Remember that first-rate plastic surgery may come high but is cheap at any price, whereas second-rate work is ruinous, at any price.

For a person who has to make a living and appear before the public, plastic surgery is often a sound solution. This is the advice I have given to people in the middle years who have taken all other measures to keep up their energies and good looks, such as intelligent eating, exercise, and sufficient rest and relaxation.

I know many, many instances in which the three following operations in particular have worked wonders for the people who underwent them: the nose plastic, the face lift, and the eye plastic. Here is what you should know about them.

The nose is the most frequent plastic operation—three to one compared with any of the others. Straightening and softening are the simplest repairs; narrowing can also be done within limits. The operation takes about one hour under local anesthetic, and it is best to remain in the hospital for a day or two. There are no scars because the work is done within the nose; and the improvement is permanent.

The face lift is the second most popular operation and a blessing to many women—men, too—who need to keep a youthful appearance. The operation tightens the loose folds of the neck by pulling the skin upward by incision behind the ears, and tightens cheeks and forehead with another incision within the hairline at the temples. It takes about three hours, under either local or general anesthetic; and the hospital stay is about three days. After two or three weeks, there is almost no sign that an operation has been performed. The improvement lasts five to ten years, depending on how well you take care of your health and your skin. The scars are hardly visible and can be covered by the hair.

Disfiguring under-eye bagginess and eyelid wrinkles may not be the result of late hours and overindulgence; they can be constitutional. Some faces have a tendency to develop small grape-sized lumps of fat under the eyes, and some skins tend to stretch and wrinkle at the lids. These repairs are two separate operations. Each takes half an hour, under local anesthetic. The hospital stay is one or two days. In a week or ten days the signs of the operation are completely gone. The only scars are thin lines at the eyelid edges, and these can be completely concealed by light make-up.

I believe in plastic surgery. I have seen mature men's lives transformed by simple reshaping of a disfiguring feature. I have seen mature women's morale and earning capacity restored by a face lift. And the psychological effect is often as important as the actual lift.

On the subject of silicone injections, which have become quite popular in recent years: silicone has been used to build up features—the forehead, the cheekbones, the chin—and to fill in the depressions of wrinkles or acne scars. Silicone is also used in the form of implants for breast reconstruction. This means that the silicone is not injected directly into the breasts but is instead enclosed in a sterile sac, which is then inserted through an incision on the underside of the breast. The F.D.A. has kept careful control over work with silicone—for good reason, since it turns out that serious infections and other problems have developed from careless use. Please do be sure to check that your doctor is fully qualified.

More Beauty Secrets

Herbs, oils, honey, salt, vinegar, milk, yogurt, yeast, and many of the things you now have in your pantry make amazingly helpful health and beauty aids. Here are some formulas and recipes I have gathered in my travels around the world. You can always be sure of the efficacy and purity of the things you prepare with your own hands, and they cost you pennies instead of dollars.

Cleopatra's Skin Peeling

It seems that Cleopatra intuitively knew about the importance of polyunsaturates for her skin and complexion. Each day she was anointed and massaged with a combination of sesame and olive oils, heavily scented with musk. After the oils had a chance to soak into the skin, one of Cleopatra's slaves, using a special tool, a strigil, scraped off the excess oil; and with the oil the dried-up old skin would also come off. These daily mild skin peelings helped make Cleopatra's complexion famous throughout Egypt.

We know that Cleopatra's mixture of perfumed oils that was massaged into her skin was rich in polyunsaturates and did help to keep her skin young and soft. But German and Swiss doctors today say that in order to stop premature aging and drying of the skin, it is also necessary to use the valuable polyunsaturated oils *internally*. (One German chemist, with a passion for statistics, estimated that the polyunsaturated fat content of a really beautiful woman amounts to about 11 percent of her total volume.) They attack this skin problem in two ways. First, they recommend at least two tablespoonfuls of vegetable oil to be used daily *internally* (the easy way is in salad dressing) and *externally* the skin should be oiled daily with the same rich polyunsaturated oils. In Switzerland you can purchase capsules of these polyunsaturates, and you can also purchase an oil ointment called vitamin F, which is to be massaged into the skin. But I believe here in the United States, where we have so many kinds of good-tasting vegetable oils, rich in the polyunsaturated acids, it is wise to use the oils in a salad dressing or mayonnaise. Make your own polyunsaturated-oil lotion from the same oils you should now have in your pantry.

IMPROVING ON CLEOPATRA'S FORMULA

Here is a combination of the world's finest and richest polyunsaturated oils. No cosmetic externally applied can do more to make the skin softer and younger-looking. It is amazing how dry, wrinkled skin will gratefully soak in this combination of pure and wax-free oils. Modern cosmetic houses already manufacture polyunsaturated combinations, but it is so easy to make your own. Simply mix in a measuring cup the following clear, natural oils:

3 tablespoons safflower oil
3 tablespoons sesame oil
2 tablespoons sunflower oil
2 tablespoons avocado oil
2 tablespoons peanut oil

1 tablespoon olive oil
1 tablespoon wheat-germ oil
5 drops oil of rose geranium or your favorite perfume

Seven drops of this combination, applied to your face, will convince you of its efficacy and purity. Use it regularly on face and neck; and if your scalp is dry, rub in a few drops there.

RICH POLYUNSATURATED MAYONNAISE UNGUENT

This is actually a mayonnaise, but it was prescribed, not for salads, but for the face, by Dr. Leo Kumer of Vienna. Facial mayonnaise has been used by many famous Austrian beauties. Here in America it was the lovely Arlene Dahl who first wrote about it in her beauty column. In response to many letters, I finally gave the recipe in *Mirror, Mirror on the Wall*. Since then many lovely ladies have prepared their own rich unguent; and they are delighted with the results.

This mixture is rich in polyunsaturates (called vitamin F in Europe). The fresh egg yolks supply a fabulous skin softener, lecithin, and vitamin A; and the vinegar, mildly acid, helps to establish the acid mantle so necessary for a glowing complexion.

Facial Mayonnaise Unguent

½ cup sunflower oil
½ cup sesame oil
1 tablespoon wheat-germ oil
2 fresh egg yolks
1 tablespoon vinegar
2 drops rose-geranium oil or your favorite perfume (so you won't smell like a salad!)

Simply mix the oils in a measuring cup. Put fresh egg yolks in a cold bowl and beat. Add oil, slowly at first; and beat with a rotary beater. Add more oil gradually; and, as the mixture thickens, add vinegar and perfume. Excellent for sunbathing, for dry, rough skin, and for removing makeup.

SALON BEAUTY MASK

One of the most luxurious beauty salons in the world kept this quick complexion pepper-upper as a deep dark secret for many years—and charged fifteen dollars per treatment. Now it is yours to keep—and to make for only a few cents.

1 tablespoon of regular toilet lanolin
1 scant tablespoon Balsam of Peru

Mix in a cup with a teaspoon until smooth and keep it in a jar, tightly covered. Apply this beige mixture over entire face and forehead. *But be careful not to apply it close to the eyes.* Allow to remain for 5 minutes only (less, the first time you use it). Later you may leave it on a few minutes longer.

This is a fabulous pepper-upper for tired faces. The glow lasts for hours. If you are a blonde with very thin skin, first apply Cleopatra's Formula (see recipe in this section) or cream and then apply the beige mask over it. Remove mask, with a spatula if you have one, or cleansing tissue. If your face feels too warm, apply a little of the Formula. *This is to be used only once a week*, so save it for the night you want to look blooming!

If your throat needs attention, you can use this same circulation treatment on it once a week, but it is best that you do the face and the throat on different days. Apply the beige mixture over throat and under chin; leave it on as long as it feels comfortable (about five minutes). Using the spatula (with upward strokes) also peels off the dead, dry skin cells (Cleopatra's secret). Incidentally, keep your throat well oiled at all times, for the skin there has fewer oil cells than the face and shows birthdays first if neglected!

New Ways to Prevent or Correct a Double Chin

Nothing destroys a woman's good looks more than the appearance of a second chin to spoil her youthful neckline. There are three main causes of double chin. First is the lack of protein foods that maintain good muscle tone. (That's why beauty farms serve high-protein diets.) The second cause is lack of exercise of the neck muscles. The third cause is the downward-forward push of the chin while reading, writing, walking, working—especially doing housework. Madame Ellene of Vienna, and now New York, has had outstanding success in treating this problem. She shows her clients how to hold the chin always parallel with the floor when sitting or walking.

There are two kinds of bad walkers, according to Madame Ellene: the *pushers* and the *hangers*. The pushers lead with the chin out; they are always ahead of themselves and in a hurry. The hangers have a collapsed, tired walk, pulling the neck in and pushing the chin *down* as if they were hiding. Both of these types develop double chins early in life. To break her clients of these bad habits, Madame Ellene makes an unusual chin strap to be worn at home while working. This band keeps the chin in the right position.

How to Stop Forehead Wrinkles

A plastic surgeon in London says he can tell a lot about a person's character by the lines and wrinkles on his face. Significant are those vertical lines on the forehead between the eyes; the deeper these are, according to the surgeon, the more intense a person you are—and he says you should learn to relax and not take yourself so seriously. I don't know whether this is always so, but I *do* know that you can prevent, and even get rid of, heavy forehead wrinkles and lines by *stopping* your habit of frowning. (Frown and the world frowns at you!) To help you stop the habit of frowning and to increase the circulation to those forehead muscles, Madame Ellene recommends that her clients wear an elastic headband for an hour each day (while taking a bath or working around the house) until they lose the habit of frowning.

Sensational Facial Sauna

For years the famous sauna bath was the secret of the hardy Finns. Now sauna baths are exported to all parts of the world.

I urge every woman who wants a clean, clear skin to take a *facial sauna* just once a week. In Austria and Germany, beauty salons give facial sauna treatments; and in Switzerland they have a special little device for home use. However, without any fancy device, you can give yourself your first facial sauna. There is nothing simpler and more effective for cleansing and purifying the complexion. Simply fill a two-quart cooking pot with ordinary water from your faucet. Bring to a boil, and add a heaping tablespoonful of your favorite fresh or dried herbs—camomile, anise, fennel, all are good. They help to make a deep, *penetrating* herbal steam. If you don't have any of these herbs on hand, go to your drugstore and buy a package of the Swiss Kriss herbs and add a tablespoon of them to the boiling water.

Now you are ready for your first facial sauna. Place the steaming herbal "witches' brew" on your kitchen table. Protect your hair with a shower cap. Cover your head and the pot with a bath towel so no steam escapes on the sides, but it all rises straight up into your face. Start with three minutes; later make it five minutes. You'll be amazed how this pleasant herbalized steam penetrates deeply and cleanses every pore. This steam is made up of the softest distilled water, free of all chemicals, as soft as rain. It makes the skin unbelievably soft.

The roses in your glowing face after a facial sauna are your own, brought about by your own rushing blood stream. The pearls of perspiration coming from every open pore loosen stale makeup, rancid oils, blackheads, and every bit of dirt. The sauna does all this in just a few minutes. After such a thorough cleansing of the pores, they are wide open; so be sure to close them with very cold water (but not ice). I cannot recommend this facial sauna highly enough. If your skin is troublesome, you might take one daily for three days; after that, just once a week. Facial saunas can keep your skin beautifully clean! A beautiful skin is a clean skin; for a flawless complexion, your skin needs more *wake up* than *makeup!*

Eye Refresher from Paris

Through my office in Paris I discovered the Hydro-Spray. When attached to an ordinary water faucet, it produces a gentle spray to massage the closed eyes with the most refreshing eye bath I have ever had. Thousands of people are enthusiastic about the way this fine spray refreshes tired, hard-working eyes. While writing this book I used it daily. After its use I felt refreshed and

I could work better. In France the Hydro-Spray is used for refreshing the whole face as well as for puffiness under the eyes.

Removing Brown Spots from Hands and Face

The quickest way to get rid of those ugly brown pigmentations, sometimes called liver spots, is to have them planed away by an experienced dermatologist. Even scars and freckles can be planed away with a fast-rotating tool that looks like a dentist's drill.

Another successful and less drastic method is deep-skin peeling. However, it should be done only by a doctor trained in this highly specialized method. It is not painful. After the acid solution is painted on, there is a slight burning. After two or three days the skin gets dark and shrivels off, and with it go the brown spots.

Dr. Jarvis has said that many brown spots can be made to disappear gradually by rubbing a few drops of castor oil into the brown pigmentation daily.

Adelle Davis attacked these blemishes from the inside. She recommended 100 units of vitamin E to be taken after each meal. This method, although slower, is longer-lasting, she said.

French Anti-Pimple Lotion

This can be a girl's (or boy's) best friend. It was given to me by a French lady ambassador famous for her flawless skin. Buy a small bottle of calamine lotion and ask your druggist to put in 1 percent of phenol. Soak a small bit of cotton in this medicated solution, and press it flat over the pimple; you'll be amazed how quickly it dries up. This treatment also discourages an oncoming pimple.

Salon Blackhead Treatment

One of the simplest and most effective treatments for blackheads (from an exclusive New York salon) is the following: dissolve one tablespoon of ordinary Epsom salts in half a cup of very hot water, and add three drops of ordinary iodine. This solution must be kept *hot;* so place the cup with solution in a bowl of *hot* water. Take a strip of absorbent cotton (not too thick) long enough to cover affected area. Saturate the cotton with the mixture and hold firmly in place. To keep maximum heat, cover with dry washcloth. When the cotton has cooled off, dip it again into solution. Apply hot solution three or four times. When finished, blackheads pop out easily. (Don't squeeze by hand; use a blackhead squeezer.)

Some Specific Anti-Gray Hair Factors

Many letters I receive are from people who tell me that with the changing of their eating habits surprising things happened. Sometimes even the gray disappears from their hair. Here is a résumé of the foods and the vitamins and minerals involved. But I must repeat, it does not work for everybody. However, should your hair-color problem be a nutritional one, give this a try. Don't expect results overnight—it is a slow process.

Follow a completely nutritious diet, with extra emphasis on liver of all kinds; eat it twice a week. Use wheat germ, brewers' yeast, yogurt, gelatin, and vegetable oils. All kinds of sea food should be included. Eat only whole-grain breads and cereals. Then, so that there is no possible chance of missing any vitamins or minerals that might help to bring back the color of your hair, let your doctor give you a prescription for the three important hair recoloring factors, and take them according to his directions:

Para-aminobenzoic acid	100 mg.
Calcium pantothenate	30 mg.
Choline	2 grams

Be patient. It might, and it might not, work for your hair. But in any case you will certainly get all the other benefits from such a nutritious diet.

Russian Wonder Cream

This old-fashioned healing combination contains four of nature's most potent soothing and healing elements for minor irritations, skin trouble, and athlete's foot. Russian soldiers massage this combination into their feet to prevent foot sores. Simply mix in a cup:

4 teaspoons anhydrous lanolin
2 teaspoons cod-liver oil
½ teaspoon pure garlic powder
½ teaspoon honey

Beat thoroughly with a fork until the honey-colored mixture turns to a creamy white. Keep it tightly covered in a jar, and use it as necessary.

How to Test Your Cosmetics

If you have the slightest suspicion that some cosmetic is causing an irritation to your eyes, scalp, face, or hands, you should make this simple test. Take a bit of the suspected preparation and press it on a small piece of gauze; tape it to the inside of your upper arm, where the skin is most sensitive. Leave the patch on for forty-eight hours; then remove it. If there is no red spot or irritation, the preparation is safe; but if there is a red spot and irritation under the patch, then that cosmetic is not for you. Should you be sensitive to many cosmetics, it is best to use only the purest of lotions and oils. There are now available several good brands of hypoallergenic cosmetics.

German Wheat-Germ Mask for Sensitive Skins

Place one tablespoon of wheat-germ *flour* and one tablespoon of yogurt into a cup, and mix until smooth as mayonnaise. Apply this soothing mixture all over face and neck and lie down and relax for fifteen minutes. When the preparation is dry, remove with warm water; then rinse with cold water. This mask is very popular in Germany, especially with people who are sensitive to soaps and detergents.

Fragrant Rose Water

You can make your own rose water if you have a rose garden. You need one pound of rose petals, the more fragrant the better, to make a quart of rose water. However, most drugstores sell rose water for about fifty cents for a good-sized bottle. With it you can flavor fruit drinks and compotes; pink grapefruit with a teaspoon of rose water is a happy surprise. But rose water is especially recommended for making delightful cosmetics, as Cleopatra did.

pH Face Astringent

To help reestablish the skin's acid mantle, and to help tighten the skin, apply this face lotion all over your face and neck before applying makeup:

¾ cup rose water
¼ cup witch hazel
1 teaspoon honey
½ teaspoon white vinegar

Pinch of alum powder
¼ teaspoon glycerin
½ teaspoon spirit of camphor
½ teaspoon extract of mint

Mix all in a bottle and shake. Apply with cotton pads.

pH Hand Lotion

This combination is one of the oldest, and still the best, of hand protectors. The skin on our hands has fewer natural oil cells than the skin on our faces and necks; therefore, constant moisturizing is necessary. In this easy-to-make formula you have two of nature's most effective moisturizers: glycerin and honey. The lotion is not sticky. Use it generously. Simply shake together in a bottle:

¾ cup rose water
¼ cup glycerin

¼ teaspoon vinegar
¼ teaspoon honey

Herbal Rinse to Darken Hair

When hair is mousy and lifeless-looking and hard to manage, make this simple hair rinse: shampoo hair thoroughly with lanolin or oil shampoo and rinse with cosmetic vinegar water (see below). Then put one heaping tablespoon of Swiss Kriss herbs into a pint of water and simmer for ten minutes. Pour through fine strainer. Apply this herb lotion all over scalp and hair with cotton pad. Do not rinse. (Blondes must never use this herbal lotion. It definitely darkens the hair.)

Cosmetic Vinegar

Dr. Culpepper, a famous English physician, wrote many books. In all of them he was full of praise for vinegar. But long before his day the old alchemists were concocting vinegar. Some of the early great beauties had their chemists prepare vinegar rinses, vinegar douches, and vinegar bath tonics. To this day you'll find cosmetic vinegar in English herb shops; and in Germany the barbers use a vinegar tonic after shaving. And today vinegar is being made popular in America by Dr. Jarvis's vinegar-honey formula (1 teaspoon of honey and 1 teaspoon of vinegar in a glass of water).

My interest in vinegar is not only because of its health value but also because it has many uses as an excellent, inexpensive cosmetic. Many women who have prepared my cosmetic vinegar have written me letters of thanks. They tell me that what they have been able to do for the looks of their hair, hands, and face is almost miraculous. Today we know that skin and scalp, when healthy, exude a mild acid that protects them against infection. Every time you shampoo your hair, every time you wash your face or take a bath, you remove that acid mantle and destroy nature's safeguard. Many scalp and skin troubles, including dry scaly scalp and dry scaly skin, could be halted by protecting the skin and scalp with its natural acid mantle. This is easily done if, after shampooing, washing, or bathing, you use a bit of cosmetic vinegar.

The old-fashioned cosmetic vinegar formula is: put two heaping tablespoonfuls of imported dried peppermint leaves into a pint of water. Let come to a boil, and simmer for three minutes. Then pour through a fine strainer. Add the peppermint infusion to a pint of pure cider vinegar.

The quick way to make cosmetic vinegar is to mix a pint of pure cider vinegar with a pint of very hot water, and add half a teaspoonful of oil of peppermint and half a teaspoon of rose geranium. (Never use straight vinegar for cosmetic purposes.)

Either solution can be applied to scalp or face with a bit of cotton; it makes an excellent face tonic. For the bath, especially for dry, itching skin, pour half a cup cosmetic vinegar into half a tubful of pleasantly warm water.

MILK PADS SOOTHE TIRED EYES

A charming nurse at the Bay City, Michigan, hospital wants to share this secret. She places cotton pads soaked in plain milk at room temperature over tired and puffy eyes and relaxes for ten minutes. She has used this many times on her patients and it really puts a sparkle into tired eyes.

13

The Beauty Farm

When you arrive at a beauty farm, you are shown to your bright and airy room. Perhaps there is an Aubusson rug on the floor, and a Renoir painting on the wall. After you have unpacked, the staff doctor comes and examines you, unless you have brought a letter from your own doctor saying that you are in good health.

The next morning your breakfast is served to you in bed by an attractive maid; and on your tray, set with very fine silver, very fine linen, and a beautiful flower, will be a bowl of fresh fruit, some scrambled eggs, and one slice of protein toast, plus coffee with hot milk (this is a modern beauty-farm breakfast—the day of coffee and fruit juice is passé).

On your tray you will also find your program of activities, your beauty menu for the day.

Right after breakfast you will be asked to put on your exercise suit, a leotard, which the beauty institutes have taken over from the ballet and dance schools. Over this you put your robe, and now you are on your way.

Before your exercise session a nurse or the exercise director—a rather determined woman—will make a record of your measurements. There will be no secrets: the exact weight and measurements will be put down in black and white, and the woman in charge will inform you just what your ideal measurements and weight should be. Then your posture is carefully noted. On California beauty farms you are asked to walk and they take a film to show you in action. After that a beautician looks over your skin, hair, and nails. Your plus and your minus points are recorded and finally the "work" begins.

One farm has a "beauty barn" where you are pommeled, steamed, oiled, and brushed. After your first workout—about eleven o'clock—you are served a cup of hot broth with an egg yolk, or fresh vegetable juice, so that you will not be too hungry by one o'clock. The time before lunch, about an hour, is your own. You can swim in the pool, where you may be given some special underwater gymnastics; some have pools with hot- and cold-water springs. If you are more than ten pounds overweight, the physical-education director will map out a walk for you of two or three miles, according to how much you have to lose. So that you will not feel sorry for yourself, one of the instructors or one of the other guests will accompany you on a lovely country road.

Mealtimes at the Beauty Farm

Lunchtime is picnic time on a beauty farm. The managers of a beauty farm in Palm Springs, California, arrange interesting picnics for their clients. They serve the finest, freshest salads, fortified with the most delicious forms of protein: chicken, lobster, eggs, fish, and always big bowls of lean cottage cheese. There is an unlimited choice of salads made with vegetable oil dressing, but only one piece of high-protein toast, whole-wheat bread, rye bread, or soya muffin is allowed. There is always steaming hot vegetable broth, hot fortified tomato juice, or Swiss broth, which is a great favorite. For dessert there are bowls full of fresh fruit. Beauty-farm beverages are clear coffee, Swiss coffee, fortified milk, tea, rose-hip tea, peppermint tea, papaya tea, fresh fruit juices, or vegetable juice. And, of course, yogurt is always available.

After lunch you are glad to retire to your room. You will be tired and you will probably take a nap. The dean of physical education suggests that every woman, before retiring or resting, should take a fifteen-minute refresher on the yoga slant and let the law of gravity put her posture into beautiful alignment. This is done on many beauty farms.

After the noon siesta, you look at your program for the day. The afternoon will be dedicated to more beautifying. There will be fragrant oil-of-rose-geranium baths or herbal facials, hair brushing under the trees, manicures, pedicures. There may be tennis or more swimming. You will be occupied every minute—there is never any time for boredom, and among the ladies there is a splendid spirit of camaraderie; they are all there for the same reason, and the favorite conversation is: how are *your* measurements: how much did you lose? There is also a friendly spirit of competition that makes even reducing easy and more like a game, and, of course, the luxurious surroundings, the beautiful service, the lean food, and the absence of family duties are other reasons for the good results.

Besides the tennis courts, swimming pools, and nearby golf courses, there are wonderful walks, and it is amazing how gladly women will walk when they have good shoes and good company.

At five o'clock you return to your own room, this time to freshen up. You are expected to change for dinner; the first beauty farms expected guests to dress, but this is no longer obligatory; they discovered the ladies often were too tired. However, the guests always change from their daytime costumes.

Ever since I introduced big glasses of fresh juices at the Main Chance beauty farm, all the other beauty farms here and abroad have started serving these "cocktails" about an hour before dinner. The most popular combination is carrot, celery, and apple juice. Some of the women are so hungry they drink two glasses in quick succession, and that is all to the good because the natural sugars of the juices raise the blood-sugar level, a sure and natural way to prevent overeating at the dinner table.

Beauty farms outdo themselves to give the guests beauty-full and satisfying dinners: broiled liver of all kinds—such as chicken livers en brochette or parsleyed calves' liver—are served several times a week; broiled chicken, broiled lobster tails, and lean sirloin steak are also favorites. There are always two green freshly short-cooked vegetables. The desserts are all delicious, with a choice of fresh fruit sherbet, apricot mousse, exotic fruits, or fruit pies made with thin shells of coconut or wheat-germ crust.

The ladies all enjoy one generous portion of everything. For the newcomers with overstretched stomachs there are always trays full of crisp, chilled finger salad made up of fresh bits of raw cauliflower, sliced green and red peppers, radishes, celery hearts, young onions, and green olives. These can be eaten freely without a bad conscience. There is never any difficulty about overeating at beauty farms. The ladies watch one another and the hostess is usually a dignified woman who keeps a watchful eye on her charges.

After dinner the women gather in the beautiful salon for cards, conversation, and perhaps some fine music. Time never hangs heavy on a well-run beauty farm. Even the evenings seem to pass too quickly. The women are naturally tired and glad to retire about ten o'clock. There is always a nightcap choice of half a dozen fragrant teas—linden, verbena, licorice, papaya—or hot Swiss broth. And then to dream in your own comfortable room.

This gives you an idea of what it is like to be a guest at one of the luxurious beauty farms; the service is fabulous, the food superb, the setting beautiful.

But there should be beauty farms for all the lovely ladies in the land, not only for millionairesses. And I predict there will be many more in the future. I hope that I can help to speed up the day.

In the meantime, let me assure you that any woman can establish her own miniature beauty farm right in her own home. You won't be pampered, you won't have your breakfast served in bed, but you also won't have to pay a thousand dollars a week!

Have Your Own Beauty Farm

It is the easiest thing in the world for you to have a miniature beauty farm in your own back yard. Even if you have only a small piece of land, you possess the important beauty-farm needs already: sun, soil, air, and water.

To let the sun caress your body, turn a sheltered corner into a suntrap with a sheltering trellis against the wind or prying eyes.

Be careful with the sun. Always oil your skin well and follow a careful sun-exposure schedule. Begin with no more than twenty minutes and turn from side to side so you will tan evenly.

You will need a yoga slant board for your beauty farm; cover it with plastic to protect it against the elements. You can get double benefits if you do your sunning in the yoga slant position and let the law of gravity work for you at the same time. But be careful not to go to sleep in the sun.

For exercise: a hanging bar for you; for your man it will be a chinning bar. Get him to put up a punching bag for himself; it is excellent rhythmic exercise for his arms and torso muscles and a first-rate tension releaser.

Iron dumbbells in different weights belong on every beauty farm. Muscles become firm twice as quickly with these; ten minutes a day strengthens your man's arms, and they are very valuable to you in keeping the bustline high. Five-pound dumbbells are best for him and two-pound dumbbells are best for you.

Add the beauty gift of water to your private beauty farm. A wonderful investment would be a small swimming pool. I believe there is nothing that can give more pleasure to the whole family. It does not have to be a big, expensive one. Investigate the round, oval, and free-form pools. There are companies that install these in one day: they bring the cement ready-mixed and blow it over a steel frame fitted into the excavation. If you say that a pool is too expensive, I say so is a second car. A pool is a much better investment for health and good looks than a second car. If a pool is out of your reach this year, then install an outdoor shower, a great comfort and wonderfully refreshing. Remember, cool water peps you up, warm and hot water relax. With a few dollars and a dash of imagination you can make a back yard into your personal beauty farm.

A Health Spa in Your Own Bathtub

If you can't go to take a cure in the hot springs of Palm Springs, Aix les Bains, or Carlsbad, you can get some of the same benefits right at home by making your own private mineral bath. You can definitely soak away tension and tiredness, and reduce rheumatism and arthritis-like pains. All you need is lots of hot water and this easy-to-make mixture of medicated minerals:

2 cups ordinary Epsom salts (magnesium sulphate)
1 cup Calgon (best water softener)
1 teaspoon eucalyptus oil
1 teaspoon menthol, 10 percent solution
1 teaspoon liquid iodine

Place salts and Calgon in a mixing bowl. Add eucalyptus oil, menthol solution, and iodine, and mix with a spoon. This makes a pale-yellow mineral-bath combination, second to none. (You can double or triple the amounts for future use.) Keep in tightly closed can. Use ½ cup to 1 cup in a tub of pleasantly warm water. Relax and luxuriate for at least 15 minutes. For complete relaxation and solid comfort, use a small rubber pillow or roll up a towel, place it behind your neck, and lean back.

Your Beauty-Farm Kitchen

Any good cook can become a beauty-farm cook.

I will go further: anyone can become a beauty-farm cook if she wants to be one.

Your cooking pots are an important key. Most women use too much water in cooking because the food burns in their ordinary pots. Avoid both the burning and the loss of essential vitamins and minerals by having heavy cooking pots with close-fitting lids that are heavy enough to stay down. You need at least two of these heavy saucepans for your vegetables. In California we use enameled cast-iron pots and lids; in New York we use heavy stainless steel. These pots are a little more expensive than thin lightweight enamel, but they last forever and are a good investment.

You will need several appliances to help you save time and valuable nutrients.

A *blender* is used on most beauty farms. This machine is by now common in most homes, but woefully underused. Your blender can make vegetable juices and can even turn nuts and seeds into delicious butters and spreads.

But rather than using your blender, why not get a modern *juicing machine* to make the important vegetable juices. (Buy a machine that can't vibrate and is easy to clean.) Every woman in search of a good skin should have a pint of carrot, celery, or apple juice each day.

A *stainless-steel vegetable shredder* is also a good investment. When vegetables are shredded they can be sautéed in five to seven minutes, as the Chinese cook them. Use a little vegetable oil or broth.

And every kitchen should have *a set of sharp stainless-steel knives* for cutting off all visible fat from all meats. Beauty-farm cookery is lean cookery.

You will also need *a fine stainless-steel strainer* to remove fat from the natural juices (fill it with ice cubes and pour the juices over them; the fat will solidify and remain in the strainer).

For making quantities of delicious yogurt you should invest in a *yogurt maker* for making fortified, plain, or fruit-flavored yogurt.

Cook with a Low Flame

I can tell a good cook by one sign: the height of the flame under her pot. Always remember, low temperatures give high quality in all cookery: boiling, sautéing, roasting; the single exception is broiling. But the most important ingredient in beauty-farm cookery is T.L.C.—Tender Loving Cooking! When the cook cares, the food remains tasty, full of beauty and health-giving goodness; it even looks good when it comes to the table. And that is as it should be. Remember, we also eat with our eyes!

Good food is everlasting pleasure that never fades. Enjoy your beauty-farm cooking and reap its benefits in health and good looks for you and your loved ones. They say that Frenchmen would rather marry a fine cook than a beautiful girl because the pleasures of good cooking go on long after other passions have diminished.

One more requisite will complete your private beauty farm. On every beauty farm there is one wise man or woman with a strong personality who gently but firmly inspires the guests and the staff with the will to accomplish what they are there to do: to redesign bodies and spirits, both within and without. On your private beauty farm that guiding, inspiring person will have to be *you!*

Foods Fit for My Garbage Can

You can't have a beauty farm until you rid yourself of empty foods. Would it shock you to know that Betty Crocker butter pecan cake mix was found to contain neither butter nor pecans? That indiscretion, among many others, was why the Betty Crocker division of General Mills was presented with the Annual Bon Vivant Vichyssoise Memorial Award at the thirty-third annual meeting of the Institute of Food Technologists in 1973.

The naïve consumer is lured through advertising and clever packaging into paying exorbitant prices for embalmed foods that are nearly nutritionally worthless. In recent years, food makers have zeroed in on the most gullible and unsuspecting market of all—children. From the TV screen, children are bombarded with stimuli to rush and ask their mothers to buy such tantalizing treats as General Mills' Sir Grapefellow or General Foods' Post Alpha-Bits. You might as well feed your growing child soda and candy for breakfast, for some of these sweet cereals contain over 40 percent sugar, not to mention artificial flavoring, coloring, and chemical preservatives. Such nutritionally empty foods not only provide many potentially harmful ingredients but also depress the child's appetite and keep him from eating healthy foods.

Recently, in a petition filed with the Food and Drug Administration by the Washington-based Center for Science in the Public Interest, the establishment of a limit of 10 percent sugar by weight was asked for breakfast cereals. The center noted in its petition that the worst offender was a cereal healthfully labeled Quaker Oats Company's King Vitaman, which contained by their calculations 50 percent sugar. This petition was supported by the American Public Health Association and the American Society for Preventive Dentistry. Dr. Eugene B. Harden, the president of the Cereal Institute, representing the manufacturers, replied as follows: "To force presweetened cereals off the market would deprive children of the nutrients they now obtain in a form they find attractive . . ." It goes without saying that if a child has developed bad eating habits, he may well prefer cookies and soda for breakfast. The whole point is to start your children early in good eating habits so that by the time they are old enough to choose for themselves, sugar-coated, vegetable-dyed, overprocessed cereal will not be the "form they find attractive."

According to Dr. Michael Jacobson, who presented General Mills with the "garbage" award, "Bad eating habits start young and General Mills spends millions of dollars a year to encourage kids to eat foods that contain a high percentage of sugar, a good deal of salt, potentially harmful artificial colorings, and refined flour from which many nutrients have been removed. Hunger, malnutrition, chronic illnesses will not be minimized in the United States until public health is accorded a higher priority than private wealth. Heart disease, tooth decay, hypertension, and intestinal cancer will be rampant as long as companies like General Mills churn out their sugary, fatty, salty, overly refined products."

This same thesis—that sugar and refined carbohydrates are at the root of many of our nutritional ills—was aired at hearings before the Select Committee on Nutrition and Human Needs, April 30 to May 2, 1973, in Washington, D.C. At one of the sessions, suitably titled "Sugar in the Diet, Diabetes and Heart Disease," Dr. John Yudkin struck a responsive chord when he said that sugar is the only commonly available food that provides calories free from any trace of nutrients. He explained that the human being can make all the glucose (blood sugar) it needs from rather small amounts of other dietary carbohydrates, mostly starches, and from parts of the protein and fat that we eat.

The lesson seems quite clear. If you rely heavily on refined carbohydrates and processed cereals, you are bound to fall into nutrition quicksand. Avoid them like the plague. Instead, use the whole-grain cereals and flours found at your health-food store. If your sweet tooth needs catering to even after you have eaten fresh fruits and vegetables, dried fruits, etc.—and your blood-sugar mechanism is functioning properly—you can add honey, molasses, or maple sugar. But use them judiciously. And instead of chocolate, use carob. You'll find it a delightful treat.

Ten Foods Fit for the Garbage Can

—White sugar
—White flour
—Greasy potato chips and french fries
—Greasy hamburgers containing nitrates
—All sugared cereals
—All cola drinks and bottled beverages made with or without synthetic sweeteners
—All artificial sweeteners, including saccharin
—All hardened (hydrogenated) cooking fats
—All frozen dinners
—All flat-tasting, overcooked food

I believe that half of the world's ills would disappear if governments would prohibit the manufacture of the above foods. Until that happy day, let's fill our bright and shiny garbage cans with these terrifying man-made concoctions. Wake up! Read labels!

Clean Out Your Pantry

Throw out all the processed foods, the hard, hydrogenated fats, white sugar, and bleached flour. Put in their place the vegetable oils, whole-grain flours, and natural sugars: honey, brown sugar, and unsulphured molasses. Also try the new sweet licorice and the delicious carob flour.

Always keep a supply of flavorsome herbs and spices of all kinds in your kitchen. By all means use fresh herbs if you have a garden; if not, use the dried ones. But be subtle with them. Beauty-farm cooking requires "a touch of poetry," and spices and herbs can give that poetic touch.

Vegetable oils all bring their own subtle and agreeable flavors. Try them all, singly, or mix two or three varieties and make your own blend.

And for more flavor and savor, you will want several bottles of wine and cider vinegar to make your own special fragrant herb vinegars, as they do in Europe. (Recipe for Swiss Herb Vinegar in chapter 23; see index.) Dr. D. C. Jarvis, in his book *Folk Medicine,* pointed out the many benefits of cider vinegar for your health.

You will always need a supply of lean milk, yogurt, the vegetable oils, and fresh sweet butter. If possible, use whipped butter; you will need less.

And now for your own cooking skills: you need to learn only how to short-cook your vegetables in a little liquid—two or three tablespoons—so that it is all gone when the vegetable is cooked. For more flavor you can use vegetable or chicken broth. Your heavy cooking pot will conserve the flavor and moisture and prevent burning. Just before serving a fresh vegetable, you add a sprinkle of vegetable salt and a bit of butter; whipped butter looks like hollandaise sauce, and you need very little. You have never tasted more delicious vegetables. And, of course, when you sauté vegetables in oil as the Chinese do, you do not need any butter.

Just One Day a Week

If you have a busy schedule during the week, one that keeps you away from your home beauty farm, you must see to it that your body is given a once-a-week break. We read in the Bible that the Lord made the world in six days, and on the seventh day He rested. The sabbath has become a traditional day of rest the world over. We owe ourselves one day completely detached from hustle and habitual routines.

I want to recommend to all wise people—regardless of income, business, family, and friends—that you declare one day of the week YOURday and make it just that. It can become the most important and valuable day of the week to you. Whether you are able to establish it for Saturday, Sunday, or a weekday, stake your claim and hold it against all odds. Make it a permanent habit and you will become richer, happier, and healthier for it. If friends and family jeer and scoff, let them; the chances are that after a while they will see what it does for you and stake out THEIRday for themselves.

YOURday is to be one completely detached from the distractions and obligations of other days, both of work and of family. On YOURday you are at no one's beck and call. Don't tell me you cannot possibly do it; the busier you are, the more you need it. The more firmly you establish the habit of YOURday as one freed from anxieties, tensions, cares, and the harassment of "what time is it?" the more easily and efficiently you will find yourself operating throughout the other days of the week. Not for nothing has it been said, "Man does not live by bread alone."

Some people have become so involved in the hectic rush of existence that they have no clear idea of how to go about using one whole day of freedom from the treadmill. If you are one of these, let me make some suggestions to get you started. We'll take the physical YOU first, then the inner YOU.

How to Spend YOURday

No alarm clock to wake you up. On YOURday, wake up naturally, easily, lazily, and relaxed. For once it does not matter what time the bus leaves. Try an oxygen cocktail before arising. Take half a dozen slow, deep breaths—inhale through your nose, exhale through the mouth. Easy does it. Don't hurry out of bed; relax awhile and enjoy the luxury of being relaxed.

Here are some ideas for the day's menus. They are generous.

Breakfast

Ready for breakfast now? Good! Give your digestive system a recuperative lazy day also. Have your favorite fruit juice, or whole fruit. (Remember, the whole fruit is preferable for reducers because it is more slowly digested and provides satisfying bulk for a stomach accustomed to being overloaded.) Treat yourself to Swiss coffee—a big cup of fresh hot coffee with fortified hot milk, mixed half and half, flavored with a teaspoonful of energizing honey. (Of course you use lean skim milk.)

Midmorning

A bracer to keep the energy high: a glass of lean milk, buttermilk, or your favorite flavor of milk shake (recipes in chapter 28; see index).

Luncheon

Now is the time to enjoy a big bowl of salad. Choose either fresh fruits or vegetables with leafy greens, plus four heaping tablespoons of cottage cheese, and sprinkle it with lemon juice and a dash of vegetable salt (and the smallest dash of light dressing, if you must have it). With your salad have one slice of whole-wheat, rye, or protein bread, very lightly buttered. For a beverage, take your choice of Swiss coffee, buttermilk, or hot tea with lemon and honey.

Midafternoon

Enjoy another refreshing snack, chosen from any *one* of the following: hot jasmine tea, or mint tea, with honey and lemon; a cup of yogurt flavored with honey; a glass of fresh vegetable juice; a glass of tomato juice spiked with a pinch of herbs and a quarter section of lemon.

Dinner

Start with something fresh, either vegetable juice or a generous green salad with light dressing. For the entree, have your choice of: a fluffy omelet; broiled liver sprinkled with parsley; broiled mushrooms; cottage cheese with chives. Add a moderate serving of short-cooked vegetable. Have a lighthearted baked potato (see recipe index) flavored with a spoonful of yogurt. Now for dessert: have a fruit compote made with any small fruits or cut-up fruits, or your choice—with honey drizzled over it. For a beverage, choose one of these: demitasse, Swiss coffee, papaya mint tea, jasmine tea, or buttermilk.

GOOD NIGHTCAP

Before retiring, soothe the inner man or woman with a glass of hot lean milk flavored with honey, or molasses, or licorice.

You will find that this one day of extra-lean eating is vastly beneficial to your digestive system, as well as to your mind and emotions.

Now let's think of other ideas for YOURday.

THE RELAXING BATH

This is a good day to treat yourself to the most enjoyable and most beneficial sort of bath. Take it any time during the day, except at bedtime. Fill the tub with pleasantly warm water and lie in it limp as a rag doll for ten, fifteen, thirty minutes, or as long as you like. Try the alternating bath (see chapter 12). Then relax in the yoga slant position (see chapter 9).

EXERCISE

YOURday is a perfect day to limber up all your body with lazy, easy exercises. You can make it a really rejuvenating day. You don't have to dress up and rush out anywhere. No hurry, no worry. Two or three times during the day, do your favorite exercises, especially the stomach lift (see chapter 9). This is YOURday to set yourself an example for simple, regular exercise all week.

SUN AND AIR

Weather permitting, do treat yourself to some sun and air on YOURday. It's a wonderful time to enjoy sunbathing and store up some "sunshine vitamins." Take a brisk walk in the park, to revitalize the circulation and give your lungs a healthy ration of good, clean oxygen. Get acquainted with the delights of walking through woods and fields, with leisure to see and to sense the beauty of the world you live in.

Take Care of the Inner Self

If you have been longing for time to putter, read, meditate and invite the spirit, or to launch some pet project, now is the day to do so. You know that the only time your conscious mind is unoccupied is when you are asleep. On YOURday, empty it of the daily routine, occupy it and refresh it with new thoughts and things.

You are an oral person, you know. That means you have a keen appetite for words. You love them: you probably can't get enough of them, in one form or another. How will you have them served to you on YOURday? That depends on your individual taste, but here is the general idea: on YOURday take your words *in the exact opposite* of the way you get them the rest of the week.

Do you spend much of your time talking to people? Then spend YOURday talking to as few people as possible. Take your words in written form—reading, dipping into the dictionary and encyclopedia, cutting and pasting clippings in a scrapbook, writing letters. Or take your words vocally, aloud. Memorize a favorite poem and recite it aloud to yourself. A well-known lecturer writes me that she spends part of HERday singing. Not that she can sing; she just likes to think she can.

Some professional talkers are gluttons for silence. I am told that one well-known news broadcaster spends HISday like a veritable Trappist monk; he sees no one, turns off the telephone, and eats crossword puzzles alive—complicated ones imported from England. A stage comedian I know spends HISday inventing cryptograms. A university professor has a taste for bird-watching; on HERday she is strictly for the birds. If you have such an appetite for silence, do indulge it on YOURday. Give yourself the greatest treat of all—the joy of sitting still and listening. Listening to what? To your own thoughts and reveries. Meditation, you know, is the nutritional element of the soul: it feeds spiritual strength and power. "Be still," the Bible tells us, "and know that I am God."

Perhaps you live and work alone. If so, on YOURday you will want the opposite of silence. "On MYday," a freelance writer tells me, "I ride on the bus, sit on park benches, eat in crowded restaurants, smiling at people (with discretion) and starting up casual conversation with anyone and everyone."

This is YOURday to pursue any new project you want to undertake. What is it? Clarinet playing? Languages? How long is it since you browsed through a library or an art gallery or a museum? You are well on your way now toward preventing or eliminating "middle-age spread" of the body. YOURday is the day to take steps against middle-age spread of the mind.

Visit a Beauty Farm

So many Americans spend their vacations traveling long distances, getting no closer to the countryside than seeing it through a car window, or perhaps from 30,000 feet above in a jet plane. Only of late have we begun to appreciate the value of getting to the country, preferably to a farm, away from noise and irritations, to eat food that comes directly from the good earth to the table.

This can do wonders, especially for tense and harassed women. Elizabeth Arden was the first to see the possibilities of this idea when she turned her nonpaying Maine farm into a beauty farm, inviting those who could afford it to come and relax for three or four weeks at a fabulous price. Now there are other beauty farms and rest resorts springing up all over the world. But they are only a drop in the bucket. There should be beauty farms in every state.

Women have discovered the beauty farms first, as they always do in matters pertaining to better looks and health. But men will follow. I predict that one day soon we shall have farms for men. They cannot come soon enough!

BEAUTY FARMS TO VISIT

Here I present an international list of selected beauty farms, spas, and health resorts. For more information, write directly to the addresses given below. For best accommodations, make reservations well in advance.

THE GOLDEN DOOR, Escondido, California. Luxurious, and most glamorous of all beauty farms. Accent on beauty, reducing, and relaxation. Ladies only. Expensive. Address: The Golden Door Beauty Resort, Highway 395, Escondido, California 92025.

RANCHO LA PUERTA, Tecate, Mexico, near San Diego, California. Modest ranch-style accommodations. Serious, somewhat cultish regime, with accent on physical and mental fitness. Caters to both men and women. The Rancho produces its own organically grown grapes and features a grape cure. Inexpensive. Information and Reservations address: Rancho La Puerta, 2107 Hancock Street, San Diego, California 92110.

MAIN CHANCE, Phoenix, Arizona. De luxe establishment with accent on beauty and glamor. Luxurious accommodations. Ladies only. Very expensive! Address: Main Chance, 5830 East Jean Avenue, Phoenix, Arizona 85018.

THE GRANGE BEAUTY FARM, Knebworth, Hertfordshire, England. About twenty-five miles north of London. Efficient establishment. All comforts, but not as luxurious as American beauty farms. Moderate prices. Accent on diet, rest, and relaxation. Caters to both men and women. Address: The Secretary, Beauty Farm, Ltd., The Grange, Henlow, Knebworth, Hertfordshire, England.

BIRCHER-BENNER SANATORIUM, Zurich, Switzerland. Pioneer diet establishment. Home of "Bircher Muesli." Serious, somewhat spartan regime. Beautiful hillside location overlooking the city. Not expensive for Americans. Address: Bircher-Benner Sanatorium, Schreberweg 9, 8000 Zurich, Switzerland.

BUCHINGER CLINIK, Überlingen, Germany. Ultramodern, semi-luxurious establishment specializing in fruit-fasts. Beautiful situation. Excellent staff of doctors, nurses, and therapists. Both men and women accepted. Inexpensive according to American standards. Address: Buchinger Clinik, 774 Überlingen-Bodensee, Germany.

A dream come true! Just before my book went to press I flew to Spain, to the island of Málaga, and discovered an amazing rejuvenation center run by the famous Buchinger family. Under sunny skies (320 days of the year) and strict medical control, you can now shed pounds and vague pains and aches. The modern equipment includes a fabulous swimming pool, scientific underwater massage, and saunas. Fruit juice, vegetable broth, and tea-fasting help remove weight the easiest and laziest way. For the ladies, there is a special beauty department specializing in organic facials and beauty masks. Prices are reasonable. For information, write directly to Clínica Buchinger, Marbella, Málaga, Spain.

I hope that with the publication of this book many more new beauty farms and health farms will spring up everywhere. Perhaps soon, too, I will be able to settle down in some spot where sun, soil, air, and water are at their best; where modern farmers will supply us with home-grown produce: fresh milk, cheese, meat, grains, fruits, and vegetables, all raised on healthy, rich soil, without harmful sprays and chemicals. I foresee beauty farms everywhere: in California, Florida, Arizona, and Nevada; also England, France, in the fertile Dordognes district, and Germany, in one of the best sanatoriums specializing in nutrition. When I find an ideal place, I will invite you to join me there.

FIVE

YOUR GOOD LIFE

14

You Are What You Think and Feel

A Philosophy of Life

Everyone must have a philosophy of life. Maybe you call it a way of living. I believe they are both the same thing. A philosophy of life is important, essential, because it is a blueprint for all our intellectual and physical activity. It helps us to train our brains to do the things we want to do, and to control our emotions so that we will be happier.

Actually, of course, no man can always do everything he wants to do. But if he has an adequate philosophy of life, he will be happy because of the things he *can* do. And an adequate philosophy of life will help you to channel your energy into productive rather than destructive channels. But in order to arrive at a good philosophy of life, one must have values, and these can be obtained only through the exercise of intellectual objectivity.

The world is a changing place. All the things in it are changing all the time. If we have values that are fixed and rigid, or that assume that the world is fixed and rigid, we are not being intellectually objective. We are not being mature. In order to use emotional energy productively we must have energy outlets. An energy outlet, if it is a good one, is a plan for the use of emotion toward a desired end. Emotion will run wild if we are not prepared for it. The person with a working philosophy of life will be hurt less by the inevitable stresses and strains of everyday modern life; he will be more elastic, more resilient.

I want to recommend a book to you—although you may have a hard time finding it. It contains, I think, the best practical suggestions for a philosophy of life that I have ever seen. But it contains much more; it is a book about managing your mind. In fact, that is the title of it: *Managing Your Mind*, by Dr. S. H. Kraines, a wise and experienced psychiatrist, and E. S. Thetford. And the subtitle of this wonderful little book is "You *Can* Change Human Nature."

I cannot recommend this book too highly. It is not a book for sick people especially. It is a book for people, for all people who have problems and want help in solving them. And that means all of us. Solving problems requires skill. It doesn't make any difference whether they are problems of piano technique or interpretation or of life. The person with skill will do a better job than the person without skill.

Laugh and Be Healthy

Laugh and the world laughs with you. Laugh and be healthy, advised the Illinois State Medical Society not long ago. Laugh and live long, said the famous Dr. Sara M. Jordan of the Lahey Clinic in Boston.

Why do these people recommend laughter? Because when we are upset emotionally, we are out of balance. And at such moments it is laughter that breaks the strain, snaps the tensions, and revitalizes the glands at their work.

The whole function of these glands is to keep our inner climate in balance. They work as partners: one set of hormones quickens your heartbeat, another slows it down. One speeds up your metabolism, another tones it down to give your system the rest it needs.

Dr. Jordan says, "There is plenty of evidence that glands like the pituitary, adrenals and others—with their hormonal secretions—exert their beneficent influence in this way."

Good wholehearted laughter is a respiratory gymnastic. It is good for the organs of the chest. We must have more laughter, and not just the twitching of nervous muscles, but deep-down hilarious laughter that shakes the whole inner man.

Garbo Laughs

One day in Hollywood my phone rang, and it was Greta Garbo asking if she could come for lunch. Now this was when Garbo was the reigning queen of Hollywood, and such a call was almost unheard of. Knowing that Miss Garbo was currently on a strict vegetarian diet, I ordered wild-rice burgers, a salad of fresh vegetables, and broiled honeyed grapefruit.

She arrived—a vision of breath-taking beauty, with her long hair and fresh, golden complexion.

Miss Garbo had heard of me through her friend Leopold Stokowski, and she came to see me because of her great interest in food. She was at that time following a diet consisting mainly of boiled vegetables and thou-shalt-nots.

In spite of her radiant beauty, this diet had had a marked effect on her vitality; she was suffering from overtiredness and insomnia and was in danger of serious anemia.

I made it my task to wean her away from strict vegetarianism, and coax her back to intelligent eating—no easy chore with a woman who has a will of steel. Finally she consented to try my suggestions. First of all, of course, I insisted on a balanced diet. The next day, when I stopped by her dressing room at lunchtime, I found that she was having her usual vegetables, in her usual privacy—but this time the vegetables were raw, in a large salad bowl, and well fortified with protein: bits of ham, chicken, cottage cheese, and wheat germ. She had begun the high-vitality program, and she quickly regained her energy.

Soon after Miss Garbo began this new way of nutrition, she accepted the leading role in the film *Ninotchka,* widely publicized with the wondrous statement "Garbo Laughs!" Many people congratulated us both on the "new" Garbo.

The Joy of Participation

A willingness to sit and let others do the thinking and entertaining for us seven days a week, as so many do before the television set, is self-destructive. A willingness to be a passive spectator and let life go by is also self-destructive.

Chronic boredom is an illness, says a distinguished psychosomaticist, Dr. Arnold A. Hutschnecker, in his book *The Will to Live*.

To let others do our reading, dancing, and playing is like engaging someone to make love for us. It is like requiring the priest or parson to say all our prayers.

> The human being who has never made love, never prayed, never danced is hardly better than the jellyfish floating in the sea.

The millions of years of life, struggling to achieve a soul, are wasted on such a person. His own fabulous body and the mind that dwells in it are wasted on him.

The "I want to be alone" theory has passed. Don't withdraw. There is no place for hermits in this century. Maintain your radius of acquaintance, and expand it. Join things, help do things that cannot be done alone. The warp and woof of your community is made up of people like yourself. Doing things will make you happy. It is an expression of love. It will bring you untold reward.

The Secret Ingredient

The highest attainment of human beings, I firmly believe, is the full love of men and women. This is something that is beyond any *individual*. It can only be achieved through mutuality. Born of attraction, bred in the flames of full passion, heightened by parenthood, and given full force by the whole life of maturity, of understanding of the pleasures and the privileges of life, love is something no man or woman can create for himself or herself. But what horrible things husbands and wives can still do to each other when they get sidetracked or derailed.

Love is anything one receives that results in the supplementation of one's own capacities with the strength, abilities, encouragement, support, and assets of others who charge no bond, ask no interest, require no mortgage, look for no advantage, and seek no profit. The pleasure of lovers, and their profit, derives from giving, helping, being of assistance, being a means of support, material or spiritual, when people they love can benefit from it or would suffer from lack of it.

Yes, love (and peace and understanding) is the secret ingredient in life. It can make every meal different, and better. It is generated by the intelligent woman who understands the nutritional needs of the human body and the spiritual needs of the human mind. No spiritual hunger can be satisfied by food. No physical hunger can be satisfied by understanding. But the mind in the well-fed body can be left wanting, just as the body of the understanding mind can be left in dire need. Into every dish, if *both* body and mind are to be well fed, must go not only the proper proteins and minerals but also love.

15

Meet Some of My People

In the course of my life I have met many People. People are my great interest, and many of them are my good friends.

In my lifelong studies I have discovered that People, whatever their talents, achievements, or position in life, have one thing in common: they make it their habit always to be at their best—to feel their best, look their best, and use their best efforts to make the world better, saner, or happier. In other words, I find that People make it their habit to control themselves and their lives instead of allowing themselves to be controlled and pushed around by circumstances.

Many of my People are in the second half of their lives. The mature person can say to himself, "I am unique. There is no one in the world who is exactly like me," and enjoy this, capitalize on it. He can say, "I love and am loved," and know what he is talking about. It is only in maturity that we have loved enough to understand and evaluate love. The mature person can say, "I am important to myself, to my family, to my community," and know wherein he is important. He can also know wherein he is unimportant; there is the great test of maturity.

Only the mature person, also, can have true self-confidence. In the first half of life, we are finding ourselves, reproducing ourselves, making a living for ourselves and our dependents. In the second half of life, we can confidently appraise ourselves, find out who we are, what we are good for, and what we were put into the world to accomplish. We have enough confidence in our strength to be able to admit and remedy our weaknesses; enough confidence in our education to want to go on learning; enough confidence in our lives to want to go on developing, expanding, *living*.

What are the attributes of youth? They are both plus and minus. The plus attributes are: courage, curiosity, excitement. The minus attributes are: ignorance, egocentricity, overconfidence.

What are the attributes of age? Again, they are both plus and minus. The plus ones: caution, objectivity, wisdom. The minus ones: timidity, intolerance, fear of change.

Check over these attributes, both plus and minus. What do you find? You find that in some respects you are still young; that in some respects you have always been old. *You have been both young and old all of your life.* Now discard all your minuses, both of youth and of age. Make a list of all the plus attributes. Resolve, consciously and deliberately, to rule out all the minus side and to develop all of the plus side (of both youth and age) for the rest of your long life. This is true maturity.

The French philosopher Henri Bergson has said, "To exist is to change, to change is to mature, to mature is to go on creating oneself endlessly."

How Does One Gain Maturity?

Just as some people are lucky enough to inherit good teeth, strong bodies, and superior digestive systems, some people also have the good fortune to be born of happy, well-adjusted parents and to inherit thereby the ingredients for true maturity.

Many others achieve maturity by instinct, often by finding, either in real life or on library shelves, some great friend, teacher, guide, or philosopher with whom they identify, whose life they use as a model for their own lives.

Many others, unfortunately, are neither "born" to maturity nor acquire it. They arrive at the second half of life still woefully immature, still fighting the old battles of their childhood against grownups who ruled or thwarted them; still tense with the insecurity and guilt of their teens; still driven by the ambitions and anxieties of their thirties. These are the "seekers," who run from one thing to another. They are looking for help but have not the maturity or the wisdom to know what they actually need. Countless such "seekers" have come to my classes, and I believe that by teaching them to strengthen their bodies, especially their nerves, I have been able to help many of them.

However, many of these people need psychiatric help or psychological counseling in order to attain true maturity. I look forward to the day when regular checkups with the family psychiatrist will be as much a matter of course as checkups with the family doctor, dentist, and oculist. Modern life grows more and more complex. There is increasing need for true maturity if, in the course of our long lives, we are to meet serenely the changes, challenges, and anxieties of the atomic era. We need equilibrium and assurance. I agree with that great philosopher Joshua Loth Liebman that "modern psychology can help normal people to maintain their equilibrium or to regain it." I also agree with Dr. Liebman when he adds that "religion can give both assurance and a spiritual purpose in life."

The famous psychoanalyst Dr. Carl Jung, in Zurich, Switzerland, once said to me, "In all the thousands who come to me for help, those who have some faith, some religion, get well more quickly."

Truly mature people, wherever you find them, are spiritual people. They may or may not live according to a specific creed or faith; the important thing is that they *have* faith—faith in themselves, in their fellow men, in the existence of a power, a universal order and purpose, that is greater than themselves. This is seldom achieved until the second half of life. Dr. Edward Bortz, a former president of the American Medical Association, claimed that *man reaches physical maturity at twenty-five; emotional maturity at thirty-five; intellectual maturity at forty-five; but that spiritual maturity comes in the later years.*

If you are falling short of true maturity, finding yourself hampered by impulses, anxieties, depressions that you cannot understand or overcome, even after you have built up your physical health and strength, then by all means consult a psychiatrist or psychologist. Dr. George Lawton, a consulting psychologist, has told us that the aim of such counseling is "to release the individual's potentialities for growth, make him more effective in the use of his energies."

Ann Astaire

I first met Ann Astaire in the 1930's when her two famous children, Fred and Adele, were starring in *The Bandwagon*. A friend took me to the Astaires' New York apartment for tea. The conversation turned to health and youthfulness, whether it was possible to remain healthy and young by will power.

I said, "Not by will power. Those are the middle-aged men in bright neckties, the women who turn girlish in their fifties and go in for bright red shoes and hats. These people are trying to look young by force, as it were. I think being youthful is a matter of *wanting* to be youthful, steadily, all day, every day."

Mrs. Astaire smiled at me. "I am supposed to need glasses," she said. "I have a prescription for them. Do you think that I can avoid wearing glasses by wanting to, steadily enough?"

I told her that there were excellent eye exercises; that if she wanted to avoid glasses enough to exercise and relax her eyes steadily—

"I'll do it," she said, with the note of quiet confidence that I like so much to hear.

I am introducing Ann Astaire to you for several reasons. One reason is that she is my very good friend. Another reason is that, although she is definitely one of my People, she is not a celebrity, a career woman, or a society leader. She is an unassuming, typically American woman, at home wherever she finds herself.

Born and raised in Omaha, Nebraska, she taught school for a time before her marriage. Her children were the center of her life; wherever they were booked to perform, she went with them and made a home. She accomplished effortlessly the transition from Omaha to sophisticated New York. When her daughter Adele left the cast of *The Bandwagon* to marry the English nobleman Lord Charles Cavendish, Ann Astaire made the transition from New York society to London society with equal ease and grace.

Her gentle, natural dignity amounts almost to nobility; she is internationally adored; members of the British royal family are her friends. As her friend, I myself was welcomed into London's most brilliant and influential circles when I went there in the late 1930's to lecture on nutrition. In that way I was able to introduce to England the Hauser way of eating, which proved to be so helpful during the bitter, deprived war years that were to follow.

During the war, Ann Astaire took over the entire management of Lismore, Lord Cavendish's huge estate in Ireland, in order to free Lady Charles Cavendish for Red Cross work. Lismore Castle, already famous for its hospitality, now became equally famous for its cuisine; short-cooked vegetables and big bowls of crisp, tossed salads were a novelty, a seven days' wonder. When food became very scarce in Ireland, fresh vegetables were still plentiful at Lismore Castle. Mrs. Astaire saw to the raising of them herself.

Now, at ninety-five, she has the same quality that she had in her fifties when I first met her—a quality not of youth but of youthfulness, of warm, young dignity.

She dresses simply, with quiet elegance, walks, gardens, enjoys her grandchildren. She is an active churchwoman, a believer in service to humanity and in the power of the mind to accomplish, little by little, the good it sets out to do.

She uses a lorgnette for theater programs and the telephone book, but she still does not need to wear glasses; she never had that prescription filled. That first day I met her, she began making a part of her life not only the eye exercises I recommended but the entire Hauser regime. With her characteristic quiet thoroughness, she has followed it ever since.

She eats intelligently; she has formed the habit of liking what is good for her, not because she must but because she wants to. She always undereats—again, not because she must but because she wants to. And she is always relaxed, for true relaxation comes from knowledge that you have yourself and your body under your own control, not because you must but because you want to have it that way.

Albert Schweitzer

I have met only two people in my life whose inner serenity is so great that in their presence I have felt at the same time humble yet inspired, relaxed yet exhilarated. One was Gandhi. The other was Dr. Albert Schweitzer.

The life and work of Albert Schweitzer, who gave up his career as a world-famous musician and theologian to found and run a hospital for the most primitive people in the heart of Africa, has long been one of my most helpful sources of spiritual refreshment. And I had long wanted to meet him, partly because I was born in the Black Forest, only an hour from his native village of Günzbach in Alsace.

One day, when I was in Paris, I learned that he had returned to Günzbach. The next day Marion Preminger and I were on our way to see him. In Strasbourg no one had ever heard of Günzbach, so we went on to Colmar. At Colmar they said, "Günzbach? Oh, you mean Dr. Schweitzer's village."

When we arrived we heard the sounds of organ music from the little whitewashed church. We entered and found Dr. Schweitzer, seated at the console of an organ built to his own design, playing Bach.

He finished the chorale, and then turned and greeted us with the warmth, kindness, and simplicity of an old friend.

"You enjoy music?" he asked. There was no need for us to reply. So he nodded and said, "Sit in the back of the church; you will hear better there."

He played the chorale "When We Are in Deepest Need." I have never been so moved and transported in my life as when the glorious music filled that little church under Albert Schweitzer's divine touch.

"You will join us for lunch?" he asked.

The meal, as I had expected, was perfectly simple and simply perfect. A green salad with tomatoes in a white porcelain bowl. Cold meats, with Swiss and cottage cheese. A basket of Alsace grapes, and a bottle of dry Rhine wine. There was one cooked vegetable, a dish of soybeans.

I asked Dr. Schweitzer whether he was a vegetarian. He answered, "No, unfortunately I am not. I realize that we need meat and fish. The higher life must live on the lower. But we must kill only as much as necessary, and never wantonly."

We started talking and I confessed a great love for dogs.

"I hope you talk to them," he said at once. "They understand. Animals, of course, do not use our language, but they understand it.

"At my hospital in Lambaréné wild animals often come, and I talk to them. A wild pig called one day and I spoke to him. So he came again. Now he is a regular visitor. He often sleeps there, though he has grown rather big and awkward. I cover him up with a rug at nights; and if he rolls out of it, I have to wake him up and put him back to bed."

Throughout the afternoon this great man talked of his hospital and his hopes for humanity, and I think perhaps the primitive buildings at Lambaréné are a symbol of those hopes. For there he established not a white-walled center of healing but a small kingdom where he ruled by love.

In that simple home, surrounded by books and pictures, by the quiet atmosphere of humane culture, I experienced a most remarkable afternoon—one that changed my life permanently for the better.

Fulfillment in Later Life

For a magnificent example of life lived to the full for almost a hundred years, read books by and about Dr. Lillian J. Martin of California. In her youth, Dr. Martin taught high-school chemistry. In her thirties, she went to Germany to study psychology (then a new science), took a professorship at Stanford University, made ten new contributions to psychological research, and then was retired, in the natural order of things, at the age of sixty-five.

Did Dr. Martin "retire"? Assuredly not. She then *began* her great work. Believing that the secret of youthfulness lay in breaking with the old and tackling the new, she launched into child-guidance work and opened the first mental-hygiene clinic for preschool children in San Francisco. Working with children, she became interested in their grandparents also. Then she opened an old-age clinic in San Francisco, now world-famous, with branches in Los Angeles and New York City.

Dr. Martin learned to type at sixty-five. She learned to drive a car in her seventies. At seventy-five she went alone to Russia. At eighty-one she toured Mexico alone in her car. At eighty-eight she made a tour of South America, including a journey up the Amazon. At eighty-nine she managed a sixty-four-acre farm (at a profit) with four sixty-year-old helpers.

Grandma Moses took up painting seriously at the age of seventy-six. She had more than thirty-five exhibitions; some of her canvases have sold for thousands of dollars. At the age of eighty-eight, she was awarded the Women's National Press Club award "for outstanding contribution to contemporary thought and achievement." Grandma Moses said (and artist friends of mine have corroborated this), "Anyone can paint who wants to. All you have to do is get the brush and paint and start in."

Frank Lloyd Wright was little known as an architect in his youth and middle life. But in his later years, he became world-famous. He was in his eighties when he received the highest professional honors from the American Institute of Architects. His comment on age was: "A creative life is a young one. What makes everybody think that eighty is old?"

Mrs. Edgar Ferry was a tiny great-grandmother when she celebrated her hundredth birthday by flying from her home in St. Paul, Minnesota, to New York. When asked about her secret for living such a long and happy life, she said, "I eat carefully and have a strong personal faith." Mrs. Ferry preferred fresh food and avoided all white flour and white sugar; honey was her favorite sweetener, and yogurt was one of her favorite foods. She gave credit to her two heroes, Gayelord Hauser and Bernarr MacFadden.

A gold medal for distinguished service to humanity was awarded to Dr. Lillian M. Gilbreth—engineer, psychologist, and author—by the National Institute of Social Sciences when she was in her seventies. She was not only an engineer, psychologist, and professor but also the mother of twelve children, the author of ten books, the recipient of nine academic degrees, and an industrial consultant presiding over her own corporation.

Clara Barton, founder of the American Red Cross, lived actively until the age of ninety-one.

Sophocles wrote *Oedipus at Colonus* shortly before his death at ninety.

Oliver Wendell Holmes started writing *Over the Tea Cups* at seventy-nine.

Titian painted his greatest masterpiece at eighty-five and lived to be ninety-nine.

The immortal Ninon de Lenclos has been called one of the most significant as well as one of the most beautiful women of the seventeenth century. A contemporary of her later years wrote of her: "Until she was over sixty she had lovers who loved her greatly and the most virtuous people of France for her friends. Until she was eighty she was sought by the best society of her time."

There is no limit to the proof that, as life goes on, energy can and does *increase*. Examples are limitless of men and women who, in the second half of their lives, have found their energy heightened, their creative powers intensified, their ability to learn doubled and redoubled. Wherever we look we find examples not just of continuing productivity but of the new flowering of gifts, talents, and abilities at forty, sixty, and beyond.

What is the secret? Let me repeat it:

>   Good health
>   A strong, vibrant body
>   A positive attitude of mind

The Fabulous Lady Mendl

Elsie de Wolfe Mendl was a good friend and faithful student of nutrition, of whom I am very proud. In the first half of her life, Elsie de Wolfe was an actress. Born in a house that stood on the present site of Macy's department store (she liked to say she was born in Macy's basement), she was educated abroad, presented at Queen Victoria's court, and moved in the inner circle of the glittering society of the Edwardian era in the United States and Europe. However, with the death of her father it became necessary to find some means of support for her mother and herself.

Elsie de Wolfe had always loved amateur theatricals, and she turned now to the professional stage for her living. She became known as the "best-dressed woman on the American stage" and was star and manager of her own company.

With her friend Elizabeth Marbury, with whom she shared houses in New York and in Versailles, just outside Paris, Elsie de Wolfe became an internationally famous hostess as well. Her parties were breath-taking; her friends were kings and queens, princesses, diplomats, poets, painters, musicians, writers, admirals, generals, and stars of opera, stage, and screen.

One day she walked from the stage, through the wings, and into her dressing room, and sat down before the mirror to remove her makeup. Suddenly she heard, clearly and distinctly, the voice of her inner self saying, "Those are the last words you will ever speak in the theater." She had always listened to her inner voice, sometimes even talked back to it. Now she said to herself, aloud, "All right. What are you afraid of?" And began to plan another career.

Ugliness in her surroundings had always depressed her. Always conscious of rooms, she knew instinctively what was right or wrong about them. Closing her eyes in an ugly room (and in those days, the more lavish the room, the uglier it was), she would mentally re-create it and make it beautiful.

When Elsie de Wolfe decided to leave the theater and become an interior decorator for the second half of her life, she was, therefore, turning back to a childhood dream. With no special training, no capital, nothing but many friends and an indomitable pioneering spirit, she became America's first woman interior decorator. Her first big assignment was the decoration of New York's celebrated Colony Club.

Stanford White, designer of the building, said, "Give the job of decorating to Elsie, and *let the girl alone*." That assignment was uphill work; American women were accustomed to living in Victorian ugliness. But gradually Elsie de Wolfe won her crusade for beauty—warm, glowing colors on walls, bright chintzes in drawing rooms, indoor "garden rooms," furniture that was beautiful, useful, and comfortable, and mirrors, mirrors everywhere.

The day in 1936 when I met this fabulous woman was one of the most interesting occasions of my life. Two of my friends took me to one of the famous "Sunday afternoons" at Lady Mendl's villa in Versailles. In the center of a group in which everybody was "somebody," I was received by a tiny lady, soignée, with shining dark eyes and platinum-white hair. She showed me her copy of my book *Eat and Grow Beautiful*. It was well marked and underscored. Across the front she had written "I *like* that man!"

Most of her life she had been interested in nutrition. As a child she had wanted good teeth and a beautiful complexion; instinctively she had avoided candy and other sweets. As the "best-dressed woman on the American stage," she had needed a perfect figure and had achieved it by teaching herself to like only fresh, vital foods, *under*eating always and cultivating the great art of relaxation. So important did she consider nutrition that for years her specially trained chef traveled with her wherever she went. Monsieur Fraise (Mr. Strawberry—a good name for a good chef) learned to prepare exactly the foods I recommended.

Lady Mendl long ago adopted my Look Younger, Live Longer principles. "I have originated modern styles in clothes and decoration," she once told me. "You have originated the modern manner of eating." In 1937 she gave a large party in my honor at her Paris apartment. Her guests were some of her favorite people. They included a number of the world's most attractive women: the Duchess of Windsor, Lady Diana Manners, Lady Charles Cavendish, Mrs. Harrison Williams, Princess Karputhala. This was the first time these women had realized the limitless possibilities of good nutrition, for themselves and for the people of their countries. I gave them the first vegetable-juice cocktail ever served in Paris and their enthusiasm was unbounded. The Duchess of Windsor, Lady Mendl, and my mother were the first three women in Europe to own the vegetable-juice-extracting machine that was then my special innovation.

"The longer I live," Lady Mendl said, "the more I realize that it is never too late to learn. I have always been eager for the new and willing to discard the old in its favor. I never think of myself as being old—I never tell my age. I am deeply interested in all of the new movements that are taking shape around me. I am an optimist.

"I have lived and laughed and loved. I have waved over my life the magic wand of self-control. I love life. I have made it an adventure. I have thrived on opposition. I rejoice that I was born with the courage to live." And live she did, fully and beautifully, to the age of ninety-four.

> Never complain—
> Never explain.
> *Lady Mendl*

Today's Beautiful People

In the 1970's many of my kind of People have a super-active life. It's no surprise that the women who are most successful are those who have also discovered the value of sound nutrition and healthful living for maintaining their stamina. Let's meet some of them. These women have achieved so much and yet never look harried or tired. They are self-disciplined People and they will take no short cuts. Their vital, glowing look isn't painted on, it comes from within.

Barbara Walters calls herself a compulsive worker, and surely no other newswoman has more television hours to her credit. Barbara spends at least two hours a day in front of the camera, starting at 4:30 a.m.! How does she do it? With relaxing cat naps whenever she can; more importantly, she doesn't smoke, drinks only an occasional glass of white wine, and pays special attention to her weight.

Cover girl and actress Lauren Hutton (over twenty *Vogue* covers to her credit) starts her day very early with a brisk freezing shower followed by a rubdown with a mixture of vitamin E oil, conch oil, and coconut oil. Next comes a high-protein breakfast including raw milk and lecithin.

In the business world, Mary Wells Lawrence is well known as a super-achiever. She is chairman of the board and chief executive officer of a leading advertising agency. What gives her the stamina to commute between a home in Dallas, a ranch in Arizona, and an office in New York, interspersed with business trips to clients throughout the country? A high-protein diet and tennis at 7 a.m. *before* work.

Historian, author, and international hostess Countess of Ramanones is absolutely iridescent at fifty-two. This American-born beauty believes there are no magic tricks to growing young, just self-discipline. Her beauty philosophy? Sleep, outdoor exercise, and no alcohol, not even wine. To keep up energy: two servings of yogurt before going out.

You may believe one is born beautiful, and no one can deny that Raquel Welch was born with a special, unique beauty, but according to her, beauty is a twenty-four-hour job. Her regimen includes eight hours of sleep, a high-protein breakfast, vitamins, and a lengthy exercise-dance routine on the beach every day.

16

Make Your Children Beautiful

One day in Paris I was visiting the Louvre with a young American woman. As we paused before Rodin's statue of *The Thinker*, she remarked wistfully, "How I wish I might be an artist! It must be wonderful to be able to create such beauty. I spend my life cooking, shopping, and nursing the children. I'm nothing but a *Hausfrau*. It makes me feel so unimportant!"

"But don't you see that you can create beauty in building beautiful children?" I asked her. "Rodin worked with clay and bronze; you work with living flesh. Just as he molded his works of art, so are you molding the bodies and the spirits of your children."

If you are a mother, you should think of yourself as a sculptor. You can be a poor artist—and create sickly, underdeveloped children; or a great artist—and mold beautiful, happy lives.

Your Infant

At birth a baby is as nearly perfect as nature can make him. Even if the mother's diet during pregnancy does not include all the substances required for baby's body, her own body tissues will be robbed to supply baby's needs.

Such perfection can be continued if you provide your baby with the proper nutrients. The best food for him is mother's milk.

Breast-fed babies have a much lower death rate and suffer less frequently from allergies, infections, and abnormalities than do bottle-fed babies. Dr. Paul Gyorgy, of the Philadelphia General Hospital, stated that breast feeding increases the infant's resistance to intestinal disturbances and to respiratory infections. However, the supply and quality of breast milk is determined by the adequacy of the mother's diet, especially in vitamins, minerals, and proteins, during pregnancy. (You should tell your pediatrician what regimen you plan for your baby; this way he will have an accurate record.)

Whether breast milk or formula is given baby, certain supplements are necessary to keep him healthy. The amount of either breast milk or cow's milk likely to be taken in a day by a newborn infant supplies only about 1,000 units of vitamin A. Twice this quantity is needed daily to keep his skin free of rashes and his resistance to infections high. The best source of vitamin A is fish-liver oil, which also furnishes vitamin D.

Perhaps the most important nutrient during infancy and childhood is vitamin D, which helps to develop a beautiful child. If vitamin D is lacking or is not absorbed into the blood, his teeth and bones may remain underdeveloped or become enlarged. Such abnormalities continue throughout life: narrow face, crooked or buck teeth, receding chin, pigeon breast, knock-knees, or bowed legs.

Liquid cod-liver oil is probably superior to all other fish-liver oils for baby because, in addition to vitamins, it contains useful unsaturated fat. However, because it is low in vitamin A, a tablespoonful (15 cc.) of plain halibut-liver oil should be added to a pint of cod-liver oil to increase its vitamin A content. Or cod-liver-oil concentrate can be followed by a few drops of vegetable oil to provide the fat needed to stimulate bile flow; this also supplies unsaturated fatty acids. In any case, the cod-liver oil should be given *after* morning and evening feedings, for only after feeding can baby's body properly absorb the vitamins in it.

If mother's diet includes adequate vitamin C, her breast milk will supply 100 milligrams of vitamin C in the amount of milk consumed in one day by a newborn baby. This amount is therefore considered ideal for baby. However, cow's milk averages only 6 milligrams per quart. Baby would require almost seventeen quarts of cow's milk to get 100 milligrams of vitamin C from it. An ounce of orange juice has only 15 milligrams of vitamin C and an ounce of tomato juice only 5 or less. The best way to ensure an adequate supply of vitamin C is to use 100-milligram ascorbic-acid tablets. One tablet can be dissolved in one teaspoonful of water and added to baby's formula or drinking water daily.

By the time baby is a week old, he should be given one tablespoonful of fresh, strained orange juice per day. This amount should be increased by one tablespoonful each week until eight ounces are being taken daily. As the amount of juice is increased, the amount of vitamin C supplement is decreased.

The B vitamins are also important, for they help to maintain normal appetite, aid digestion and elimination, encourage sound sleep, and help prevent skin rashes and eczema. A teaspoonful of brewers' yeast, mixed with baby's formula, will supply B vitamins. Later, wheat germ, added to cereal or fruit, will provide more. Wheat germ can be softened in hot milk.

Water in which short-cooked vegetables have been steamed will supply many valuable nutrients. A little iodized vegetable salt added to it will supply iodine, often neglected in baby's diet. But do watch your baby's salt intake. Commercially prepared baby foods are often loaded with salt.

Sunbaths should be given daily whenever possible. Start with three to five minutes and gradually increase the time up to a half hour. Be sure to coat baby lightly with a vegetable oil, such as avocado or peanut oil, before the sunbath. Leave the oil on until it is completely absorbed.

Late in the fourth month, baby can be introduced to solid food. Start with no more than a half teaspoonful, and gradually increase the amount each time it is offered. Thus, if any food upsets him, the upset will not be severe. This method of introducing new foods also allows baby to grow gradually accustomed to new tastes and textures.

Whole-grain cereal, cooked in milk, can now be introduced. Wheat germ, added to cereals or fruit, should continue to be given daily. Baby can also have the yolk of a hard-boiled egg, mashed with a little milk or formula. (Soft-cooked egg and egg white are difficult for him to digest and sometimes cause an allergy.)

Dark-green and orange or yellow vegetables, such as carrots, broccoli, chard, and squash—as prepared for the family table—are now suitable for baby. Of course, they should be mashed or puréed; with a blender or liquefier, this can be done in just a few minutes.

By the fifth month, baby is ready for applesauce, very ripe mashed bananas, steamed and blended prunes and apples, or any fruit pulp. (Never, never add any white sugar.) He can also have cottage cheese and baked Irish or sweet potato.

Your Growing Child

When your child is five or six months old, new foods can be introduced rapidly. But there is no place in baby's diet for any refined foods; and such foods as crackers, melba toast, and zwieback should be completely avoided. Let him cut his teeth on such foods as raw carrot sticks, raw turnip sticks, and celery. He can now be given bite-size pieces of whole-grain bread and larger portions of salad, raw vegetables, and fruits.

At about the age of nine months, he should be ready to eat most of the foods prepared for the family—provided, of course, that the table holds no food that does not build health.

When the child is about a year and a half old, he should receive daily a tablespoonful of powdered food yeast, and this amount should continue to be given as he grows up. He should also have about six ounces of citrus juice daily, and two tablespoons of wheat germ. The fish-liver oil should also be continued daily until the bones and teeth are completely developed. And vitamin D is also needed to keep his teeth and bones healthy.

Many mothers, anxious to provide all the nutrients they know their children need, try to overstuff them. A child will quickly learn that, by eating very little or not eating at all at regular mealtimes, he gets extra attention—which he finds pleasant. If the mother is overanxious, this situation can snowball; so don't make an issue over his not eating, but proceed with the meal. What he fails to eat at one meal he will make up at the next (unless he is ill or lacks vitamins). Lack of appetite can be caused by illness, excitement, emotional upset, or some other condition in which the child is better off not to eat very much. Continue to put small portions of proper food before him and, of course, permit between-meal snacks of natural foods. He will soon get over his eating problem. If the problem continues, you should of course consult your pediatrician.

If this method of feeding is continued as the child grows up, he should be able to reach maturity without digestive upsets, constipation, tooth decay, skin abnormalities, malformation of bones, nervousness, and dozens of other disturbances experienced by most children. He should have beauty and boundless energy. The mother-artist should take pride and pleasure in molding such a child.

Your Teen-ager

Some people think teen-agers are terrible. I think they're terrific. But anyone that knows teen-agers will agree: they are terribly hungry. This is natural. During the teens the permanent foundations of bony structure, organic soundness, resistance to disease, nervous stability, and lifelong well-being (or ill-being) are laid. For teen-agers good nutrition is, literally, the most important thing in life. Therefore when I am asked what to *do* about them, my answer is, first of all, *feed 'em.*

Obviously, proteins, vitamins, and minerals are necessary for the growing body. But growing emotions and growing minds must also be fed.

Teen-agers may receive all the necessary proteins, carbohydrates, fats, minerals, and vitamins and still hunger for the most essential nutrient of all—love. But love can have a two-way action. Enough of it means sturdy emotional and mental growth; too much can create emotional and mental overdependence. So the full answer to what we are to do about our teen-agers is: *Feed 'em. Love 'em. And leave 'em alone.*

In spite of the fact that our nation's standard of living is at an all-time high, nearly half our teen-agers are gravely undernourished. An investigation at Pennsylvania State University showed that about three fourths of them are not getting enough energy foods, such as whole-grain flours and cereals and natural sugar from fresh fruits and vegetables, to run the body efficiently. About half fail to get enough protein foods (meat, fish, cheese, eggs, milk) for building and repairing body tissues.

They do not get enough essential minerals—calcium and phosphorus for good red blood. Their diets are lacking in B vitamins, required for proper growth and nervous stability; in vitamin C, important to health of gums and healing of injuries; in vitamin A, essential to proper growth, clear skin, good vision.

What can we do about this?

If we give our teen-agers the well-balanced meals and the well-balanced love they need for physical and emotional growth, we have equipped them for freedom. Give them the independence they crave—they'll thrive on it. Give them your confidence—they'll respect it.

17

The Man in the Family

Some of the world's greatest chefs are men, yet in most households throughout the world cooking is done by women. But times are changing. More and more men are venturing into the uncharted territory of the kitchen out of necessity or curiosity. Lacking the know-how that has passed traditionally from mother to daughter, it is initially a difficult task. The simple act of deciphering a recipe is for some men a mystifying ordeal. If you are a man, don't let failure discourage you. There are a number of "kitchen guides" that take the mystery out of what pot to use for what and also tell you what it means to blend, sauté, cream, and so on. Why deny yourself the creative outlet, not to mention the praise from friends and family, that cooking brings just because "Mother never told you"? If you are a woman, encourage and assist when help is needed, but don't direct.

Men have often left the whole area of food to women, so it is not surprising that their knowledge of nutrition is often limited. The best advice a woman can give to the man in her life is on what he can do for his very special dietary needs.

Your man may have minor complaints, aches and pains, a creaking body that is no longer joyfully active. He may have poor digestion, possibly ulcers. (Nothing is clearer in science than the connection between food and the emotions.) He may take an extra drink somewhat too often. Dr. Roger J. Williams, who has done brilliant work in biochemical research, has told us that alcoholics are hungry, malnourished people. He said that in our American diet of highly saturated fats and overrefined starches and sugars, the hypothalamus—that center in the brain that guides the appetite—is starved for the relatively large quantities of minerals, vitamins, and amino acids that it requires. He believes that much alcoholism could be prevented, as well as cured, by sound nutrition. Should you be so unfortunate as to have an alcoholic problem in the family, I strongly suggest you read Dr. Williams's book, *Alcoholism: The Nutritional Approach*.

You may see your man constantly tired, sleepless, anxious, irritable. He may be troubled about a seeming loss of his masculine powers; this is a profound anxiety. Yet this is often a result of tension, lack of energy, and deficient nutrition.

Finally, you may be worried about his heart. What wife today is free of this worry?

It is not surprising that bachelors have a shorter life expectancy than married men. Certainly a man without a woman to love and care for him is not the best candidate for a happy, long life. Yet, from the thousands of questions married men ask me, it is evident that they face many problems. No doubt the strains and tensions of our competitive way of life are to blame, and to change all that is a large order for one lone woman!

I believe that married partners must look out for each other. They must provide that extra bit of will power or caution that the individual lacks.

I have found that women—despite all the jokes about their unrealistic thinking—are the realistic, practical members of the human race. Men are the adventurers, the gamblers, often the self-deluders. Women are the ones who recognize a fact when they see it—they seem to have an extra sense! So, women, look out for your husbands.

Our country enjoys the highest living standard in the world. Yet, in other countries, men live longer past the age of forty-five than they do in the United States. The increase in heart-disease deaths among young American men—the "epidemic," as the medical world is beginning to call it—can be traced directly to changes in living habits—the rise in the consumption of hard fats (which increases as the standard of living goes up) and the use of processed, overrefined foods. "Lack of exercise, coupled with rich snacks in front of television screens, may be a major factor," reported Dr. David M. Spain, pathologist of Beth-El Hospital and Columbia University College of Physicians and Surgeons.

There you have the man-killing American "way of life," pinned down to a few facts as simple as your own grocery list!

Three Gifts Every Man Wants

In the fairy tales that we loved as children, there were always three magic gifts by which the prince made his way through perilous adventures and returned to his princess, to live happily ever after. Here are the three magic gifts every man wants.

A new heart, one that will enable him to work and reach life's goal.

A new waistline, his youthful looks and vigor restored.

Last, but most important, *a new you,* transformed within and without by good nutrition and exercise.

The Epidemic of Heart Disease

The crucial combination of factors in heart disease and hardening of the arteries are these: sedentary occupation, overweight, high cholesterol, and the stress and strain of modern living.

Dr. Harold Thomas Hyman pointed to the "lush American diet," and as the immediate causes of arteriosclerosis he listed: "Sustained and prolonged hyperalimentation [overeating]; excessive salting of foods; and undue dietary dependence on concentrated carbohydrate foods and on saturated fats which, in the process of refinement, have lost certain essential amino acids, minerals, fatty acids, and vitamins."

Most doctors now test for cholesterol level in the blood, and if the level is above normal, they prescribe a diet low in cholesterol-producing foods, mainly the saturated fats. If you are at all worried about your husband's heart, I strongly urge you to discuss this test with his doctor. As Dr. Hyman says in his textbook for physicians, it is especially valuable to the doctor in general practice because it gives him a way of detecting, *in advance,* those "overtly healthy individuals" who are *prone* to arteriosclerosis.

The Sedentary Man

The second step, both to trim looks and good health, is exercise.

Men were hunters before they were farmers, and farmers before they were businessmen and desk-sitters. The human body, Dr. Laurence E. Morehouse has told us, was built for the rigors of the hunt. This professor of physical education at the University of California reminded us of what I have already mentioned in urging you to exercise for your own sake:

"Movement of the skeletal muscles in man not only performed his external work in primitive days, but also acted as supplemental heart muscles in moving fluids through the body. The modern sitting man relies on his heart muscle alone to pump fluids which support the internal environment of the body. The heart cannot do the job of circulation without the aid of other muscle pumps and sitting man soon begins to suffer."

Sitting man soon begins to suffer. Mighty important words, these, and the shouting will become louder and louder, because movement or exercise is important not only for your man's heart but for every part of his body—even his hair!

From many years of experience, however, I have learned that you cannot force a tired, flabby body to exercise. How many mechanical exercisers, stretchers, bicycles, and rowing machines are gathering dust in attics and basements! Many homes have one or two in the storeroom. All these appliances cost money, and they were bought with the most earnest resolutions.

But resolutions are not enough. First of all, new energy is needed. The body must be built up to meet the demands of exercise, so much that exercise will become a pleasure.

Million-Dollar Secrets for the Kitchen

For a new way of eating, start preparing tasty, delicious meals, rich in proteins, vitamins, minerals, fatty acids; low in sugars and starches and especially lean in saturated fats. Replace refined sugars with natural sugars, full of their own good minerals and vitamins, and replace refined starches with the whole, natural variety. Replace the killing, hard fats with liquid vegetable oils that contain the lifesaving, essential fatty acids. If polyunsaturated fats are substituted for animal fats, scientific research has shown the blood cholesterol level is reduced 10 to 20 percent. Stop oversalting, oversugaring, overcooking; and instead flavor food with delightful spices, herbs, and flavors.

With even a single menu change, the change from hard fats to vegetable oils, you can protect the health of arteries and at the same time rid the waistline of extra inches. And with the change of the whole spectrum from empty foods to sound nutrition, you have new vigor and zest for living. Morale will rise along with metabolism.

So throw away the hardened hydrogenated fats that you have been using as shortening, even if they are vegetable fats. Look at the label on your margarine; make sure it is not the hydrogenated kind. Have your butcher trim the fat off the meat you buy, or sharpen your best knife and trim it off yourself.

Soya oil, which the Japanese use; sunflower oil, which the Soviet Ministry of Nutrition is devoting thousands of extra acres to produce; peanut, sesame, avocado, and wheat-germ oils are all insurance for a better heart and general health. (See also the discussion of fats in chapter 2.)

Something exciting has been discovered about wheat-germ oil and wheat germ. Experiments with athletes show a direct connection between this little heart of the wheat and the stamina of the human heart. At the Physical Fitness Laboratory of the University of Illinois, fitness scores were higher with wheat germ or its oil added to the diet than with exercise alone. Just one teaspoon of wheat-germ oil taken daily increased athletes' physical capacity and endurance by as much as 51.5 percent.

Wheat germ is rich in vitamin E, and there is one school of thought that considers vitamin E a specific vitamin for the health of the heart. Whether it is this vitamin in the wheat germ or some other factor, it is clear that this food element provides something that gives men added endurance under physical stress. Yet this very precious substance is refined out of American bread and cereals. But you, performing your magic in the kitchen, can easily learn how to restore it. You simply add some golden wheat-germ oil to your salad dressing. Sprinkle wheat-germ kernels over salads and cereals. You can even make a delicious wheat-germ piecrust. (Recipe for Honeyed Wheat-Germ Piecrust in chapter 26; see index.)

How to Fight Baldness

Next to loss of sexual potency, a man worries most about losing his hair. Most men do not admit it, but it is one of the questions I am most often asked at my lectures before men's clubs, and today there is a booming business in hairpieces for men. Medical science, as a whole, pays little attention to this problem. Yet I think it is important, otherwise men would not spend millions of dollars on useless hair tonics.

The whole question of baldness is confusing. There are many theories. Some researchers claim that men lose their hair more often than women because an excess of male sex hormones affects the quantity or quality of the oil produced in the sebaceous glands of the skin and scalp. The laboratory evidence for this claim is that when the oil was rubbed on the bodies of mice and rabbits, all the rabbits and many of the mice lost their hair in ten days.

When female hormones were injected into bald men they stopped losing their hair; but they also began developing breasts, so obviously that was not the solution. A good endocrinologist can determine the cause of falling hair.

A more drastic, but seemingly successful, treatment for baldness has come into the spotlight. Dr. Norman Orentreich, Associate Clinical Professor of Dermatology at New York University, has been able to transplant healthy hair from the sides of the head to the bald spots. The treatment is given in the office, under local anesthetic. Ten to fifteen small circular pieces of scalp, each containing six to ten hair follicles, are taken from the base of the neck, where the hair is thickest, and transplanted into the bald spots. While this is a drastic and expensive way of adding hair to a bald pate, it is most welcome to actors and other people whose jobs depend on their looks. Dr. Orentreich has done thousands of these transplantations, and 90 percent have been successful. Women who have lost their hair have also benefited from this operation. But never forget that all hair, transplanted or otherwise, gets its proper nourishment via the blood stream.

Ancient Secrets for Sexual Strength

Can a man strengthen his sexual powers with food?

Some years back I wrote an article for *Esquire* on the care and feeding of executives. It won a tremendous response and brought me many invitations to lecture to men's clubs. I remember especially a luncheon at the Athletic Club in Philadelphia. As usual, I answered all kinds of questions on diet and health, on how to relax, on how to get rid of tiredness.

Then there was a lull, in which I could plainly hear some snickering from a table at the end of the room. Finally a small, slight man stood up and blurted, "Is there any connection between food and sex, and what should a man eat when his love life is on the blink?"

The whole room shook with laughter, but I admired that courageous little man. He looked tired and worried, but he was the only one who had dared to ask the question that haunts most men past the age of forty, and even some who have not reached that fortieth birthday. I answered him in all seriousness. I told him that of course there is a relationship between a man's diet and his sex drive. I said, "I only wish I could give you one potent recipe, food, or formula to make you a romantic, carefree lover, but unfortunately, it is not that simple."

I went on to tell him what I now want to tell you. The search for a more satisfying sex life has been going on ever since Adam found the first gray hair in his beard. The ancient Greeks and Romans had books full of strange formulas for waning sex powers. Some of them contained dangerous poisons—the Roman poet Lucretius died of one of these "love philters."

And some were frankly based on magic. For instance, the early Greeks swore by onions and garlic because both of these root vegetables have the shape of male testes. Another favorite was wine made from the mandrake root, simply because this two-legged root looked rather like a miniature man.

But strangely enough, many of those ancient love potions contained such highly nutritious foods as eggs, snails, and fish, all of which are full of vitamins and minerals; liver, the richest source of iron and the B vitamins; wild game, which we know today ranks higher than domestic meats in many vitamins and is also much leaner. Among the vegetables they recommended were cabbage, a fine source of the B vitamins and vitamin C, and peas, which are high in vegetable protein. High on the ancient lists of love foods was honey, one of nature's finest sugars.

Listen, now, to a two-thousand-year-old tip on foods for sexual prowess: wild honey, ginger, vinegar, wild garlic, shallots, cinnamon, nutmeg, wild seeds, pepper, and all heat-producing spices.

Today we laugh at such concoctions. But do you recognize in this list some health-giving foods? Of course you do. As for the spices, we know today that they stimulate the stomach to produce gastric juice and thus promote good appetite.

The Prostate Gland

It is estimated that one third of all men will be affected by an enlarged prostate by the time they are fifty. The prostate gland is the male sexual organ where semen is secreted and is located at the base or neck of the bladder. Because of this close proximity, symptoms of enlargement are frequent urination, especially during the night; low-back pain; and uremia if stagnant urine accumulates. As the enlargement progresses, the bladder becomes weak and it is increasingly difficult to discharge urine.

The cause of enlargement of this gland is not known. There seems to be no connection with sexual practices or infections of the genitalia. We do have a clue, though, that one aspect of the disorder may be nutritional. The prostrate gland contains more zinc than any other organ in the body. Men who subsist largely on white flour and processed carbohydrates (during processing zinc is removed and it is never replaced during the so-called enrichment process) are deficient in zinc. In 1974 the Food and Nutrition Board of the National Academy of Sciences listed zinc for the first time as an essential mineral. Its recommended dietary allowance is 15 mg. of zinc per day for males.

Men who suffer from this painful disorder should eat foods naturally rich in zinc, such as fish, shellfish, liver, egg yolk, oatmeal, brewers' yeast, and all seeds, especially pumpkin seeds.

Pumpkin Seeds, a Man's Best Friend

During my lectures at the Titania Palast in Berlin, it was my pleasure to meet an unusual man, Dr. Devrient. He was a medical doctor who specialized in nutrition. Dr. Devrient complimented me on my work, but he said, "Hauser, you neglect telling your students about one of nature's most potent foods, the seeds. Seeds have been used since biblical times, and they are an excellent food. They contain protein, vitamins, and minerals, and some of them contain hormones." Then the Berlin physician gave me a copy of an article he published in the German journal of health *Androgen:* "Hormonal Curative Influence of a Neglected Plant." In this article he said:

"Only the plain people knew the open secret of pumpkin seeds, a secret that was handed down from father to son for countless generations. No matter if it was the Hungarian gypsy, the mountain-dwelling Bulgarian, the Anatolian Turk, the Ukrainian, or the Transylvanian German, they all knew that pumpkin seeds preserve the prostate gland and thereby, also, male potency. In these countries people eat pumpkin seeds the way they devour sunflower seeds in Russia, as an inexhaustible source of vigor offered by nature."

How to Cook a Husband

A good many husbands are utterly spoiled by mismanagement in cooking and so are not tender and good. Some women keep them constantly in hot water; others let them freeze by their carelessness and indifference. Some keep them in a stew with irritating ways and words. Some wives keep them pickled, while others waste them shamefully. It cannot be supposed that any husband will be tender and good when so managed, but they are really delicious when prepared properly.

In selecting a husband, you should not be guided by the silvery appearance as in buying a mackerel; nor by the golden tint as if you wanted salmon. Do not go to the market for him as the best ones are always brought to the door. Be sure to select him yourself as tastes differ. It is far better to have none unless you will patiently learn how to cook him.

Of course, a preserving kettle of the finest porcelain is best, but if you have nothing better than an earthenware pipkin, it will do—with care. Like crabs and lobsters, husbands are cooked alive. They sometimes fly out of the kettle and so become burned and crusty on the edges, so it is wise to secure him in the kettle with a strong silken cord called Comfort, as the one called Duty is apt to be weak. Make a clear, steady flame of love, warmth, and cheerfulness. Set him as near this as seems to agree with him.

If he sputters, do not be anxious, for some husbands do this until they are quite done. Add a little sugar in the form of what confectioners call kisses, but use no pepper or vinegar on any account. Season to taste with spices, good humor and gaiety preferred, but seasoning must always be used with great discretion and caution. Avoid sharpness in testing him for tenderness. Stir him gently, lest he lie too flat and close to the kettle and become useless. You cannot fail to know when he is done. If so treated, you will find him very digestible, agreeing with you perfectly; and he will keep as long as you choose unless you become careless and allow the home fires to grow cold. Thus prepared, he will serve a lifetime of happiness.

ADVICE TO WIVES

If all else fails in your plans to remake your husband, you may wish to try the preceding recipe, which comes from a hundred-year-old English cookbook.

A Man-Size Diet

Eating in the modern manner means *cutting down* on hard fats, starches, and sugars, and *increasing* the protein foods. Men should be just as diet-conscious as women. Also, include as many fresh fruits and vegetables as possible. You may have difficulty at first changing your eating habits—do it gently and gradually. By all means begin by eating a good protein breakfast, because this greatly determines whether the day ahead will be hectic or whether things are taken calmly. Follow the menus given in chapter 4 for a healthful, high-protein daily meal plan.

A Malnourished President

President Lyndon Johnson was probably the most poorly nourished of our recent leaders. (President Ford's and ex-President Nixon's famous cottage cheese and ketchup lunches sound awful, but at least they are high in protein.) LBJ was frequently hospitalized and many of the disorders definitely had nutritional overtones. He was a heavy smoker during most of his life and drank lots of coffee. He was very fond of sweets; there was a standing joke about his fondness for tapioca pudding. A restless man, he often did not sleep well, usually had only coffee for breakfast, and sometimes skipped lunch because he didn't have time to eat. The evening meal was generally late at night, when, having starved most of the day, he would eat voraciously. Meals were repeatedly interrupted by phone calls so that he could seldom enjoy his food leisurely. In her book, *A White House Diary* (Holt, Rinehart and Winston), Lady Bird Johnson refers to the President's demanding schedule and his bad eating habits.

It comes as no surprise that President Johnson was hospitalized regularly. In 1937 he had appendicitis; in 1948 he was hospitalized for kidney stones and bronchial troubles; in 1955, while Majority Leader of the Senate, he had a heart attack; in 1965 he had his gall bladder removed. In between were bouts with laryngitis and respiratory infections. During his last days he was plagued by overweight, diverticulosis, chest pains, and other disorders. Finally he succumbed to a massive heart attack.

One of President Johnson's doctors, Lawrence E. Lamb, recently wrote a book downgrading the high-protein, low-carbohydrate diet many experts recommend. Dr. Lamb's suggestion for weight reduction is to count calories. Judging by President Johnson's abysmal health history, Dr. Lamb's book is not one that I would recommend. It apparently never occurred to Dr. Lamb and other medical advisors to investigate what the President was eating. Consequently, he was malnourished and afflicted with so many of the degenerative diseases that are a direct result of a lifetime of improper eating.

We have no way of knowing whether or not President Johnson took diet supplements. My guess is that he probably did not. With his hectic schedule and constant stress, it would have been prudent for him to have taken a good all-in-one vitamin capsule, vitamin B_{12} when tired and under stress, and certainly vitamin B_6 for better sleep. The heavy smoking depleted what little vitamin C he got from his meals. Vitamin E would have been useful in strengthening his heart muscles and circulation. Extra calcium would have also been helpful. Of course, good balanced meals, especially a high-protein breakfast to start his hectic day, would have kept his blood-sugar level functioning normally and might have prevented the subsequent overeating at night. Some exercise, rest, and relaxation would have rounded out an ideal regime. Presidents unfortunately lead rather sedentary lives. Only President Truman, with his legendary walks, apparently exercised regularly. No doubt this was a contributing factor to his long life.

President Ford, however, may well revive the idea of physical fitness in the White House. He is an avid swimmer (forty laps a day), he skis, and he enjoys many outdoor activities with his family. Perhaps this good example at the top will bolster nationwide interest in physical fitness.

SIX

INTELLIGENT DIETING

18

Reduce and Rejuvenate

Make Reducing a Pleasure

Once I wrote an entire book on reducing: *New Guide to Intelligent Reducing*. I did many years of research on that book. In it I explained why so many people overeat and described their physical and emotional problems. I gave recipes galore, diets and low-calorie menus, all worked out to perfection. I received hundreds of letters, in many languages, telling me that somehow, when excess pounds disappeared, feelings of depression and inferiority also disappeared; and all who wrote me agreed that they felt and looked much younger. Naturally, I was delighted that through this book, which is now in paperback, I could help so many people.

But looking back over the years, and talking to thousands of people here and abroad, I discovered that there is something wrong with all reducing diets and books of the past—including mine. Men and women the world over have developed a deep hatred for all prescribed diets and the pains associated with reducing. The chores of following a severely restricted diet are the greatest obstacles to slimness. Why, you ask? Let me remind you of what that wise man Sigmund Freud said: "The most powerful urge is to seek pleasure and avoid pain." This is the pleasure-pain principle, a biological and psychological truth.

Dieters and doctors, nutritionists and dietitians, all must remember that pleasure-pain is the most basic motivation of men and women; and unless we can turn the pains of reducing into pleasure, the most scientifically planned diets are of no avail.

Why Most Diets Fail

Let us be absolutely realistic. Every month, hard-working beauty editors beat the bushes for a new diet or exercise regime to take off pounds and inches. How many of them have you tried? How many have been successful for you? And how long has it taken you to get back to your old weight and measurements?

Quick-reducing schemes are all deceptive. They often show sensational results. But they do not change your eating habits. And so the quick miracle is a mirage. It cannot last; the pounds come back.

The Simple Arithmetic of Weight-Losing

Once and forever, let us look squarely at the mathematical facts of gaining and losing. The food that you take into your body each day is fuel. Your body uses up as much as it needs for the day's activities. What it does not use, it stores.

The body has three levels of storage. A certain amount it keeps in circulation as glucose—blood sugar—for immediate use. The next level of storage is in the form of body starch, called glycogen, and it is stored in the liver.

The third, the long-term fuel storage form, is body fat. This is the most compact form of stored energy. Any food that you eat in excess of your body's needs, especially the overrefined starches and sugars, eventually ends up as stored energy in the form of body fat.

These are the mathematical facts. There are no other explanations, no alibis. And don't blame your glands!

Women especially have a tendency to retain fluid in the body tissues, and this adds both weight and inches. These pounds and inches are the first to come off when you begin a reducing regimen, and that is why the results of a quick-reducing program seem so gratifying. But the moment the program ends, and you return to your normal eating and activity, the fluid seeps back into the tissues; and there you are, right back where you started.

The biggest handicap is that you try to lose weight without ever knowing *how* you gained it. You feel guilty, dissatisfied with yourself, obsessed with the question of just what to eat. But you have no real guide to how you can achieve your best contours *permanently*, until you know how you gained weight in the first place.

Let us check up a little. Compare your weight today with your best weight since your twenties. What did you weigh on your wedding day? What was the size of the dress or suit you wore at your wedding?

Now consider: what has changed in your way of life since then? Are you eating more? Or are you using your body less?

For Those Who Find It Hard to Reduce

One hundred years ago, an Englishman named Banting, who, incidentally, was an undertaker, made a marvelous discovery. He was short—five feet, five inches—and he was vain; his bulkiness made his life miserable. When he became so fat (202 pounds) that he could no longer see his feet, Banting became frantic. He visited one doctor after another. They all told him he was eating too much and put him on very low-calorie diets. These made him feel even more miserable; his whole life seemed a hopeless battle against his excess layers of fat. Then a new misery descended on Banting. He started to lose his hearing. Friends sent him to a fine ear surgeon, who obviously was a wise man. Instead of ordering surgery, this doctor put Banting on a diet different from any other he had ever followed. This time he did not follow a 1,000-calorie restricted diet; he ate foods he liked. In less than a year the hard-to-reduce Banting lost 50 pounds and 12 inches around the middle. But what made Banting happiest was that his hearing came back. So elated was Banting that he put his experiences in a booklet called "Letter on Corpulence." Today we know this as the high-protein, low-carbohydrate diet. In it he reported just what he ate and drank. Here was his daily fare:

Breakfast:	4 ounces beef, mutton, kidney, liver, fish, or cold meat (no pork); 1 slice of toast; cup of tea without sugar
Luncheon:	5 ounces fish or meat (no pork), or any kind of poultry, especially game; choice of any vegetable (no potato); 1 slice of toast; fruit for dessert; 1 glass of claret, sherry, or Madeira wine (no beer or champagne)
Teatime:	2 or 3 ounces fresh fruit; 1 slice of toast; tea without sugar
Dinner:	Same as luncheon
Before Retiring:	If wanted, a glass of grog or a glass of sherry

As you can see, the Banting regime was very high in calories. Thus it could *not* have been low caloric intake that did the reducing; it was the low, low amount of carbohydrates, as Banting himself wrote in his book—and which every modern nutritionist, dietitian, and doctor should write in *his* book: "I can now confidently say that quantity of diet may be safely left to the natural appetite and it is the quality only which is essential to abate and cure corpulence." Banting stuck to his diet. He omitted concentrated starches and sugars and kept his weight down to normal. He lived a comfortable and long life.

MORE SCIENTIFIC PROOF

In 1950 another distinguished Englishman, Sir Charles Dodds, before the Royal Society of Medicine in London, threw a monkey wrench into the well-established low-calorie-diet theory. He tested both men and women who had kept their normal weight for years. He now had them eat two or three times as much food as they were accustomed to. All of them stuffed themselves, yet none of them gained weight. It was discovered that the body metabolism of these normal-weight people was automatically increased; or, in simple language, the body fires burned brighter and did away with the excess food.

Then Sir Charles picked another group of men and women. This time he selected those who had weight problems and whose weight constantly fluctuated. These people were also asked to eat much more than usual. Of this second group, all gained weight and inches. Obviously, their metabolism did not rise; the extra foods were not burned and were turned into fat.

Here, then, was scientific proof of what happens to people when, sitting at the same table, eating the same meals, some gain weight and others stay slim. People blamed glands, nerves, disposition, digestion—but now, with the help of isotopes, scientists have been able to tag many food and chemical substances; and we no longer need to guess. The action of the isotopes can be watched and followed throughout the body. The metabolism of the foods we eat—the proteins, carbohydrates, and fats—is no longer a mystery. What Banting found out the hard way, scientists can vouch for today: it is the large group of carbohydrates, especially the denatured, overrefined ones like white sugar and white flour, that are the real troublemakers. They are the real enemies of the millions of men and women who gain weight easily but have difficulty losing it.

If you are that type, you should remember that your body obviously is not equipped to handle carbohydrates—the starches and sweets. For that reason, shun the empty flours, sugars, and cereals, and use even the whole, natural carbohydrates in modest amounts. According to Dr. Briggs of the University of California at Berkeley, even normal diets should have no more than 80 grams of carbohydrate. The "low-carbohydrate" diet now in vogue calls for 60 grams or less. At this rate you should lose weight.

Turning Point

As is so frequently the case, this new idea of not counting calories was not easily accepted. The doctors in England did not like to give up their established ideas that overweight is caused by overeating and that the way to correct it is to count calories and eat less. No one wanted to admit that Banting was right, until Drs. Kekwik and Pawan published their scientific tests of Banting's diet carried out in London's Middlesex Hospital. They announced: "The composition of the diet can alter the expenditure of calories in obese persons, increasing it when fat and proteins are given, and decreasing it when carbohydrates are given."

In 1951 Dr. Pennington went one step further. He wrote an important report based on his research with fat and high-protein diets: "The Use of Fat in a Weight-Reducing Diet." In it he had the courage to say: "Contrary to the claims of the low-calorie school of thought, low-calorie diets have failed." Dr. Pennington also insisted that "the ability of tissues to oxidize fat in contrast to carbohydrates is unlimited."

He also discovered that some people can burn only small amounts of carbohydrates—and any excess is turned into fat. At long last there was scientific proof of what Banting already knew and applied a hundred years ago: *Carbohydrates are the fat person's poison!*

Easy Does It

And now, instead of giving you a neatly worked-out 1,000-or 1,500-calorie diet, with dry toast, half squares of butter, vegetables without salt, and a carefully measured piece of fish or liver, let me pass on to you another important and almost forgotten biologic secret (especially if you are sick and tired of calorie charts and regimented eating): there is an easier, relaxed, and sure way to get back into shape. It has proved to be the best and shortest short cut to most reducing problems. You need only to remember these four major points:

Eat slowly, in a relaxed atmosphere.
Enjoy first-class proteins with each and every meal.
Cut carbohydrates (starches and sugars) to a minimum.
Chew your food twice as long; you will have twice the pleasure, it will help your blood sugar to rise, and you will feel nourished and satisfied with less food.

It sounds too simple to be true. Yet it is the simplest possible rule to follow. And it works—for reasons that are not quite so simple. If you would follow your natural appetite, and if your foods came to you directly from the fields instead of the supermarkets, it would be very simple: you would eat only what your body needs, and you would never weigh one extra ounce. *I am really more concerned with what you eat rather than how much. If your foods were truly full of their natural nourishment, you probably would never overeat.* And you would not have to count your calories, for calories *alone* don't count.

GET MORE PLEASURE FROM YOUR FOOD

We do not eat only to appease hunger. We also eat for satisfaction and pleasure. But most of the time we miss the pleasure. We gobble our food absent-mindedly, not knowing what we are eating. This gulping of food is an ugly habit, not only because lumps of food are harder to digest, but also because so much more food must be eaten before hunger is appeased. Long before I talked about this, Robert Burton, in his book *The Anatomy of Melancholy*, stressed the importance of *slow, conscious eating and careful chewing. In that way the appetite is thoroughly appeased with only half the usual amount of food.*

Our teeth, our jaws, our facial muscles were all made for chewing. According to Dr. Frederick Stare, chairman of the Department of Nutrition at Harvard's School of Public Health, "A certain amount of vigorous mastication is good for the teeth, gums and tongue, as well as for aiding digestion and hence nutrition." In his book *Eating for Good Health* he also recommends as I do, "foods that require chewing, such as raw fruits and vegetables." But what benefits most of all from chewing is the mind. When you chew twice as long, you also taste your food twice as long, and it gives you twice the pleasure.

Last, but not least, masticating your food slowly gives the blood-sugar level a chance to rise so that it can send signals to the appetite-control center (in the hypothalamus) that your hunger has been really satisfied. You automatically lose the urge to overeat. You will no longer need to diet. You can throw away all reducing books, including mine, because your psychological appetite, as well as your physical appetite, will be satisfied. That,

I believe, is the real million-dollar secret to most reducing problems.

When my friend Martha Deane, in New York, interviewed Carl Sandburg, the earthy and outspoken American poet said: "People eat too fast; they don't take time to appreciate their food."

Stop Stretching Your Stomach

A woman of average size has a stomach that can hold a quart of food. Yes, just one quart. A large person, a six-footer-plus like myself, has a stomach capacity of one and one-half quarts. Those are normal capacities. But a habitual overeater, a real *Fresser* as they say in German, or a *gourmand* as they say in French, can stretch his stomach to hold as much as six quarts! And once he has stretched it to that size, it will clamor for that quantity of food—until he disciplines it and reduces it to normal.

An overloaded stomach groans, prolapses, and eventually goes on strike. You do not have a six-quart stomach—far from it. But you can easily stretch your stomach by eating until it groans. You do not need all that food; you cannot possibly use it all up. But your thrifty body will not waste it. Your digestive system will process it, your liver will convert it, and your body will store it away—as body fat.

Seven Secrets for Smart Eating

1. *Chew,* slowly, pleasantly. The longer you chew, the less you will eat, as thousands of my students have proved.
2. *Enjoy* and appreciate every bit consciously. No more absent-minded eating that stretches the stomach.
3. *See* what you eat. We eat with our eyes, too (no TV dinners in the dark).
4. *Taste* what you eat. Satisfy your need for pleasure in eating.
5. *Refuse* to eat anything that does not satisfy your body's needs. No more empty carbohydrates.
6. *Take time* to eat. Satisfy your psychological need for unhurried pleasure in food, and give your blood sugar a chance to rise.
7. *Eat only for eating's sake.* Find other remedies for boredom, tenseness, and emotions. Thousands have done it.

Your Ideal Weight

Most people are at their best weight between the ages of twenty-five and twenty-eight. After thirty, with a general lessening of movement and exercise, weight seems to pile on gradually.

The following weights for both women and men have been painstakingly tabulated by the Society of Actuaries, an organization of experts, after studying five million policyholders. The Metropolitan Life Insurance Company has prepared these charts. Compare your weight with these new figures, according to your height and the size of your body frame. If you have difficulty ascertaining whether you are small-, medium-, or large-boned, let your doctor help you.

Remember that your ideal weight should be figured out according to these new findings, regardless of your age.

*Ideal Weight for Women**

	SMALL BONES	MEDIUM BONES	LARGE BONES
4'10"	92–98	96–107	104–119
5'0"	96–104	101–113	109–125
5'2"	102–110	107–119	115–131
5'4"	108–116	113–126	121–138
5'6"	114–123	120–135	129–146
5'8"	122–131	128–143	137–154
5'10"	130–140	136–151	145–163
6'0"	138–148	144–159	153–173

*Ideal Weight for Men**

	SMALL BONES	MEDIUM BONES	LARGE BONES
5'2"	112–120	118–129	126–141
5'4"	118–126	124–136	132–148
5'6"	124–133	130–143	138–156
5'8"	132–141	138–152	147–166
5'10"	140–150	146–160	155–174
6'0"	148–158	154–170	164–184
6'2"	156–167	162–180	173–194
6'4"	164–175	172–190	182–204

* Heights for women: with shoes, two-inch heels; heights for men: with shoes, one-inch heels.

Nonregimented Reducing Regimen

(HIGH-PROTEIN, MEDIUM-FAT, LOW-CARBOHYDRATE)

Have a Good Breakfast

I cannot repeat this often enough: breakfast is the most important meal of the day. Start with a glass of fruit juice, preferably fresh (but canned and frozen juices are permissible, provided they are unsweetened). If you are tired and irritable in the morning, drink your juice as soon as you get up. As your blood-sugar level rises, your spirits will also rise, and the world will look brighter. For your all-important protein, you can choose from the following: fresh eggs, preferably boiled, scrambled, or poached, with bacon; plain omelet; cheese omelet; chipped beef; or a quarter pound of your favorite lean meat: ground beef, liver, chops, steak, mixed grill; or ⅔ cup of cottage cheese. With any one of these you can enjoy *one* slice of bread, whole-wheat, gluten, or rye, toasted if you like, buttered lightly, or still better, spread generously with sunbutter (recipe in chapter 2; see index). Large cup of fresh or instant Swiss coffee. While reducing, it is best to forgo ready-to-eat cereals. If you like, you may have a cooked whole-grain cereal, but it should be cooked in skim milk and sprinkled with a tablespoon of toasted wheat germ.

Let your conscience and your waistline be your guides. Eat lots of protein, some fat (vegetable oils or sunbutter), and be a miser with carbohydrates (starches and sugars).

So that there is no possible chance of missing any important nutrient, take your vitamin-mineral concentrate at breakfast and be fortified for the day ahead.

Luncheon Time Should Be Salad Time

Heap a generous portion of your favorite protein food on a bed of green salad leaves (other vegetables such as tomatoes, cucumbers, radishes, and green peppers are permitted, but green leaves are more important). Take your choice of: hard-cooked eggs, lean meat, lean fish, Swiss cheese, soybeans, cottage cheese, or yogurt cheese. Salads should be mixed with a tablespoon of French mayonnaise or vegetable-oil dressing. For office workers, a pint of milk, yogurt, or buttermilk, or two hard-cooked eggs, with an apple or orange, makes a nutritious and satisfying lunch.

Midafternoon, If Hungry

Your choice of a large cup of yogurt, buttermilk, or egg tonic (recipe for German Egg Tonic in chapter 22; see index). For office workers, a handful of unsalted almonds or pumpkin seeds.

Dinnertime Is Relaxing Time

A half hour before dinner, enjoy a tall cool Vitality Drink—your choice of fresh vegetable juice or a glass of Hi-Vi tomato juice (see recipe for Hi-Vi Booster in chapter 4). Take your time, relax and unwind, and give your blood-sugar level a chance to rise. Then, enjoy a large portion (at least half a pound) of lean meat, fish, fowl, or cheese; a large green salad mixed with a tablespoon of vegetable oil or mayonnaise; and one short-cooked green vegetable with a teaspoon of sunbutter, vegetable oil, or margarine. Once a week, a Lighthearted Baked Potato (recipe in chapter 24; see index). Dessert should be fresh fruit, although nuts or lean cheese may be substituted.

One piece of bread (toasted only if you must), spread generously with sunbutter, may be eaten at each meal (but only if wanted). Milk drinks or Swiss coffee are the best mealtime beverages, taken at the end of meals. Under no circumstances should water be drunk while eating—only between meals.

These suggestions offer you a diet that provides a wide choice of foods and a chance to eat freely of the foods you like best. Anyone can plan tasty, balanced meals following the above outline. With a high-protein, medium-fat, and low-carbohydrate diet, you should not only lose fat but gain in health and vitality.

> "Any nobleness," says Thoreau, "begins at once to refine a man's features." This is especially true of overweighters who take the great step forward to reclaim their normal body.

Sample Menus for Reducing

Here are some menus to get you started. You can follow these or make up your own. But remember, lots of protein and fresh foods; use at least 2 tablespoons of vegetable oil each day; and go easy on carbohydrates.

Menu One

Breakfast: ½ grapefruit; 2 poached eggs; 1 slice whole-wheat bread, with sunbutter or margarine; Swiss coffee or tea; *best time to take your vitamins*

Luncheon: Salad bowl with ½ cup cooked shrimp, vegetable-oil dressing; 1 slice gluten bread or toast; 1 glass buttermilk

Dinner: Green salad with vegetable dressing; large lean beefburger, broiled; short-cooked green vegetable; fresh fruit in season; demitasse

Menu Two

Breakfast: Sliced orange; 2 scrambled eggs with fresh sliced mushrooms; 1 slice gluten bread, with sunbutter or margarine; Swiss coffee or tea; *best time to take your vitamins*

Luncheon: Salad bowl with ½ cup cottage cheese, vegetable-oil dressing; 1 slice rye bread; 1 cup yogurt

Dinner: Fresh vegetable juice; ½ broiled chicken; short-cooked green peas; fresh fruit in season, demitasse

Menu Three

Breakfast: Grapefruit juice; chipped beef simmered in milk; 1 slice rye bread, with sunbutter or margarine; Swiss coffee or tea; *best time to take your vitamins*

Luncheon:	Salad bowl with ½ cup lean ham and Swiss cheese, vegetable-oil dressing; 1 slice whole-wheat bread; 1 glass buttermilk
Dinner:	Green salad, with vegetable-oil dressing; broiled lean steak; short-cooked string beans; fruit gelatin; mint coffee

> GOOD NEWS: Russian doctors discovered that the constantly hungry and overweight man or woman should not despair on a reducing diet. With every pound of fat that is lost, the appetite will also decrease; the more you lose, the faster you will lose the desire to overeat.

You will not be hungry if you eat slowly and chew your food well; the longer you chew, the less food your appetite-control center, or appestat, demands. You can always eat celery, carrot sticks, radishes, and green and red ripe peppers to your heart's content; these are wonderful appetite trainers, and they keep an overdemanding stomach filled.

Should you be hungry between meals, have a cup of yogurt, buttermilk, or Hi-Vi milk. These help to feed the friendly "flora" in the intestines. Do not tolerate constipation; use natural laxative herbs—never mineral oil or synthetic laxatives. Office workers can satisfy any between-meal hunger with one or two apples. Before retiring, check up on your protein intake. Make up any deficiency with a glass of Hi-Vi milk, hot or cold.

19

Reducing Plans from All Over the World

How the French Reduce without Tears

Some of the most elegant people in the world come to our Centre Gaylord Hauser at 4 faubourg Saint-Honoré in Paris, where, under the direction of chic Colette Lefort, thousands of men and women have been shown how to eat intelligently.

The French are special people. They do not fall for fads and trick reducing schemes. For one thing, good food and pleasurable eating are probably more important to the French than to any other people in the world. Any diet that takes away the pleasure in eating is doomed from the start.

The 900-calorie liquid diet that fooled millions of Americans had no success in France whatsoever. Neither did the "Safflower Capsules and Fried Food" diet have any success there, because no Frenchman would live on such a one-sided, rich, oily, fried-food diet. Every Frenchman knows that rich fried foods are bound to play havoc, especially with the liver (the French are the most liver-conscious people in the world). French homemakers would never give up serving their butter, the sweetest in all the world; nor would they deny themselves their delicious fruits and fruit juices.

The thousands of French ladies and gentlemen who come to or write to the Life and Beauty Center in Paris are told to forget their reducing regimens, to throw away their calorie charts and scales, and, instead, to concentrate on one thing only: building up health and vitality. This means *stepping up* the basal metabolism—making the body fires burn more brightly—with the foods that do it best: the first-class proteins. For about a month, or until the ideal weight is reached, they are invited to eat freely of lean fish and sea food; fowl, preferably wild; and lean meat, especially liver, kidney, and other organ meats, including tripe, which is a great favorite in France. These meats are never fried, but broiled, baked, or stewed (with any excess fat removed).

Green Salads Are Most Important

The French love their salad greens, the greener the better. Fortunately they never heard of iceberg lettuce, the palest and least nourishing of all. Instead, escarole, endive, Bibb lettuce, romaine, and watercress are piled high in all the farmers' markets, and every homemaker takes pride in making a tossed salad that looks like shiny green gold. Such a salad, the bigger the better, is eaten with a good helping of meat or fish for lunch and for dinner. This protein and green-salad combination helps immeasurably to pep up lazy metabolism, and the green leaves help to balance the high acid content of the meats.

Vegetable Oils Burn Brightly

In Provence, where people cook predominately with fresh oils, they have fewer metabolic disturbances and overweight than in Normandy, with its rich cream cookery, or in Alsace-Lorraine, bordering on Germany, where the majority still cook with lard and goose grease.

A crude example of the burning qualities of animal versus vegetable fats is known to every cook. If you put animal fat in one pan and vegetable oil in another, you can see with your own eyes that the vegetable oil cooks cleaner and smokes less. In order to get all the benefits of vegetable oils, they should be fresh and cold-pressed. Use them not only for cooking but also in the form of salad dressing and mayonnaise. Most French women still make their own mayonnaise, which is utterly delicious and has no fillers or artificial preservatives. The favorite French salad and cooking oils are: olive oil, peanut oil, poppyseed oil, walnut oil, sesame oil, sunflower oil, and pumpkin-seed oil.

Remember: meat and fish proteins, eaten with a green salad tossed with a rich oil dressing, are ideal for pepping up basal metabolism and getting rid of unwanted weight without going hungry.

To prevent monotony, the following protein foods may also be eaten: eggs, not more than two a day (try a delicious omelet made fluffy in 40 seconds with the French thermo omelet pan). French yogurt, the best in all the world, made with lean milk, can be eaten two or three times a day, plain or with unsweetened fruit. This custardy milk food plays an important part in reducing and is easily made at home. Short-cooked vegetables, especially the green leafy kind, can be added to meals if the large green salad is not enough. Fresh fruits make the best desserts. Lean milk or decaffeinated coffee and milk is the ideal mealtime drink while building up vitality and losing weight.

Foods That Dampen Body Metabolism

These troublemakers should *not* be used if you want to get your body back to normal: all cereals, with the exception of wheat germ; white sugar and white flour in all forms; white bread (you are allowed one slice of 100-percent whole-wheat or gluten bread at each meal); cola drinks and all other soda pops; all hard and hydrogenated fats, with the exception of a tablespoon of sweet butter or nonhydrogenated margarine to be used on bread or toast.

Remember: These foods put a damper on body fires. Many people cannot metabolize them completely, so they are responsible for excess weight, which destroys health and good looks.

Vive la Différence!

The difference between the dynamic French diet and the many starvation diets is immense. First of all, you can eat generous portions of first-class proteins, plus green salads with at least one tablespoon of fresh vegetable-oil dressing. This mixture satisfies even an overdemanding appetite more than any other combination because it stays with your stomach longer than any so-called reducing food which "guarantees" that you lose a pound each day (but which you will gain back as soon as you start eating normally). These high-protein and salad meals will step up your basal metabolism and thus increase your energy. Men and women on both sides of the Atlantic report that this way of eating eliminates "that tired feeling" and re-creates a natural urge to exercise. The loss of weight is gradual—and permanent. Best of all, eating these natural, wholesome foods retrains the appetite so that the craving for foodless starches and sweets is gone forever. This is as it should be.

> When first-class proteins keep the blood sugar at an all-time high, false cravings stop automatically; your reducing problem is solved for a lifetime.

MOST POPULAR FRENCH REDUCING SECRET

Superlevure, a high-protein, high-vitamin, good-tasting brewers' yeast, has become a tremendous success. It can now be purchased, in powder form or in compressed tablets, all over France. Even supermarkets there carry it. The French take this Superlevure regularly, much as Americans take their vitamins. When on a reducing diet, the Superlevure is taken ten to fifteen minutes *before* each meal. Two teaspoonsful of the powdered yeast are taken in a little fruit juice or tomato juice; or four compressed yeast tablets can be swallowed with some water. Thousands of French men and women who have reduced successfully insist that regular use of their good-tasting yeast has kept them from being hungry and helped them to normalize their appetite. Since brewers' yeast is rich in both protein and B vitamins, it also helps to prevent tiredness while reducing.

FRENCH REDUCING MENUS

Here are three menus that will help you be as slim as a French mannequin.

Menu One

Breakfast: 10 minutes before eating: Superlevure (food yeast); orange juice; 2 tablespoons fresh cream cheese with a little honey; 1 slice high-protein bread, buttered lightly; *café au lait* or tea

Lunch: 10 minutes before eating: Superlevure; broiled lean fish with tomatoes; watercress salad, vegetable-oil dressing; 1 slice high-protein bread, buttered lightly; *café au lait* or tea

Dinner: 10 minutes before eating: Superlevure; fresh vegetable-juice cocktail; French omelet with cheese; 1 slice high-protein toast, buttered lightly; melon or fresh berries; *café au lait* or demitasse

Menu Two

Breakfast: 10 minutes before eating: Superlevure; pineapple juice, unsweetened; yogurt with honey; 1 slice high-protein bread, buttered lightly; *café au lait* or tea

Lunch: 10 minutes before eating: Superlevure; large endive salad with vegetable-oil dressing; large veal chop, broiled; 1 slice high-protein bread, buttered lightly; *fraises des bois* (strawberries) sprinkled with honey, or melon in season; *café au lait* or tea

Dinner: 10 minutes before eating: Superlevure; large green salad, olive-oil dressing; slice of lean broiled ham; braised celery; 1 slice high-protein bread, buttered lightly; fresh fruit; *café au lait* or demitasse

Menu Three

Breakfast: 10 minutes before eating: Superlevure; sliced orange with 3 heaping tablespoons fresh cottage cheese; 1 slice high-protein toast, lightly buttered; *café au lait* or tea

Lunch: 10 minutes before eating; Superlevure; breast of chicken, broiled; mixed green salad with vegetable-oil dressing; 1 slice high-protein toast, buttered lightly; *café au lait* or yogurt

Dinner: 10 minutes before eating: Superlevure; vegetable soup; boiled beef with carrots and leeks; French mustard; fresh fruit salad with yogurt; *café au lait* or demitasse with honey

The Truth about Cellulite

The dreadful word *cellulite* (not to be confused with *cellulitis,* a very painful inflammatory condition) has finally arrived from France, but the condition has existed since women began to sit down more, exercise less, and eat more starches and sweets.

Cellulite in plain language is nothing else but stagnating waterlogged tissues on the upper thighs and derrière. In more polite language, French women speak of it as *"cascade,"* which is exactly what it is—waterlogged, fatty tissues hanging in cascades from the derrière.

Just as a river deposits its debris where the current is slow, so is the debris of fat cells deposited where circulation is poorest. Notice you will never see cellulite on a swimmer, tennis player, or bicycle rider.

I believe cellulite can be prevented by more movement, a high-protein diet, cutting down starches and sweets to a minimum, and all the vitamins you can afford, especially vitamin C, which prevents capillaries from enlarging and causing sluggish circulation, varicosities, and that ugly dark color.

Beware the miracle cure. The massage devices presently sweeping Europe are worthless. You must work from the inside.

How the Russians Fight Bulging Waistlines

While in Moscow, I could see for myself that the Russians also have a serious overweight problem. After watching them eat, it became clear that one reason for their overweight is their shortage of good proteins. The average Russian diet is made up chiefly of grains, potatoes, and cabbage. Meat is expensive, and so are eggs.

Their best and cheapest sources of protein are cottage cheese, milk, and yogurt. Russian doctors emphasize exercise more than diet. After two conferences with Dr. Menshikov in his nutrition clinic, I learned how the Russians fight bulging waistlines.

Dr. K. M. Bykov, one of the most respected researchers, claims that basal metabolism is controlled by the brain, which in turn is influenced by the muscular activity of the body. The idea of overweight being caused by being starved for love or security is ridiculed. Millions who lack love and security are skinny, and millions of overweighters are happy with their mates and their jobs. According to Bykov and Pavlov, *the most important thing in reducing weight is the effect our muscles have on the brain and the whole body. Muscular activity, they say, rules metabolism.*

In reducing menus they stress raw vegetables, fresh fruits, lean milk, meat, yogurt, and kumiss; they permit one slice of dark rye bread with each meal.

Russian nutritionists agree with American nutritionists that you should not feel hungry while reducing, and suggest that you eat raw vegetables and fruits for bulk and satisfaction. They ask you to go easy on vitamin B_1 because it stimulates the appetite, and, above all, avoid the slightest case of constipation. To Russian doctors, this is a major necessity in every reducing program because an active bowel helps to get rid of cholesterol. They also stress having a big meal for breakfast, a midmorning snack, the main meal in the afternoon, and a light supper at night. The before-going-to-bed snack should be milk or an apple. Weight should be lost slowly—about one to one and a half pounds a week.

Russian Unloading Day

After you reach the proper weight, Russian nutritionists recommend an "unloading day" each week to prevent excess weight from creeping back. On an unloading day you can choose from different kinds of foods, but it is best to stick to one or two basic foods.

Milk Day: This is a popular one-day diet. On it, you may drink a quart and a half of fresh milk. If you are more than ten pounds overweight, use skim milk. If you are suffering from constipation, use yogurt in place of milk.

Apple Day: This is probably the most popular unloading day. It is made up of apples and apple juice. You can eat about three pounds of apples a day. The juicier the apples, the better.

Salad Day: On this day you can eat great big bowls of salad all day long. The more green leafy vegetables you use, the better. Always serve salad with simple vinegar-oil dressing, spiked with dill or your favorite herbs.

Fruit and Meat Day: On such an unloading day, you are permitted to eat two pounds of your favorite fresh fruit, and for your noonday meal you are permitted half a pound of lean meat, any way but fried. A cup of tea or coffee (nothing added) is permitted with meals.

On unloading days it is suggested that you space your meals two or three hours apart, such as eight o'clock, eleven, two, four, seven, and nine. Remember, these are just one-day-a-week diets.

Exercise Breaks, Not Coffee Breaks

The Russians believe that exercise such as walking, swimming, bicycling, and dancing, done willingly and with pleasure, brings joy to the body and stimulation to the brain and nervous system and peps up metabolism. The real control of body weight, according to Russian scientists, is physical exercise—or, as they call it, "muscular joy."

Each and every day of the week there are morning and afternoon "exercise breaks," when millions of workers stop what they're doing and twist and bend and stretch. Millions could be made happier with such cheerful exercise breaks, instead of those coffee breaks and foodless sweet rolls!

They say that a man or woman climbing a mildly sloping hill can burn up to six ounces of excess weight; climbing 300 yards on a fairly steep hill can burn up ten ounces of excess weight; climbing a hill for just two miles can burn up twelve ounces. The favorite form of exercise in Russia is bicycling (few people can afford cars); going to and from work they can burn up four ounces of body weight. I know that these figures seem greatly exaggerated to us in America. But in any case, muscular joy, or good sensible exercise in the fresh air, is of tremendous value in keeping the body fires burning brightly (increased metabolism). I only wish that more people would go in for more muscular joy.

> Combating overweight by diet alone is like fighting with one hand behind your back. Exercise is the other fist that enables us to deal the knockout punch.
>
> Dr. Jean Mayer
> Harvard University

The Thrifty Swiss Apple Diet

A short time ago the Swiss Fruit Association, in cooperation with Dr. Edouard Jenny, introduced an apple diet to the thrifty Swiss people. It proved eminently successful. Nothing was actually forbidden to the participants; only the over-all daily intake was restricted. The Swiss nutritionists emphasized a point that is important to every dieter the world over: that the dieters could eat the foods they were accustomed to eating. But to overcome the feeling of hunger between meals, they recommended eating apples.

Apples are low in calories, as everyone knows; but what most people do not know is that apples quickly satisfy the appetite, which obviously makes them an ideal food for a reducing regime. The apple diet was more popular and more successful than any other diet the Swiss people had ever followed. More than thirty thousand men and women who followed the diet wrote glowing reports to the Swiss Fruit Association. (Of these thirty thousand participants, 78 percent were women and 22 percent were men.) The diet became so popular that many hospitals and more than six hundred Swiss doctors recommended it. As a whole, the men had greater success than the women—and those who followed their doctor's advice had the greatest success of all.

Swiss doctors were delighted to discover that an extra bonus resulted from the apple diet: *people with high blood pressure, after a few weeks on the apple diet, found their blood pressure had become normal, without their having taken any additional medication.*

Dr. Ancel Keys's research in the United States proved that it is the rich content of pectin in apples that is responsible for the lowering of blood pressure. In these experiments, 15 grams of pectin were given, which equals the amount of pectin in about two apples. (The apple peel contains the greatest amount; therefore apples should not be peeled, only thoroughly washed.)

My students who eat apples when hungry between meals have discovered the following: apples seem to satisfy hunger more than any other fruit. Apples are cheaper and taste better than those between-meal preparations that come in cans. Three apples a day seem to give extra-soft bulkage, which improves bowel elimination. No rigid menu planning is necessary; the usual foods are eaten. And apples between meals seem to prevent overeating at the next meal, especially if the apples are chewed well.

The weight loss is gradual—no hectic seven- or ten-day diet—but it's a pleasant way of eating and retraining a spoiled, overdemanding stomach with a vitamin-, mineral-, and pectin-rich fruit that is easily obtainable. Slow and pleasant weight reduction avoids the tiredness, loose skin, and wrinkling so characteristic of "crash" diets. Homemakers do not have to prepare different diets for each member of the family. The diet remains a pleasant one, with sufficient proteins, vitamins, minerals, unsaturated fats, and carbohydrates of the wholesome kind—no empty starches or sugars!

One medium-sized apple contains:

vitamin A	50 I.U.
thiamine	0.04 milligram
riboflavin	0.02 milligram
niacin	0.1 milligram
vitamin C	3.0 milligrams

plus minerals, especially calcium, phosphorus, and iron

Eating apples when you are hungry between meals will also help to train your appetite away from sweets such as candies and colas. Most people do not realize that one candy bar has sugar value equal to that of about twelve apples. Our normal appetite control (appestat) automatically prevents us from overeating on apples; but it doesn't know how to deal with the highly concentrated sweets, because they confuse a normal appetite. Cutting out sweets and other harmful snacks, and substituting apples whenever hungry between meals, can within a few weeks help to normalize the craving for concentrated sweets.

APPLE DIET AS SERVED IN SWITZERLAND*

Breakfast: Large cup Swiss coffee; 1 slice rye bread, buttered lightly

Midmorning: 1 large juicy apple

Luncheon: (The Swiss take their main meal at noon) large cup clear broth; 1 veal chop; large helping red cabbage, cooked with apple; 1 potato boiled in jacket; green salad with vegetable-oil dressing

Midafternoon: 1 large juicy apple

Evening Meal: 2 hard-boiled eggs or Bircher apple muesli; 1 slice rye bread, buttered lightly; clear tea or Swiss coffee

Before Retiring: 1 large juicy apple, or glass of apple milk

APPLE DIET À L'AMÉRICAINE

Not too many people will follow such frugal fare, so here is an adapted Swiss Apple Diet.

Breakfast: Your favorite fruit or fresh apple juice; your choice of eggs, cheese, fish, or meat (once a week have the Bircher apple muesli sprinkled

---
* Recipes follow diet menus.

	with fresh wheat germ); 1 slice whole-wheat, rye, soya, or gluten bread, buttered lightly (toasted, if you like); large cup Swiss coffee
Midmorning:	Good-sized juicy apple, peel and all, and eat it s-l-o-w-l-y
Luncheon:	Salad bowl (be sure it contains a good helping of fish, lean meat, cheese, chicken, or egg, with vegetable-oil dressing); 1 slice of good bread, buttered lightly; clear tea or Swiss coffee
Midafternoon:	1 juicy apple, peel and all, and eat it s-l-o-w-l-y
Dinner:	Apple juice, fresh vegetable juice, tomato juice spiked with lemon and herbs, fruit cup, or salad with vegetable-oil dressing; good helping of lean meat, liver, fish, or eggs; 1 or 2 short-cooked green vegetables; twice a week, a Lighthearted Baked Potato (see index); fresh fruit or five-minute applesauce; demitasse or tea
Before Retiring:	Another juicy apple, glass of apple milk, or apple juice

This is how one day's menu would look:

Breakfast:	Sliced orange or glass apple juice; soft-boiled eggs, spiked with herbs; 1 slice rye, whole-wheat, or gluten toast; Swiss coffee
Midmorning:	1 juicy apple—eaten s-l-o-w-l-y
Luncheon:	Large cottage cheese and apple salad, vegetable-oil dressing and parsley; 1 slice rye bread, lightly buttered; tea or Swiss coffee
Midafternoon:	One juicy apple—eaten s-l-o-w-l-y
Dinner:	Waldorf salad, vegetable-oil dressing; broiled lean meat, liver, or fish; short-cooked spinach; Lighthearted Baked Potato; fresh berries or melon; demitasse or tea
Before Retiring:	1 juicy apple, apple milk, or apple juice

USE DIFFERENT KINDS OF APPLES

For variety's sake, try different kinds of apples. It would be ideal if you could get the fresh, home-grown variety, but not many of us are so lucky. The best-tasting apples, and richest in vitamin C, are: Pippin, Northern Spy, Yellow Newton, Baldwin, Golden Delicious, and Winesap. These can be stored in a cool, dry place without refrigeration. (The Swiss keep them all winter long in their attics.) Ease of storage is a special advantage for those who spend their days in an office.

Swiss Apple Milk

Cut one medium-sized apple into one cup of skim milk. Add one teaspoon of honey, and mix in blender until smooth.

Bircher Apple Muesli

For thirty years this simple apple dish has been the mainstay at the Bircher-Benner Sanatorium in Zurich, Switzerland. It is served for breakfast and dinner. When prepared correctly, the muesli is creamy and delicious. Simply soak overnight one level tablespoon of whole cereal (at the sanatorium they use oatmeal) in two tablespoons of water. Next morning, add the juice of half a lemon and one tablespoon of condensed milk, and mix. Quickly shred or grate one large unpeeled apple into the mixture, and stir in a tablespoon each of honey and fresh wheat germ. Serve at once. To increase the protein content you may also add a tablespoon of chopped walnuts, almonds, or sunflower seeds. Thousands of thrifty Swiss are thriving on this simple and nutritious dish. This wonderful food can readily be prepared from the commercially available Familia or Alpen. Just add fresh apples, and milk, if you like.

FRESH APPLE JUICE

Many people have never tasted this delightful nectar made from fresh ripe apples. Now that Dr. Ancel Keys has reported his amazing results with pectin in apples (normalizing high blood pressure), no doubt many people will eat and drink more juicy ripe apples. When eaten slowly, apples give bulk and fill up an overdemanding stomach. Fresh apple juice, with its vitamins, minerals, and pectin, gives a natural lift when taken between meals and curbs an unruly appetite when taken twenty minutes *before* meals, due to its natural sugar content. Since most of the pectin is in the peel of the apple, when making juice you simply cut the fruit into quarters—peel, seeds, and all—and put it through your rust-proof vegetable juicer. Drink this foamy white apple juice immediately; or add a few drops of lemon juice to prevent it from turning dark, refrigerate, and serve chilled.

Tip to the apple growers of America: millions prefer the milder acid of apple juice to citrus juices. Why not serve it in every bar and corner drugstore? The benefits would be tremendous.

There is a terrific new book out called *The American Cider Book*, written by Vrest Orton. In it Orton celebrates the healthful, pleasureful qualities of fresh, unadulterated apple juice, cider, and vinegar. I recommend the book highly; it will make you look at the humble apple with a new respect.

Fresh Raw Applesauce

Shred unpeeled juicy red or yellow apples on medium shredder or grater. To prevent the apples from turning dark, sprinkle with lemon juice. Sweeten with honey, if you wish. Serve at once in sherbet glasses.

Five-Minute Apple Dessert

Shred apples as above; sprinkle with lemon juice. Heat some butter and some vegetable oil in equal proportions in heavy skillet, to prevent burning. Mix apple shreds with enough butter and oil to moisten and heat. When thoroughly hot, flavor with honey and a tablespoon of toasted sesame seeds. Serve hot. A good substitute for apple pie.

The Japanese Way to Health and Longevity

In Japan, fish and soybean products are the main sources of protein; milk, eggs, and meat are terribly expensive. There are many fresh vegetables; these are always short-cooked, in vegetable oil, and they are used to stretch the small amounts of meat, as in a mainstay, sukiyaki.

More than any other people, the Japanese cultivate the sea— not only for all kinds of fish, but also for sea greens. In a Japanese market you may find a dozen varieties of sea kelp, sea lettuce, sea bulbs, and sea herbs. These are eaten daily, fresh or dried. A typical Japanese breakfast consists of a bowl of brown rice, a piece of tofu (a cheese made from soybeans and dried sea greens), and a cup of tea.

It is well known that all food coming from the oceans is rich in minerals, especially iodine, plus the many trace elements. But Japanese scientists claim that certain seaweeds are the best source of vitamin K, the vitamin discovered by the Danish chemist Henrik Dam.

Dr. Shichiro Goto, M.D., Professor at Kyushu University, has written a booklet explaining the virtues of seaweeds, stressing their high content of vitamin K. Dr. Goto, after reading my book *Look Younger, Live Longer,* sent me his book *A Way to Health and Longevity.* He quotes many Japanese scientists who stress the importance of undereating, rather than overeating, as a means of staying slim and young. In the Mishi Health Program, which is very popular in Japan today, the scientist Kondo, of the University of Tohoku, insists that the diet of long-lived individuals consists of large quantities of seaweeds and vegetables that are rich in vitamin K. According to these investigators, vitamin K has many functions in human nutrition. Goto claims that vitamin K regulates the functions of the liver, adrenals, and reticuloendothelial system, and has potent detoxifying and antihistamine action. They even claim that a lack of vitamin K is one of the underlying causes of heart and kidney disorders. Goto also points out that the rich supply of fish and seaweeds eaten by the fishermen and fisherwomen who cultivate the sea farms and dive for their living is responsible for their superior strength and long life.

I hope that scientists of the Western world will investigate and verify some of the claims Japanese scientists are making for sea foods. Is it the iodine or is it vitamin K that makes the Japanese so active and slim? These and many other questions need to be answered by our biologists.

Here are the nine vital points in Dr. Goto's Japanese-type rejuvenation and road to long life:

1. Have regular habits, avoiding mental and physical overwork.
2. Stop drinking and smoking.
3. Avoid physical and mental work under direct sunlight or in high temperatures. (Overheating is definitely aging.)
4. Ventilate your living and work areas, and cool them as much as possible without discomfort. Clothes and bedclothes should be light.
5. Do not take overhot baths. It is better to take baths of low temperature, even cold, especially in summer. If possible, rub down with a *cold* wet towel every morning.
6. Do not eat to excess. (Taking meals only twice a day is of significance.) Follow a diet rich in vitamin K, especially seaweed and green leafy vegetables. If sufficient fish is eaten, eggs and milk are not especially needed. It is better to take meat in small quantities, and *no* animal fat. When large quantities of meat are eaten, large quantities of leafy vegetables should be taken at the same time in order to neutralize the acidity caused by meat.
7. Drink fresh water on an empty stomach, especially in the morning, instead of boiled water (as in coffee or tea).
8. Regulate bowel movements. If help is needed, use only natural herbal laxatives.
9. Vitamin K, taken daily in small doses by mouth, is recommended to prevent disorder to cardiac function due to physiological decrease of vitamin K in older people.

20

My Seven-Day Elimination Diet

I created this, which is probably my best-known diet, in 1922, when I started my first food clinic in Chicago. This was one of the most interesting periods in my long career. People came to me from all over the country—rich and poor, fat and thin, young and old. They were sick. They had "been everywhere, tried everything." Now they came to me as a last resort. Many were skeptical about trying "food science," as I then called it. I had to work fast to convince them, do something basic to help all these overfed and undernourished people—overfed with foodless starches and sugars, undernourished in proteins, vitamins, and minerals.

Like all overfed and undernourished people, they were burdened with excess fat, while the tissues and fluids of their bodies, in varying degrees, were starved of vitamins and minerals.

My Seven-Day Elimination Diet is a seven-day housecleaning, a putting in order of one's physical house. It restores to the tissues and fluids of the body much-needed vitamins and minerals and affords an opportunity for the body to eliminate accumulated waste products.

What it does is to give the "inner man" a much-needed rest from past dietetic mistakes, and give nature a perfect opportunity to exert her marvelous capacity to rebuild the body.

You can go on this Seven-Day Elimination Diet (actually it is a feast) whenever you feel the need for a thorough cleansing. Springtime is ideal, for the first vegetables and fruits coming from the garden are especially rich in vitamins and minerals. But here in America, where we have fresh fruits and vegetables the year round, the diet can be taken at any time of the year. I and thousands of my students go on the Seven-Day Elimination Diet twice a year: before Easter and again in the fall. I am convinced that such periodic cleansings and removal of body wastes can prevent much suffering and premature aging.

Here, then, are the foods which you can eat to your heart's content for seven days and at the same time give your body a seven-day housecleaning:

Breakfast: Upon arising, after brushing your teeth, drink a large glass of fruit juice, preferably fresh orange, grapefruit, pineapple, or apple juice. In addition to fruit juice, you may have one or two cups of fragrant herb tea such as peppermint, strawberry, or papaya. These can be flavored with a little honey and a slice of lemon. It is best to do without coffee. However, if you simply cannot get along without it, have one cup of fresh coffee and drink it black. Should the fruit juice and a hot beverage not satisfy you, you might add some fresh or stewed fruit sweetened with a little honey.

Midmorning: If you want something more substantial, have a cup of yogurt, plain or flavored. You could also have a finger salad consisting of celery sticks, carrot sticks, slices of green pepper, or bits of cauliflower spiked with vegetable salt. If chewing is a problem, have a glass of vegetable juice.

Luncheon: One cup of Hauser Broth (recipe in chapter 22; see index), a fresh fruit or vegetable salad, a dish of yogurt, and hot tea with lemon.

Midafternoon: A glass of your favorite fruit or vegetable juice, fresh if possible. If something hot is wanted, one cup of peppermint tea with lemon and honey.

Dinner: A cup of broth, one short-cooked vegetable, a fresh green salad, and a cup of herb tea or demitasse.

Before Retiring: Take a twenty-minute warm relaxing bath. If bowels have not been moving freely, take some mild herbal laxative. If hungry, have some fresh fruit, fruit juice, or fat-free yogurt.

You can make up your own menus from the lists of fruits and vegetables that follow, or you can follow the menus. *The pint of yogurt which I have added to the daily menu is of great help, but do not use more than a pint if you are overweight, and be sure to use low-fat yogurt.*

Here Are the Fruits to Choose From

First Choice: Oranges, grapefruit, pineapple (whole or in juice form), lemon and lime juices in water

Second Choice: Apples, peaches, grapes, pears, apricots, and all berries

Third Choice: All melons, also papayas, pomegranates, and persimmons (no bananas during this week)

Here Are the Vegetables to Choose From

First Choice: Celery, carrots, spinach, parsley, beet tops, watercress, and okra

Second Choice: Celery roots, cucumber, asparagus, green and red peppers, bean sprouts, and eggplant

Third Choice: Red and white cabbage, sauerkraut, cauliflower, beets, zucchini, and young peas

Cooked vegetables can be spiked with herbs or soy sauce, not butter.

Don't let yourself get hungry. If you are working, take some fresh fruit, or some celery and carrots, to the office so that you will have something to eat during the morning and afternoon.

AND HERE ARE YOUR SAMPLE MENUS

Menu One

Breakfast: Large glass of orange juice or grapefruit juice; Hot beverage: your choice of peppermint, papaya, or strawberry tea with a little honey; black coffee, if you must; If still hungry, you may add some fruit such as melon, berries, peaches, or apples, or pears, fresh or baked

Midmorning: Your choice of any *one* of the following: fresh fruit in season or fruit juice (no bananas); raw vegetables in season or vegetable juice; tomato and sauerkraut juice (equal amounts mixed—an excellent reducing cocktail); yogurt (not more than a pint through the day); if you prefer something hot, your choice of hot Hauser Broth, hot tomato juice, hot herb tea (peppermint, papaya, strawberry), weak tea with lemon—sweetened only with a little honey or brown sugar; black coffee, if you must

Luncheon: Hot Hauser Broth or tomato juice; yogurt—1 cup; salad: cucumber, lettuce, green pepper (or your own combination), with yogurt dressing; choice of hot beverage as above

Midafternoon: Same as midmorning

Dinnertime: Hot Hauser Broth; spinach, or other greens, steamed with thin slices of onion; yogurt; baked apple; choice of hot beverage as above

Before Retiring: Same as midmorning

Check on your elimination. Take a simple herbal laxative when needed.

Menu Two

Breakfast: Large glass orange or grapefruit juice; hot beverage: your choice of peppermint, papaya, or strawberry tea with a little honey; black coffee, if you must; if still hungry, you may add some fruit such as melon, berries, peaches or apples, or pears, fresh or baked

Midmorning: Your choice of any *one* of the following: fresh fruit in season (no bananas) or fruit juice; raw vegetables in season or vegetable juice; tomato and sauerkraut juice (equal amounts mixed—an excellent reducing cocktail); yogurt (not more than a pint through the day); if you prefer something hot, your choice of 1 or 2 cups hot Hauser Broth, hot tomato juice, hot herb tea (peppermint, papaya, strawberry), weak tea with lemon —sweetened only with a little honey or brown sugar; black coffee, if you must

Luncheon: Hot Hauser Broth or tomato juice; yogurt—1 cup; salad: pineapple, carrot, and raisins; choice of hot beverage as above

Midafternoon: Same as midmorning

Dinnertime: Hot Hauser Broth: steamed cauliflower; salad: celery hearts and strips of green peppers; yogurt; fresh or broiled grapefruit; choice of hot beverages as above

Before Retiring: Same as midmorning

Check on your elimination. Take a simple herbal laxative when needed.

Menu Three

Breakfast: Large glass orange or grapefruit juice; hot beverage: your choice of peppermint, papaya, or strawberry tea with a little honey; black coffee,

	if you must; if still hungry, you may add some fruit, such as melon, berries, peaches, or apples, or pears, fresh or baked
Midmorning:	Your choice of any *one* of the following: fresh fruit in season (no bananas) or fruit juice; raw vegetables in season or vegetable juice; tomato and sauerkraut juice (equal amounts mixed—an excellent reducing cocktail); yogurt (not more than a pint through the day); if you prefer something hot, your choice of: 1 or 2 cups hot Hauser Broth, hot tomato juice, hot herb tea (peppermint, papaya, strawberry), weak tea with lemon —sweetened only with a little honey or brown sugar; black coffee, if you must
Luncheon:	Hot Hauser Broth or tomato juice; salad: cabbage and pineapple with yogurt dressing; yogurt; choice of hot beverage as above
Midafternoon:	Same as midmorning
Dinnertime:	Hot Hauser Broth; broiled eggplant (inch-thick slices) or summer squash; salad: sliced cucumbers; yogurt; fresh or stewed fruit; choice of hot beverage as above
Before Retiring:	Same as midmorning

Check on your elimination. Take a simple herbal laxative when needed.

21

More Million-Dollar Secrets

Purely Personal

For the past forty-five years I have followed my own teaching—eating intelligently most of the time. Twice each year I have gone on a week's housecleaning diet. Thousands of my students and I can vouch for the great benefits of such a regular housecleaning (see my Seven-Day Elimination Diet). Some years ago I learned about the many diet sanatoriums where people from every walk of life go to take tea, vegetable juice, and fruit fasts. I have always been one of my own guinea pigs, so I decided to take a fourteen-day trial. I wanted to see what happens when one stops eating solid food for two weeks.

I had the first surprise when I registered at one of Germany's most famous fasting sanatoriums. I was impressed with the elegance and cheerfulness of the place. There were 150 sunny rooms and every room was occupied. After an examination by the head physician, I was put on a fruit day. I could eat two pounds of fresh fruit—peaches, apples, and plums. This seemed meager fare after my vacation in Taormina.

The next day the head nurse brought me a pitcher with a pint of hot *Bitterwasser*, a terrible-tasting laxative drink—and that pretty nurse stayed right there to see that I drank every drop of it. When I thought I could not take another swallow, she gave me a spoonful of sweet raspberry juice. Eventually I emptied the whole pitcher of *Bitterwasser*. (I knew, of course, that this *Bitterwasser* was a terrific laxative, so I stayed close to my room.)

What surprised me most of all was the fact that I was not hungry that whole day—nor was I hungry throughout the rest of the fourteen days. During these two weeks, the nurse brought me a cup of mint tea for breakfast, a cup of clear vegetable broth for lunch, and in the afternoon, at teatime, a cup of herb tea with honey. In the evening there was always a large glass of fruit juice. This is absolutely all I had for two weeks—and I repeat, I never was hungry. When I entered Dr. Buchinger's sanatorium, I weighed 205 pounds; after two weeks I weighed 190 pounds and felt like a million dollars. Since I am six foot four inches, Dr. Buchinger decided that I was about at my ideal weight and suggested that I stop the fast. He recommended a one-week transition diet, consisting of fresh salads, fruits, cottage cheese, and yogurt, which I carried out in my own home.

I speak of this personal experience only to show you that the body can get along on very little food. Actually the diets in this book are banquets, and you need not ever feel sorry for yourself when you restrict your food intake *temporarily*. Naturally, all such strict dieting and fasting should be supervised by a sympathetic doctor. I definitely do not recommend that you, my reader, go on such strict fare for more than one day. Fasting, if done for more than twenty-four hours, requires supervision by a physician specifically trained in this branch of the healing arts—and a physician who knows your physical background and present condition.

Dr. Buchinger and his son are both medical doctors, but they have specialized in scientific fasting for many years. So far, they have successfully supervised the fasting of more than thirty thousand men and women, and the results they are achieving in all sorts of so-called incurable conditions are absolutely amazing. I would not have believed it if I had not seen the results with my own eyes. Tired, overweight, toxic, rheumatic people, with all sorts of vague pains and aches, looked brighter and lighter and seemed to take a new lease on life after a few weeks of fasting.

If you or your doctor are interested in juice-fasting, I suggest you write directly to Dr. Buchinger's sanatorium: Buchinger Clinik, 774 Überlingen-Bodensee, Germany.

Two American doctors seem to agree that fasting isn't a fad. (How could it be?—people fasted in biblical times.) They are using it successfully, especially on the hard-to-reduce and grossly overweight people. Dr. Walter Lyon Bloom, in Atlanta, Georgia, made his first experiments in 1958. He placed nine chronically obese men and women in the Piedmont Hospital and put them on short fasts, lasting from four to nine days, with excellent results. Dr. Bloom noticed especially that these patients were not depressed, and they were most enthusiastic about their weight losses. And, at the Pennsylvania Hospital in Philadelphia, another group of doctors, led by Dr. G. Duncan, has used fasting therapy with amazing success. One woman who had tried all sorts of low-calorie diets lost twenty-five pounds in ten days and never felt hungry. Dr. Duncan, a specialist in weight reduction, had this to say about fasting: *"This may prove to be one of the most significant breakthroughs in obesity therapy in the last twenty-five years."*

A Few Reducing Tips

Don't bore your friends with the intimate workings of your body while reducing. Keep those secrets between yourself and your doctor; he will listen patiently and advise you professionally.

Before starting to reduce, make up your mind not to feel sorry for yourself. You will still get plenty to eat. In fact, millions would consider your rations a banquet.

Loving wives, while cooking, should remember that all solid fats tend to settle not only on hips but also in a husband's arteries.

Sugar and cream in your coffee is a passé habit. Waistline watchers thrive better on Swiss coffee. The milk gives added protein and keeps the stomach contented longer.

Tiredness while reducing is often due to a lack of B vitamins and protein. Brewers' yeast is rich in both; the more you use, the better you feel and the more active you become.

According to a Hollywood psychiatrist, feelings of inferiority and even emotional conflicts seem to melt away with the rolls of fat.

If you have many pounds to lose, do not be discouraged. Promise yourself that you will lose just five pounds. That's easy! When you have accomplished that, promise yourself just five more. With this accomplished, you experience one of life's greatest thrills, the feeling of victory. Now nothing can stop you!

A wise husband can greatly help his wife to reduce by buying her an expensive and beautiful dress in the size she was when he fell in love with her. This works like magic for two reasons: the beauty of the dress and the fact that he *cares!*

A craving for rich, sweet foods is no manifestation of body need. It is a bad habit. Habits can be broken. Within thirty days you can replace your fondness for fattening sweets with a preference for fresh fruits.

Protein foods, with their specific dynamic effect, are 35 percent less fattening than starches or fats.

Lean meats, fish, and hard-boiled eggs keep the diet varied and flavorful and prevent that feeling of hardship while reducing.

Yogurt remains in the stomach longer and prevents between-meal hunger pains.

Chilled raw vegetables (see finger salad, chapter 5) help to retrain an overstretched, overdemanding stomach by keeping it filled longer.

Taking a balanced vitamin-mineral concentrate in the morning makes reducing easier.

Advice from Doctors and Researchers around the World

Dr. Herbert Pollack, of New York University, has said: "You can lose ten pounds a year by simply walking one mile each day."

Dr. D. T. Quigley, M.D., said: "We overeat on carbohydrates because they have no self-limiting action on our appetites."

Dr. Herman Friedel, M.D., English author of *Slenderness through Psychology*, said: "Get to understand the reason why you reach for a sweet . . . and you've taken the first and most important step toward slenderness."

Dr. Margaret Mead says that the American way of "dieting" and "slimming" by counting calories has something of the same pathetic rigidity that accompanied early bottle feeding. Eventually bottle feeding was modified according to the needs of self-demand or self-regulation.

Dr. L. M. Morrison, M.D., author of *The Low Fat Diet,* discovered that soya-lecithin is very effective in reducing blood-serum cholesterol and, therefore, weight. He also discovered that adding brewers' yeast and wheat germ to the daily diet was helpful in the prevention of heart trouble.

Dr. Hilda Bruch, M.D., has said: "Within every fat person is buried the real person, signaling frantically to be let out."

Dr. William Brady, M.D. and beloved newspaper columnist, urges his patients and readers to speed up their metabolism and lose their blankets of fat with a daily iodine ration. His favorite prescription is a tablet of dry sea vegetables that contains as much organic iodine as a large fish. Dr. Brady also points out a fact that is well known to dermatologists: dry skin and dryness, thinness, and poor growth of hair are often signs of iodine deficiency.

Dr. O. K. Alieva, as head of the U.S.S.R. Institute of Nutrition, tested four different fats on a hundred patients who had atherosclerosis and who had suffered from heart attacks. Patients were divided into four groups according to the fat consumed in their daily diets. The fats tested included sunflower oil (most popular in Russia), cottonseed oil, corn oil, and butter. The men and women eating straight butter had the least favorable results. Some improvement was reported by those eating cottonseed oil; those eating sunflower oil had still better results; but the best results were reported by those using cold-pressed corn oil exclusively.

Dr. Charlotte West, M.D., in her book *Ageless Youth* said: "Constipation is probably so little heeded because it rarely gives rise to actual pain. It does give rise to a vast amount of health and beauty defects. Who can be attractive with an offensive breath, a muddy skin, dull eyes, a listless manner and dullness of mind?"

Dr. Paul Dudley White, famous heart specialist, said: "Physical activity is just as necessary to life as food, air and water. People live by activity. It helps to keep your muscles in tone . . . it aids respiration, digestion, blood circulation and the elimination of body wastes. It is a law of nature that your organs as well as muscles grow stronger with use, weaker with disuse."

Dr. M. K. Horwitt, associate professor at the University of Illinois College of Medicine, presented evidence at a conference in Switzerland that an increased amount of polyunsaturated fats calls for increased amounts of vitamin E.

Dr. Laurance W. Kinsell, as Director of the Institute for Metabolic Research in Oakland, announced: "We feel the evidence is sufficiently strong to advise people to use a low-fat diet and take vegetable oils . . . oils like safflower, corn, and cottonseed tend to dissolve cholesterol spots and lower the cholesterol level in the blood." Dr. Kinsell believes the cholesterol count should be maintained below 180. He also explained how we can get the important linoleic acid in our breakfast eggs; when chickens are given safflower oil, the linoleic acid in their eggs is increased up to 30 percent.

Dr. Anton J. Carlson, a professor at the University of Chicago, used to say: "On the whole, we can trust nature further than the chemist and his synthetics."

Dr. A. S. Church, in the *New York State Journal of Medicine*, stated that there were serious evidences of malnutrition in over 80 percent of the 750 boys tested in a correctional institution; they were living on the worst possible diet of canned and processed meats, white bread, white sugar, jam, and soft drinks. When the diet of these delinquents was changed to include fresh fruits, fresh vegetables, nuts, salads, fish, cheese, and honey instead of sugar, these youngsters quickly became less aggressive and less quarrelsome. Their bad habits gradually disappeared. The most significant part of the experiments was that the difference in their *behavior* was amazing.

Dr. G. Lehmann, of the Max Planck Institute in Dortmund, Germany, discovered a million-dollar secret for those who tire easily. Instead of relaxing for half an hour at the end of the day, Dr. Lehmann suggests six short relaxation pauses of five minutes each. This prevents exhaustion at the end of the day.

Dr. Royal Lee, D.D.S., of Milwaukee, Wisconsin, said that chalky teeth, as a rule, can be converted into normal teeth by the use of calcium lactate and vitamin F.

Dr. Melvin E. Page, D.D.S., said it was well known in the medical and dental professions that sugar is not essential in the diet as an energy food. The general public suffers from the misconception that sugar is essential because of misleading advertisements.

Follow the Stars

Cary Grant believes that seeing yourself slim in your mind's eye helps you to develop a dislike for all fattening foods. It seems to work for Cary!

Bob Hope keeps fit with a balanced protein diet prescribed by his doctor. He also does specific muscle-tensing exercises and takes sauna baths. When Bob is asked about his secret for staying young, he says: "I lie about my age."

Ann Delafield, the ageless beauty who directed Elizabeth Arden's beauty farm, swore by a high-protein diet, plus two half-hour relaxing periods on the yoga slant board.

Queen Elizabeth II of England transformed herself into a glamour queen by eating frugal, balanced meals predominating in proteins.

Greta Garbo, a reformed vegetarian, learned to enjoy lean beef, even steak tartar, and lean lamb with dill sauce. Dinner starts with a huge salad and ends with fresh fruit. She is a champion walker (in earth shoes) one hour each day, rain or shine.

Mrs. Kingman Douglass, the vivacious Adele Astaire, trained her cook to prepare her favorite Southern dishes—but minus the hard fat and grease. Such delightful meals are kind not only to one's waistline but also to one's guests.

Lydia Lane, beauty editor of the *Los Angeles Times,* through her syndicated column helps millions of women to achieve their heart's desire. She believes that beauty is an inside-outside job and writes with enthusiasm about beauty-full eating and scientific body care. In her words: "A woman's beauty is not imprisoned by her skin; it permeates her entire home, creating warmth, love, and harmony . . ."

Julia Meade is a protein-breakfast enthusiast. She always starts her day with a glass of unsweetened fruit juice, and she boosts her vitality during the day and before performances with protein snacks. She loves yogurt and Hi-Vi tomato juice.

Anita Loos, famous author of *Gentlemen Prefer Blondes* and *Kiss Hollywood Good-by*, still has her tiny ninety-pound figure. Her favorite foods are broiled meats, especially calf's liver, plus huge salad bowls with golden olive-oil dressings, spiked with fresh garden herbs.

Mae West, the endurable one, does not smoke or drink; she keeps her body beautifully fit. Her secret? Daily exercise. Says Sexy Mae, "My father was a muscle man, and I learned it from him."

Princess Grace of Monaco enjoyed her mother's delightful German cuisine until she came to Hollywood, where she learned to diet. Now she eats a nourishing breakfast, a light luncheon, and a well-balanced dinner with lean meat. To banish between-meal hunger, there is always French yogurt in the palace refrigerator, as well as unlimited amounts of fresh raw vegetables and fruits. And see what a beauty her daughter Caroline has grown into. A healthful diet surely had some effect there.

Paulette Goddard is a high-protein enthusiast. She not only insists on lean broiled meats but also has taught her cook in Porto Ronco to make protein bread and soy muffins. Her favorite sport, waterskiing on Lake Garda, also provides an outlet for her tremendous verve and vitality.

SEVEN

RECIPES AND FORMULAS

22

Fabulous Proteins Build Beautiful Bodies

Today there is a new movement among intelligent people for food that is honest, wholesome, and healthful. Everywhere they are revolting against puffed-up white bread, foodless precooked cereals, ready cake mixes, artificially colored fruits, foodless white sugars and bleached flours, and all the highly touted hydrogenated fats that settle on hips and in arteries. Millions of people have gone back into their kitchens to try to re-create the wholesome dishes they enjoyed as youngsters. Many even bake their own bread. Fortunate indeed is such a family where someone practices the fine art of *tender loving cooking*.

I believe all who care about their own well-being and the health of their family can prepare delicious meals in the modern manner if they apply these five common-sense rules:

1. Undercook rather than overcook.
2. Learn to be more generous with the good proteins.
3. Be extravagant with fresh living foods, especially green growing things.
4. Use carbohydrates modestly, and only the natural whole-grain variety.
5. Be a miser with animal fats; in their place, use vegetable oils and spreads.

If you keep these five common-sense pointers in mind you can continue to cook your favorite dishes, with a tremendous increase of health and well-being. In the following pages you will find some old stand-bys, but you will also discover some new nutritious dishes that I hope will add to your eating pleasure.

At the moment, I am finishing my twenty-first book. *Tender Loving Cooking* is a new kind of cookbook. It contains more than a thousand utterly delicious recipes from all over the world that are full of nourishment and the most wholesome ingredients. To live a good health life, this is the only cookbook you need. Watch for it at your favorite health-food store or bookshop.

Let us start with our most important group of foods, the important proteins, our valuable meats and fish. Any cut of beef, veal, lamb, or poultry can be used, provided always that you cook it lean. The only products of the pork family I can recommend with good conscience are the smoked ones: lean ham and lean bacon (although there has even been some worry here about the harmfulness of the nitrate additives used to make the meat look pinker). Organ meats of all kinds, and especially liver, are super-proteins and should be used much more frequently. Also, fish and all foods coming from the sea should be enjoyed several times a week.

Learn to Like Liver

I know that fresh raw liver is not particularly appetizing to the novice or squeamish cook. It has a consistency more like gelatin or aspic than like steaks or chops. But once it is properly cooked—and that means very briefly—it takes on a delicate firmness that is quite pleasing to the eye and to the palate.

Liver contains first-class protein, is the best source of iron, and is a treasure house of vitamins. Old-fashioned cookbooks still tell you to soak all the good out of the liver and then fry it like shoe leather. But, actually, the less liver is cooked the more beneficial it is. Modern chefs know that tender calf and chicken and turkey livers should be quickly washed and quickly cooked—only until they change color. Beef liver, also an excellent food, is a little tougher, but it can now be tenderized. Lamb's liver, one of the cheapest kinds, is just as good nutritionally as the more expensive kinds. A fine old American custom is to have golden-brown onions with all livers. For variety's sake have some apple slices with your liver occasionally. To convince you of the amazing nutriments contained in one of the cheapest of all, lamb's liver, let me give you a comparative analysis.

	EXPENSIVE CALF'S LIVER (3 OZ.)	INEXPENSIVE LAMB'S LIVER (3 OZ.)
Protein	16.2 gm.	17.8 gm.
Fat	4.2 gm.	3.3 gm.
Carbohydrates	3.4 gm.	2.5 gm.
Calcium	5.0 mg.	7.0 mg.
Phosphorus	292.0 mg.	309.0 mg.
Iron	9.0 mg.	10.7 mg.
Vitamin A	19,130.0 I.U.	42,930.0 I.U.
Thiamine	0.18 mg.	0.34 mg.
Riboflavin	2.65 mg.	2.79 mg.
Niacin	13.7 mg.	14.3 mg.
Vitamin C	30.0 mg.	28.0 mg.
Vitamin D	45.0 I.U.	20.0 I.U.

Broiled Liver

If you can afford calf's liver, you are lucky. If you use beef liver, sprinkle it on both sides with an easy-to-use tenderizer, and let it stand for 30 minutes at room temperature. Then take ½-inch-thick slices and brush them lightly with a little vegetable oil. Place on broiler pan and broil 3 inches from the heat. This takes only 3 minutes on each side. Place on hot platter, season with herbs, and trim with parsley or watercress.

Enjoy Liver This Way

Take any fresh tender liver. Cut in noodle-like strips. If at all tough, sprinkle with a natural tenderizer and let stand for 10 to 20 minutes. Then put just 1 tablespoon of vegetable oil or margarine in a heavy, heated skillet. Sauté 1 large sliced onion to a golden brown. Add the strips of liver and sauté for just 3 minutes. Sprinkle with a bit of vegetable salt and serve at once. This is my favorite recipe for liver, and many liver-haters enjoy it when prepared this way.

Liver Loaf

1 pound beef liver	1 tablespoon minced celery leaves
3 tablespoons vegetable oil	2 tablespoons minced parsley
½ cup minced onion	1 tablespoon wheat germ
¼ cup diced celery	1 teaspoon vegetable oil
4 tablespoons finely chopped green pepper	¼ teaspoon paprika
1 pound ground beef	2 fresh eggs
1½ cups chopped carrots	

Have the liver cut in ½-inch slices. Heat the vegetable oil in a heavy skillet and sauté the liver a few minutes. Remove the liver from the pan and put it through a food chopper, using the fine blade. Add the onion, celery, and green pepper to the hot skillet, adding more oil if necessary, and sauté for 3 minutes or until the onion is golden brown. Combine all ingredients and mix thoroughly. Place in a well-oiled dish or casserole, cover, and bake 30 minutes in a moderate oven (375° F.). Uncover and bake 15 minutes longer or until the top is brown. If your family leaves any of this delicious dish, your dog will gobble it up.

Chicken Livers

¾ pound chicken livers	2 cups sliced mushrooms
1 tablespoon butter or margarine	2 tablespoons sliced onions
1 tablespoon vegetable oil	½ teaspoon vegetable salt
	Dash of paprika

Wash livers and cut into small pieces. Heat butter and oil in heavy skillet and sauté the livers, mushrooms, and onions over low heat for about 4 minutes, stirring occasionally. Add seasonings and serve.

High-Potency Tonic for the Heart, Liver, and Kidneys

Up to now it has been impossible to eat raw liver; but with that clever invention the blender, raw liver can be easily transformed into a palatable drink with the livery taste entirely eliminated. I highly recommend this Hi-Vi tonic to all who need nourishment quickly and in the most concentrated form. This liver tonic can win the *grand prix* every time for making rich red blood and rosy complexions within a few days' time.

Put half a cup of vegetable broth or chicken broth into the blender. To this add a tablespoon of fresh parsley and a slice of mild onion. Spike with vegetable salt and a dash of soy sauce. Turn on blender, and when the mixture is puréed, add one tablespoon of the freshest raw liver obtainable (chicken, calf's, or very young beef). Continue puréeing until the mixture is smooth; then pour into a cup of hot tomato juice or chicken broth. Stir and drink at once.

P.S. Not only liver but heart, kidney, and other inner organs can be prepared the same way; and they are also highly recommended by nutritionists. Raw organ meats are loaded with vitamins, hormones, and as yet undiscovered substances. Thousands of years ago Chinese doctors ordered their patients to eat young hearts for strengthening the heart. Who knows? Scientists may yet discover that specific organ meats help to nourish specific organs.

Calf's Liver with Avocado

1 pound calf's liver (¼-inch slices)
vegetable oil or margarine
1 large ripe avocado, sliced
¼ cup vegetable or chicken broth
Lemon juice
Vegetable salt to taste

Sauté the slices of liver slowly in the oil over medium heat. When browned on both sides, remove liver to serving platter and keep warm. Brown the sliced avocado in the same pan and put slices on top of the liver. Add hot vegetable or chicken broth to the pan and briskly boil down, stirring constantly. When reduced by half, pour over the liver and avocado. Sprinkle with lemon juice, add vegetable salt, and serve immediately.

Beef—a Favorite Protein

For Americans particularly, beef has long been the favorite meat. Properly cooked, all cuts of beef offer flavor and high nutrition, especially if the visible fat is removed. A low oven temperature for roasting prevents shrinkage and loss of vitamins. If you are cooking with moist heat (stewing), a small amount of acid (lemon or vinegar) acts as a natural tenderizer. When pan-frying or broiling, a little vegetable oil prevents meat from sticking to the pan.

Broiling Is Best

When you want a steak for broiling, ask the butcher for his most tender cut, 1½ inches thick. Ask him to remove all visible fat.

Preheat the broiling oven 5 to 10 minutes, at 400° F. Brush the steak lightly with a little vegetable oil. Then brush the broiler rack with oil. Place the steak on the rack about 2 inches below the heat. Sear it on both sides, then reduce the heat and continue cooking. (Usually the door of the broiling oven is left open, unless directions for your range specify otherwise.)

For a rare steak, 1½ inches thick, broil 12 to 15 minutes; for a 2-inch steak, 15 to 18 minutes.

One of the most important steps in preparing a steak is to make sure it is seasoned delicately, yet adequately. Have a platter of the right size hot and ready. To season the underside of the cooked steak, add about 1 tablespoon of vegetable oil to the hot platter, 1 teaspoon of vegetable salt, and 1 teaspoon of chopped parsley. Stir. Place the hot steak on this seasoning. Season the top of the hot steak lightly and quickly, adding a little chopped parsley. Pour any lean juices from the broiling pan over the steak. Garnish the platter with parsley.

Inexpensive Beefburgers

1 pound lean chopped beef
2 tablespoons wheat germ
½ cup water
1½ tablespoons nonfat dry milk

2 tablespoons chopped onions
2 tablespoons chopped parsley
1 tablespoon chopped celery

Mix all ingredients and make into 4 flat patties, ¾ inch thick. Put into a heavy pan with vegetable oil or margarine and brown quickly on both sides. Beefburgers may also be broiled on a lightly greased rack.

Budapest Goulash

Meat tenderizer
1 pound lean beef cut in small cubes
1 pound veal cut in small cubes
2 tablespoons vegetable oil
4 large chopped onions
2 cloves garlic, chopped
1 teaspoon vegetable salt
1 teaspoon paprika
1 bay leaf
½ teaspoon caraway seeds
2 cups puréed tomatoes
2 cups scrubbed, unpeeled, cubed potatoes

Sprinkle natural tenderizer over meat cubes; let stand for 20 minutes at room temperature. Then heat oil in heavy iron kettle or Dutch oven on top of the stove, and brown the meat with the chopped onions and garlic. Add salt, paprika, bay leaf, and caraway seeds. Heat tomatoes and pour over meat. Cover tightly and simmer about 1½ hours. If the mixture begins to dry, add more tomatoes or tomato juice. Add the potato cubes ½ hour before meat is to be done.

Beef Stroganoff

Meat tenderizer
2 pounds lean beef cut into small cubes
2 tablespoons whole-wheat flour
2 tablespoons vegetable oil
1 medium onion, sliced
½ pound sliced mushrooms
2 cups vegetable or chicken broth
2 tablespoons chopped parsley
½ pint thick yogurt
½ teaspoon vegetable salt
Paprika to taste

Sprinkle natural tenderizer over beef cubes; let stand for 20 minutes at room temperature. Then dredge beef cubes in whole-wheat flour. Pour oil in heavy iron kettle or Dutch oven and heat. Brown the meat on all sides. Add the onions and mushrooms and cook until golden. Add the broth, cover the kettle, and let simmer over low flame for about 1 hour. Remove cover during the last ½ hour and let liquid cook down to half its quantity. Ten minutes before serving, add parsley and yogurt. Season to taste with vegetable salt and paprika.

German Beefburger

1 cup ground raw carrots
1 cup ground unpeeled raw potatoes
2 tablespoons chopped onion
2 tablespoons chopped parsley
1 pound ground lean beef
½ cup chopped celery
1 beaten egg
¼ cup milk
¼ cup wheat germ
2 teaspoons vegetable salt

Mix all together, then form into patties, place them on lightly oiled shallow pan, and bake in hot oven (400° F.) for 20 minutes.

Veal

Picadillo—a Delightful Party Dish

2 pounds ground veal*
Vegetable oil
4 medium onions
2 green peppers, diced
1 clove garlic, mashed
1 cup sliced olives
½ cup raisins
½ cup blanched sliced almonds
Dash nutmeg
1 tablespoon chopped fresh basil (or 1 teaspoon dried)
1 teaspoon honey
3 ripe tomatoes, quartered
Vegetable salt
Bananas (optional)

Sauté the ground veal in a heavy skillet with just enough vegetable oil to cover bottom. Cook until all red disappears. Put veal into large pot or Dutch oven. In the same skillet sauté the onions, peppers, and garlic, adding a small amount of oil, until soft and golden but not brown. Add vegetables to veal in the pot. Add olives, raisins, almonds, nutmeg, basil, and honey. Combine well. Cover and simmer until all ingredients are blended. Remove from flame and hold until serving time. Just before serving, add quartered tomatoes and reheat. Salt to taste. Serve with fluffy rice. Fresh sliced bananas are often served on top of the picadillo.

*If veal is too expensive, you can substitute ground beef.

Chicken at Its Best

Roast Chicken

For this delicate, wonderfully flavored low-fat dish of chicken, select a bird not less than 3½ pounds, or a capon of about 5 pounds. Rub the bird inside and out with a little vegetable oil and lemon juice. Place the chicken breast side up in an uncovered roaster. Roast in a hot oven, 450° F., about 20 minutes, or until brown. Reduce the heat to moderately slow, 325° F., and roast, allowing 18 to 25 minutes per pound. For a plump chicken, roast a little longer, to be sure it is well cooked through and not red around the bones.

While the chicken roasts, baste it at intervals with beauty-farm basting sauce (see below). When the chicken is nearly done, turn it breast side down and let the underside brown evenly. To test a chicken for doneness, insert a two-tined kitchen fork into the thickest part of the breast and the second joint of the leg. If the juices do not run red, the chicken is done.

Some prefer the moderate-temperature method of roasting. (Protein is coagulated by heat, so as with meat, chicken is more tender when cooked at low temperature.) For this, heat the oven to 350° F. Roast the chicken at that temperature for 25 to 30 minutes per pound. (A 4-pound chicken requires 1 hour and 40 minutes to 2 hours.)

For a good poultry stuffing, mix about 3½ cups cooked brown or wild rice, add 4 chopped cooked prunes, and 1 chopped whole orange (seeds removed). Stuff and bake as described, allowing a few minutes more per pound.

For the added pleasure of eating herbed roast chicken, add 1 teaspoon each orégano and sweet basil to the stuffing; or add these herbs to the hot oil and water with which you baste the chicken, or to the beauty-farm basting sauce.

Delicious Beauty-Farm Basting Sauces

You can prepare a delectable roast chicken or turkey without using any fat, even in the basting. Prepare the whole fowl, or separate pieces such as breast and legs, for roasting. Roast as usual, but baste every 20 minutes of roasting time with the following sauce:

2 chicken or vegetable bouillon cubes
1 cup boiling water
1 cup orange juice
¼ cup lemon juice
½ teaspoon vegetable salt

Dissolve the bouillon cubes in the boiling water. Combine with the fruit juices. Add salt and mix well. Use for basting with spoon or pastry brush.

For roast *lamb,* skim the fat from the roaster continually during the cooking period. Baste the roast frequently with a warm mixture of white wine, bouillon, and a few chopped fresh mint leaves.

Blend tomato juice with bouillon. Add a crumbled bay leaf and a dash of dried rosemary. Heat slightly, and use to baste *veal* as it cooks. Wonderful flavor in the roast when you carve it onto warmed dinner plates.

Baste roasting *chicken, turkey,* and other fowl with a warm mixture of orange juice, lemon juice, and bouillon, flavored lightly with orégano and a little dried rosemary.

And, for superlative flavor in any roast, rub the meat thoroughly with vegetable salt before it goes into the oven. Basting washes some of the seasoning off, so add a light sprinkling of vegetable salt over the top of the roast after the last basting.

Modern Oven-Fried Chicken

½ cup vegetable oil
1 teaspoon vegetable salt
1 clove garlic, crushed

½ teaspoon sweet paprika
½ cup wheat germ
2 1½-pound broilers, quartered

Mix the oil, vegetable salt, crushed garlic, and paprika. Apply to the chicken pieces with a pastry brush. Roll chicken in wheat germ and place, skin side down, in a shallow baking dish coated with remaining oil mixture. Bake for approximately 1½ hours in a 350° F. oven. Turn skin side up after 45 minutes.

A NOTE ON FATS

Always remember that the younger the chicken, the less fat it contains. A spring broiler contains only about 10 percent fat, but an old stewing hen can contain as much as 40 percent fat. This is hard fat, remember. Don't you dare serve such a stew without skimming off the fat.

Turkey is another favorite and an excellent protein food. The fat content of turkey depends upon whether or not the turkey was fattened for the market, but most fowl contains only 10 or 15 percent fat. If you are lucky enough to go hunting for wild fowl, I envy you. All wild game is richer in nutrients and has much more muscle than fat, a good example of the shining effect of exercise. If you enjoy wild duck, pheasant, quail, or grouse, remember not to spoil these by serving greasy gravies.

Eat Fish and Live Longer

That's the slogan the Fishery Council coined after it was discovered that the fats and oils in fish help to reduce cholesterol; and, of course, fish contains the same first-class protein that meat does. Shellfish are slightly lower in protein because of their high water content. Fish is also richer in phosphorus and has the added beauty-giving mineral iodine. The fat content of our beloved steaks is as high as 40 percent, whereas the fat content of fish is only about 15 percent—and of the friendly unsaturated variety. Do not use a lot of fat in fish cookery. Just a bit of one of the nonhydrogenated vegetable margarines or, still better, your favorite vegetable oil, will seal in the flavor and nutrients. In Sicily they prefer straight olive oil; sophisticated Romans cook with half oil and half butter; the French, with their clever fish poacher, can cook fish with *no* fat, which is ideal. Short-cooking is the key to preparing tasty fish, especially when broiling. Overcooking causes fish to dry out very quickly. You know it's done just enough if it flakes when tried with a fork.

Here are a few unusual and delightful fish recipes, some from the sunny Mediterranean countries. Try them all.

Sesame Halibut Steaks

3 halibut steaks, 1 inch thick
1 teaspoon vegetable salt, about
3 teaspoons oil or margarine, about
2 cups soft whole-wheat bread crumbs

3 tablespoons toasted sesame seeds
½ teaspoon thyme
3 tablespoons melted margarine

Put steaks in an oiled baking pan; sprinkle with a little salt and pour 1 teaspoon of oil or margarine on top of each steak. Combine bread crumbs, 1 teaspoon salt, the sesame seeds, thyme, and a little more margarine, and spread on top of steaks. Place in oven preheated to 350° F. and bake uncovered for about 30 minutes, or until fish flakes easily.

Baked Bluefish

1 bluefish (approximately 4 pounds cleaned)
4 strips lean bacon
Chopped parsley
Lemon wedges

Split the fish and place on an oiled baking sheet, skin side down. Top with bacon slices and bake in preheated oven (425° F.) for about 25 minutes, or until fish flakes when fork-tested. Sprinkle fish with parsley, and garnish with lemon wedges.

Grilled Salmon Steaks with Herbs

4 salmon steaks, ¾ inch thick
½ cup dry vermouth or white wine
½ cup vegetable oil
1 tablespoon lemon juice
Generous pinch of thyme
Generous pinch of marjoram
1 tablespoon minced parsley
Small pinch of sage
½ teaspoon vegetable salt

Put the steaks in shallow pan. Mix the other ingredients and pour over the steaks. Marinate for 2 hours, turning once. Lift steaks from marinade and place on preheated, oiled rack and place in hot broiler. While cooking, brush several times with the marinade. Turn once, after 7 or 8 minutes. Cook until tender (flaking easily with a fork), in all about 15 minutes.

Broiled Lobster Tails

If you use quick-frozen African lobster tails, follow directions on package. Usually one package makes two servings.

Oil broiler pan or grid with a little vegetable oil. Place lobster tails on broiler, flesh side up, and season with a bit of vegetable oil. Broil in moderate oven (325–350° F.) for about 8 minutes (see directions on package). Baste twice during broiling period with a mixture of 1 tablespoon fresh lemon juice and 1 tablespoon vegetable oil. Then turn lobster tails over, shell side up, and broil for 2 or 3 minutes more, basting once more with lemon and oil mixture. Remove from broiler. Serve lobster tails flesh side up, with membrane cut for easy eating, and sprinkle with a tablespoon of finely chopped watercress or dill. Serve at once.

Lobster tails can be served hot with a hot hollandaise sauce, or chilled, with cold hollandaise sauce.

Delicious Meatless Protein Dishes

When eggs, milk, brewers' yeast, wheat germ, seeds, or soy products are mixed with vegetable protein they become much more nutritious. Such combinations can be enjoyed, not only by vegetarians, but by all those wishing for more variety in their menus.

Walnut Loaf

2 cups walnuts, chopped
2 cups whole-wheat bread crumbs
2 tablespoons soy flour
2 eggs, beaten foamy

1 medium onion, chopped
½ green pepper, chopped
1 cup Hauser Broth (see index)

Put all ingredients into bowl, mix thoroughly, and put into a loaf pan. Place in a moderate (350° F.) oven and bake for about 40 minutes.

Georgia Pecan Loaf

1 cup pecans, chopped
½ cup cooked brown rice
½ cup whole-wheat bread crumbs

1 medium onion, chopped
1 tablespoon parsley, chopped
1 egg, beaten foamy

Put nuts, rice, bread crumbs, onion, and parsley into bowl. Add beaten egg. Mix all ingredients thoroughly. Put in loaf pan and bake in moderate (350° F.) oven for about 40 minutes.

Savory Nut Loaf

¾ cup finely chopped nut meats
1¼ cups cooked tomato
1 cup celery, chopped
⅓ cup parsley, chopped
½ cup onion, finely shredded
1 egg, slightly beaten
1 teaspoon vegetable salt
½ teaspoon savory
1 cup dry whole-wheat bread crumbs
2 tablespoons vegetable oil
2 tablespoons wheat germ

Combine first six ingredients and mix thoroughly. Add the remaining ingredients and mix again. Pack into a well-oiled loaf pan. Bake in a moderate (350° F.) oven about 40 minutes, or until firm. Serve with lemon wedges, parsley butter, or tomato sauce.

Golden Carrot Loaf

¾ cup raw carrot, grated
1 small onion, minced
2 tablespoons parsley, chopped
1 stalk celery (including some leaves) diced
½ cup chopped nuts
2 tablespoons dry whole-wheat bread crumbs
2 tablespoons cream
1 egg, slightly beaten
1½ teaspoons vegetable salt
2 tablespoons vegetable oil
whole-wheat bread crumbs
2 teaspoons margarine

Mix thoroughly all ingredients but the last three. Coat the inside of a loaf pan with vegetable oil and dust oiled surfaces with remaining bread crumbs. Pack mixture into loaf pan, dot with margarine, cover pan, and bake in moderate (350° F.) oven about 35 minutes. Invert on serving platter. Serve with your favorite sauce.

Celery Loaf

½ cup celery, chopped
½ small onion, chopped
⅜ cup nut meats, chopped
¾ cup thick tomato juice
½ teaspoon grated cheese
1 teaspoon vegetable salt
1 tablespoon margarine, melted
⅔ cup dry whole-wheat bread crumbs
1 egg, well beaten
2 tablespoons vegetable oil
Chopped parsley
Tomato wedges

Put celery, onion, and nut meats through food grinder, using medium blade. In a bowl, thoroughly mix celery, onion, nut meats, tomato juice, cheese, salt, margarine, and all but 2 tablespoons of the bread crumbs. Add egg and mix lightly. Coat inside of loaf pan with vegetable oil and dust with remaining bread crumbs. Pack the mixture in pan, and bake in moderate oven until firm, about 40 minutes. Loosen sides with knife and invert loaf onto serving platter. Sprinkle with chopped parsley and garnish with fresh tomato wedges.

Oven Baked Beans—Inexpensive Protein

1 cup dried beans (kidney, lentil, navy, lima, or pea)
5 tablespoons vegetable oil
4 tablespoons molasses (or honey, or 3 tablespoons brown sugar)
1 onion, cut into wedge-shaped pieces
1 teaspoon vegetable salt
Juice of ¼ lemon
2 tablespoons brewers' yeast
Parsley

Rinse dry beans thoroughly, and soak 4 to 6 hours (or overnight). Pour into casserole, and add oil, molasses, onion, and salt. Add hot water *almost* to cover. Cover casserole, and bake in a slow oven (250° F.), stirring occasionally. Add more hot water as needed to keep beans almost covered until nearly done. Then add lemon juice and yeast, and return casserole to oven uncovered. Allow top to brown. Serve in casserole, garnished with parsley.

Special suggestions: Lima beans are delicious seasoned with garlic. Lima beans and lentils require no sweetening. Lentils are better with twice the above amount of lemon juice. Stewed tomatoes make a delicious vegetable accompaniment for any baked beans.

Quick Baked Beans—an Excellent Party Dish

There are many varieties of legumes, such as beans, peas, and lentils, that are canned in a wholesome manner. They can save you much time. But you may find them too bland for your taste. Here is an utterly simple and delicious way to make canned baked beans better:

1 tablespoon prepared mustard
1 tablespoon cider vinegar
2 tablespoons unsulphured molasses
2 1-pound cans of baked beans
1 sliced tomato
1 sliced onion

Mix mustard, vinegar, and molasses, and stir into beans. Pour in a pan or skillet. Top with tomato and onion slices. Heat slowly, stirring occasionally, until heated through (about 15 minutes).

These beans are especially delicious when served with Virginia bacon (the Duchess of Windsor's favorite). Place lean strips of bacon in a pan. Dribble 2 or 3 teaspoons of unsulphured molasses over the top. Place in moderate (350° F.) oven for 5 minutes, or until molasses starts to bubble.

Wild Rice Nutburgers

2 cups cooked wild rice	½ cup coarse chopped nuts
1 egg, slightly beaten	(pecans, hazelnuts, walnuts, or peanuts)

Combine ingredients. Form into patties, using 1 heaping serving spoonful for each; or drop from the spoon directly into a well-oiled hot skillet or griddle. These are for special occasions—wild rice is expensive. However, you can substitute whole brown rice, which is equally nutritious and also quite tasty.

Quick Wild Rice

½ cup wild rice	½ teaspoon vegetable salt
1½ cups boiling water	1½ teaspoons margarine

Add rice to boiling salted water. Cover and cook over very low flame, without stirring, for 15 minutes. Remove cover and dot the margarine over the top. Let stand for a few minutes in a barely warm oven or on an asbestos mat over a very low flame to dry out the grains.

The Wonder Vegetable

Soybeans—the meat without a bone. That's what millions of Orientals call this high-protein legume. Actually, this unassuming little bean is the only vegetable that contains a complete protein and can actually take the place of meat. It is also a good source of calcium, pantothenic acid, and vitamin B_1 (thiamine). So highly do Orientals regard this meat without a bone that wars were fought over the Manchurian fields where the finest soybeans grow to this day. Americans and Europeans so far have not profited by using soybeans, perhaps because they were once difficult to prepare. But now there are easy-to-cook soybeans grown in

America and Europe, so no doubt more soy products will be used by people of the West.

Everybody knows that soybean oil is an excellent vegetable oil, containing 53 percent of the valuable linoleic acid. Most people do not know that soy flour is as nutritious as egg yolks; and too many people have never tasted baked soybeans—a real stick-to-the-ribs protein dish costing pennies instead of dollars. Toasted soybeans are a delight; and they can take the place of expensive nutmeats. Soybean milk, on which millions of Oriental babies thrive, is a godsend for those of our babies who are allergic to cow's milk.

With soy milk it is possible to make yogurt and a nutritious cheese called tofu, or bean curd, but the real million-dollar secret is that sprouted soybeans are a superfood, containing protein, vitamins A, B, and C, enzymes, and auxins (a type of vegetable hormone). Soybean sprouts are indeed a "living" food. Everybody should learn to grow them. Use them fresh in salads. Use a handful when making potent vegetable juices. Short-cook them as for chop suey. As emergency rations, a sack of soybeans could keep a person alive and chipper for weeks, so versatile and potent is the honorable little bean.

Grow Your Own Vitamins

Simply cover the bottom of a glass baking dish with a layer of soybeans—the small Mung variety are best. Cover with lukewarm water and let soak overnight. Next morning, pour off excess water, rinse, and add fresh water to cover. Cover glass dish with its lid or another dish of the same size and place where the beans will have even room temperature. Twice each day, pour off stale water, rinse, and add fresh water to barely cover. Young, tender vitamin sprouts will appear the second day, and they are usually ready to eat by the fourth day. The shells of the beans can easily be removed. These bean sprouts are an amazingly rich source of vitamin C. You derive greatest benefit from them when they are eaten raw in salads or sandwiches. They are also excellent sprinkled over cooked vegetables, and wonderful when mixed into chop suey. Bean sprouts are indeed a wonder food. After you have learned the secret of sprouting soybeans, you should also learn to sprout whole-wheat kernels and lentil and alfalfa seeds.

Baked Soybeans (oven baked)

Baked soybeans can provide a welcome change. They are a fine and inexpensive protein. (If you are too busy to cook soybeans, I recommend ready-cooked canned ones.)

1 cup dried large soybeans	1 onion, thinly sliced
3 cups water	1¼ teaspoons vegetable salt
Hot vegetable broth	Juice of ¼ lemon
4 tablespoons vegetable oil	¼ lemon cut in thin slices
2 tablespoons unsulphured molasses	Chopped parsley or green onion tops

Wash the soybeans and put them in a kettle in which you can boil them next day. Pour 3 cups of water over them and soak overnight. Next day, bring to a boil in the same water. Reduce heat and cook slowly, adding hot vegetable broth as needed to keep the beans almost covered. Simmer for 2 hours, or until the beans are a light tan. Transfer to a casserole, and add the oil and molasses. Cover casserole. Bake in moderate oven (325° F.) for 30 to 40 minutes. Stir occasionally. During the baking, keep the beans barely covered with liquid. Remove from oven, add the onion, salt, lemon juice, and lemon slices. Return to oven, uncovered, and bake another 30 minutes, or until the liquid is almost absorbed and the top is brown. Serve from casserole dish, garnished with chopped parsley or green onion tops. Makes 4 servings.

Baked Soybeans (quick method)

You can save yourself time and work by buying canned soybeans. They are delicious and nutritious.

2 1-pound cans baked soybeans	1 tablespoon vinegar
¼ cup unsulphured molasses	1 tomato, chopped
1 tablespoon prepared mustard	1 onion, chopped

Pour the soybeans into a deep, heavy pan. Add the remaining ingredients. Heat over low flame, stirring occasionally, until thoroughly hot and bubbly (about 15 minutes). Makes 6 delicious servings.

Soy Flour Adds Protein

This is one of the most nutritious, least expensive foods of all. It contains protein, choline, and inositol. One tablespoon of soy flour has approximately the same food value as an egg. Soybean flour (available at health-food stores) can be added to muffins, biscuits, pancakes, waffles, and breads. Eating such soybean-enriched products for breakfast makes it easy to get sufficient proteins into this most important meal.

Soy Grits Save Money

These are made by chopping up raw soybeans in your blender until they are the consistency of finely chopped nuts. In this way soybeans are much faster to cook. Soy grits can be mixed with many other foods. They give a nutlike flavor to hamburgers, casseroles, and meat loaves. They can also be mixed with cereals. One tablespoon of soy grits gives an added 6 grams of protein to any dish. Actually, soy grits have formed the main part of the food supplies our government distributes to many needy nations. Soy grits are available at any health-food store.

How to Make Soy Milk

This vegetable milk is used by millions of Orientals. When milk causes allergies, soybean milk makes an excellent substitute. It can now be bought in cans, but you can make it at home as follows:

Soak 1 cup of large soybeans in 3 cups of water for 24 to 48 hours. *Pour off water in which beans have been soaked.* Grind the beans through a meat chopper, or put them in a blender until chopped very fine. Add 5 to 6 cups of warm water, and boil for 30 minutes. Strain through fine strainer; add a pinch of vegetable salt and 1 tablespoon honey. This milk can be used exactly the same as cow's milk.

Tasty Soy Treats

Delicious and nutritious as toasted almonds are these easy-to-make soy treats. Simply cover ½ cup of big dry soybeans with 1½ cups warm water and let soak overnight. Next morning, dry the soaked beans with a towel. When dry, put beans into a heated heavy skillet and stir until beans are a golden brown. Just before removing from skillet, add 1 tablespoon of vegetable oil or sunbutter (see recipe in chapter 2) and sprinkle with ½ teaspoon of vegetable salt. A great success when served fresh and hot at cocktail parties!

Eggs—a Wonder Food

More and more nutritionists feel that fertile eggs are preferable to eggs produced on the assembly line. The protein content of eggs is slightly lower than that of meat, poultry, and fish, but they do contain all the essential amino acids in such ideal proportions that they are often used as a standard in the laboratory for evaluating the protein content of other foods. Eggs are a treasure house of vitamins A and B_2 and iron. However, raw eggs should not be used habitually. The raw egg white can cause all sorts of skin difficulties and allergies because the avidin in the white combines with the biotin, one of the B vitamins, and so prevents it from getting into the blood stream. Biotin deficiencies can be responsible for many ugly skin conditions.

Eggs are nutritionally at their best hard-cooked, or at least cooked until the white is firm. Contrary to popular belief, hard-cooked eggs are not hard to digest. Each one contains seven or eight grams of first-class protein. Cook a few extra at breakfast-time to keep in the refrigerator for the next day or two. They have tremendous satiety value eaten with or between meals. They help to satisfy an overdemanding stomach. All healthy people should enjoy one or two eggs a day. *They are high in cholesterol, but they are also high in lecithin and the B vitamins that help to keep cholesterol on the move.* Unless your doctor has specifically forbidden you to eat eggs, I hope you will enjoy them daily. Eggs are also wonderful fortifiers of other foods. Always get the freshest eggs available, preferably (if possible) from a nearby farmer who has a rooster and lets his chickens walk on the fresh earth.

EAT EGGS IN EVERY FORM

Have eggs soft-cooked, hard-cooked, poached, scrambled, occasionally raw, and even fried (but use the friendly vegetable oils, such as sesame oil, which has a delightful flavor). Eggs fried hard in butter are definitely detrimental to good health and good looks.

Low temperature and short cooking maintains the delicate, tender texture of eggs. They should be kept refrigerated until the moment they are to be used *except* when they are to be used in a batter or when the whites are to be stiffly beaten. Eggs that are allowed to warm to room temperature will blend better, and chilled egg whites cannot be beaten satisfactorily.

Quick Pep Breakfast

Beat 2 fresh raw egg yolks into a glass of orange juice or any other unsweetened fruit juice. This makes an ideal breakfast or lunch for those poor souls who have to eat and run!

German Egg Tonic

Beat 1 fresh raw egg yolk into ½ glass of sherry. Sip through straw. German doctors consider fresh egg yolk the richest source of lecithin and prescribe this brain and nerve tonic for a quick pickup.

Henrici's Egg Pancake

½ cup fresh milk	3 tablespoons nonfat dry milk
3 fresh eggs	2 tablespoons vegetable oil
½ cup whole-wheat flour	½ teaspoon vegetable salt

Mix all ingredients in a bowl, or preferably a blender; then pour into oiled pie tin (be sure it is cold). Bake at high heat (about 450° F.) for 10 minutes, then lower heat to about 350° F. Bake for 10 more minutes. Such a puffed-up pancake is a delight. It makes an ideal Sunday breakfast served with lean ham or bacon. The chef at Henrici's in Chicago kept this delightful recipe a deep, dark secret for many years. Now it is yours!

Protein Soups—a Meal in a Cup

When meats and eggs are expensive, it is quite a problem for the homemaker with a large family to get 20 to 30 grams of protein into each person at each meal. Here is where fresh and powdered skim milk can be most helpful. With them you can make many delightful soups. If you have a blender in your kitchen, there are dozens of cream soups you can make on a moment's notice. One cup of such a gourmet soup can give each member of the family 30 grams of good protein.

Potage au Crème

The million-dollar secret of a French chef's *potage au crème* is the gentle sautéing of finely cut-up or grated vegetables in mild butter or vegetable oil. Leek and onion soups are great favorites in France, but any vegetables—spinach, parsley, watercress, carrots, celery, mushrooms, young peas, and avocados—singly or in combination, make a meal in a cup in a matter of minutes. A level tablespoon of good-tasting brewer's yeast adds another 6 grams of good protein to each cup. Here is what you need for one serving:

½ cup shredded or grated raw vegetables (carrots, celery, spinach, parsley, etc.)
2 teaspoons grated onion
1 tablespoon vegetable oil or margarine

1 cup fresh milk (8 grams of protein)
⅓ cup nonfat dry milk (22 grams of protein)
1 tablespoon brewers' yeast (6 grams of protein)

Sauté the chopped or grated vegetables and the onion in the heated oil or margarine. Be sure to use low heat; do not allow the margarine to get brown. Stir constantly. Put the sautéed vegetables, the liquid milk, the dry milk, and the dry yeast into the blender. Blend for about 15 seconds. Pour into a double boiler and cook for 2 minutes; do not allow to boil. Season to taste before serving. The onion improves the taste for most people, but it may be omitted. When using celery, remove the outside "strings."

Potage Hippocrates

If you are allergic to milk drinks of all kinds, learn to make nourishing soups and broths with meat stock, chicken broth, bouillon cubes, or dry brewers' yeast. The oldest of all vegetable broths was created about four hundred years before Christ by Hippocrates, the wise Greek physician. He recommended that a rich mineral broth be made with carrots, celery root, parsley, and especially leeks. Here is the ancient formula:

1 cup chopped or grated carrots   1 cup chopped leeks
1 cup chopped or grated celery root   ½ cup chopped parsley

Put all vegetables into 1½ quarts of water and simmer slowly for 30 minutes. This makes a rich combination of the water-soluble vitamins B and C. When Americans make potage Hippocrates they add some onion, tomato, and other flavorsome vegetables, and season it with vegetable salt. On beauty farms they add a tablespoon of celery-flavored brewers' yeast and call it their complexion broth.

Hauser Broth

This is the most popular of all the "alkaline broths." When I created this in 1922, it was called potassium broth. This clear broth was based on the Hippocrates formula, which he recommended to all those who felt "under par." My broth is now used on many beauty farms. It is also a part of my Seven-Day Elimination Diet (see chapter 20), which has become extremely popular as a one-week "housecleaning." Thousands of my students the world over take this diet in the spring, when all nature turns green and glad and when vegetables are at their best.

1 cup finely shredded celery,   1 cup tomato juice
 leaves and all   1 teaspoon vegetable salt
1 cup finely shredded carrots   1 teaspoon honey or brown sugar
½ cup shredded spinach   1 tablespoon chopped parsley
1 quart water   or chives

Put all shredded vegetables into a quart of water. Cover and cook slowly for 30 minutes. Then add thick tomato juice (or tomatoes), vegetable salt, and honey or brown sugar. Let cook for 5 more minutes. Strain and serve. A sprinkle of chopped parsley or chives will add vitamins, minerals, and color. You may add any one of your favorite vegetables or herbs. If you have no facilities for making this broth, you can get it in powder form at your diet and health shop.

Quick Avocado Broth

4 cups chicken broth (can be made with cubes)
1 large or 2 small avocados
Curry powder (optional)

Heat the broth to boiling point. Transfer to blender and add the peeled and pitted avocado. Blend for 15 seconds. Serve immediately in heated bowls. A sprinkle of curry powder is a delightful addition.

Giuseppe's Nutritious Broth

Into each bowl of hot clear vegetable or chicken broth, stir 1 fresh egg yolk. Sprinkle with finely chopped basil or orégano. When unexpected guests arrive in my home, my clever chef fills them up with a cup of this delicious broth. It always makes a big hit.

Silemi Lemon Soup—Exciting and Delicious

When Mr. and Mrs. Joe Lambert, of Dallas, Texas, visited my new home, Casa Silemi, in Sicily, the lovely Mrs. Lambert kindly offered to make lunch for me and my guests, after she saw all the fresh things growing in profusion in my garden. This delicious and unusual lemon soup was only the first course. It was followed by Picadillo (see index), which makes a delightful party dish—guests always rave and want the recipe.

12 cups chicken stock
8 medium cucumbers
10 lemon wedges (including rind)
Vegetable salt
Yogurt

Prepare chicken stock in advance, or use cubes or concentrate. Peel and remove all seeds from the cucumbers and cook them until soft in barely enough water to cover. Pass the cucumbers through mixer. Then add the cucumbers to the chicken stock and mix thoroughly. Pass the mixture through blender again, adding 1 lemon wedge for each cup of the mixture. Blend until lemon is thoroughly minced. Spike with vegetable salt and chill before serving. Just before serving, top each cup of soup with a teaspoon of yogurt. Makes 10 servings.

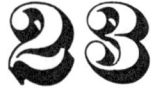

Sunlit Food

"*Un giorno senza verdura è come un giorno senza sole.* A day without green things is like a day without sunshine." That's what they say in the sunny Mediterranean countries, and how right they are! It's the fresh green growing things that are loaded with sun energy. The sun makes them "living foods," which are of greatest importance in a high-vitality diet. American food scientists emphasize, and rightly so, the importance of more protein in our daily meals; but some of them neglect to stress the importance of the fresh green things. European food scientists insist that *Frischkost*—fresh leaves, fruits, and seeds—contain the greatest health potential of any foods, and should be the mainstay of a healthy diet.

Forty years of research, teaching, and traveling all over the world has convinced me that the secret of any successful diet lies in its balance. And in balance there is strength.

Fresh, tender salads should be eaten as a first course. In this way they protect us against overeating, against vitamin-mineral deficiencies, against constipation, against overweight; and they are the best insurance against excessive acidity. *If the alkaline-tablet slaves would eat a good salad at the beginning of the meal, they could say goodbye forever to their alkalizers!*

At the beginning of the meal, appetite is keenest; and the

salad makes a good foundation for the meal to follow. Just make sure that salad vegetables are fresh and crisp. The green leaves, whether you use lettuce, escarole, or Bibb, should be washed *and dried.* The salad should be prepared just before the meal, and dressing added at the last minute.

French and Italian chefs are masters in making delicious salads. They consider it an insult to their guests if the salad dressing does not adhere to the leaves. This is their secret: after the salad leaves are washed and broken (by hand) into small pieces, they *must* be dried. If you have traveled abroad you may have seen French peasants swinging wire baskets filled with lettuce, escarole, watercress, field salad, etc., shaking off every bit of water. (You can, of course, buy such wire baskets in the United States.) Salad oils will cling to dry leaves, sealing in the chlorophyll, preventing the leaves from wilting, and keeping the salad fresh and crisp.

If you are lucky enough to have your own herb garden, cut some fresh mint leaves into half a cup of finely chopped chives, parsley, and young green-onion tops. Put these in your wooden salad bowl with lettuce or romaine. Splash with your favorite vegetable oil and toss with a wooden spoon and fork until the salad shines like green gold.

Instead of always using the loud-mouthed garlic, spike your salad bowl with a tablespoon of minced fresh basil, watercress, chopped green pepper, or fragrant mint leaves.

> Put the green leaves and other vegetables in the salad bowl, add the oil, and toss the greens until they are coated with oil. It is this tossing, lifting, and mixing of salad vegetables with the oil, which takes only a few seconds, that makes a salad a delight instead of a punishment. Then add the vinegar or lemon juice (the French use three parts oil to one part vinegar), and the salt, spices, and herbs. Toss lightly once more, and serve immediately.

Dress all salads well with vegetable oils. Season with vegetable salt and serve at once—while the herbs are still speaking to you.

Try These Delicious Salad-Bowl Combinations

    Leaf lettuce, Bibb lettuce, watercress
    Head lettuce, escarole, and Belgian endive
    Tomatoes, green peppers, parsley, and avocado
    Cucumber, artichokes, radishes, and watercress
    Apples, cabbage, celery, and fresh mint
    Carrots, celery roots, and field greens (dandelion greens, wild onions, etc.)
    Chopped red cabbage and red apples
    Chopped young beets, green peas, and onions
    Chopped romaine lettuce, grated cauliflower, and radishes
    Chopped carrots, green peppers, parsley, and celery
    Chopped fresh or unsweetened pineapple, red cabbage, and parsley
    Chopped Swiss chard, grated carrots, and onions
    Young spinach, cabbage, and watercress
    Thinly sliced Spanish onion, chicory, and spinach
    Green apples, radishes, and watercress
    Cucumbers, tomatoes, and avocados
    Chopped endive, sliced beets, and watercress
    Cabbage, carrots, celery, and finocchio (fennel)

These salad-bowl combinations are especially good when served with meat or other good proteins. Or combine the proteins and the fresh, green, growing things in one dish. Such salad bowls are available at all good restaurants, but you will also want to make them at home. Always make a bed of greens, breaking them into bits by hand. Add vegetables, raw or cooked, and chopped fine. Then add any of your favorite proteins, depending on your taste and pocketbook—half a cup or more of tuna fish, salmon, lean ham, Swiss cheese, chicken, hard-boiled eggs—all make delightful luncheon dishes. Or you can use any leftover meat or, still better, use cottage cheese or homemade cream cheese. The protein in these cheeses is just as valuable as that in meat. Mix your protein and salad greens with at least a tablespoon of vegetable-oil dressing. All you need with such a salad is one slice of wholesome bread—whole-wheat, soya, or rye. A glass of milk, buttermilk, yogurt, or Swiss coffee, and you have a nourishing luncheon, fit for a king!

To make a delightful salad dressing, you may want to combine several oils. Safflower oil alone is a great favorite, but it becomes rancid quickly. The other oils seem to be more stable. Sesame oil is mildest in flavor. Sunflower oil is probably the easiest to keep. In Germany linseed oil, which is quite strong-flavored, is very popular; and in France people prefer olive oil mixed with cold-pressed peanut oil. Please make your dressings fresh and keep them refrigerated. Last, and very important, *the use of vegetable oils increases the need for vitamin E, so be sure to add a tablespoon of fresh wheat-germ oil whenever you make a batch of vegetable oil dressing or mayonnaise.*

Swiss Herb Vinegar

Put your favorite herbs into pure cider or wine vinegar. The Swiss prefer a mixture of dill, mint, and tarragon. (Remove leaves from stems.) To get a full-bodied delightful *Krauteressig*, just put 1 cup each of fresh dill, mint, and tarragon leaves in a gallon of vinegar. Place bottles in a warm and sunny place and cork tightly. After 3 or 4 weeks, strain; put into clean bottles and cork tightly.

Fabulous Salad Dressing

½ cup sunflower oil
½ cup peanut oil
½ cup olive oil
½ cup cider, wine, or herb vinegar

1 tablespoon wheat-germ oil
2 teaspoons honey
2 teaspoons vegetable salt
1 clove garlic

Place all ingredients in a covered jar and shake vigorously. Store in the refrigerator. You can give it a different flavor every time you use it by adding your choice of: 2 tablespoons of chopped fresh parsley, fresh chives, fresh mint, mild onion, or dried herbs; ½ teaspoon of orégano or curry powder; 1 teaspoon dried mustard; 2 tablespoons Roquefort cheese; 2 tablespoons chopped ripe olives. Use your imagination. There is absolutely no limit to the number of delightful salad dressing combinations you can enjoy. *The million-dollar secret of this dressing is that it contains* everything—*all the essential fatty acids, plus lecithin and vitamin E—and it tastes delicious.* Should it be too rich for your taste or your pocketbook, do not hesitate to use some of the less expensive oils; but do be sure they are cold-pressed and fresh. Look for them in your health-food store.

French Fourteen-Carat-Gold Mayonnaise

½ cup olive oil
½ cup peanut oil
1 tablespoon wheat-germ oil

2 fresh egg yolks
1 tablespoon wine vinegar
½ teaspoon vegetable salt

Mix oils in a measuring cup. Place fresh egg yolks in cold bowl and beat. Add a little oil very slowly and beat with rotary beater or a whisk. Gradually add more oil. As mixture thickens, add vinegar and salt. Beat until thick and golden.

French Yogurt Dressing

Mix 4 tablespoons of yogurt with 4 tablespoons of French Fourteen-Carat-Gold Mayonnaise. Beat to consistency of heavy cream. Add a tablespoon of finely chopped carrots or parsley. This is particularly good with freshly chopped raw vegetables.

Avocado Dressing

1 cup avocado pulp
1 cup thick yogurt
1 tablespoon honey
1 tablespoon vegetable oil

¼ teaspoon vegetable salt
Dash of favorite herbs
1 tablespoon lemon juice

Place all ingredients in blender for 1 minute. This mixture is especially delicious with citrus and fruit salads.

SUNLIT APPETIZERS

That is what they call their fresh young vegetables along the balmy Mediterranean. You and your guests can eat these with good conscience. They are not only healthful, they are the most beautiful and sophisticated appetizers or hors d'oeuvres you can serve. A plateful of raw vegetable tidbits is served with a bowl containing a nutritious dip made from fresh yogurt, cream cheese, or cottage cheese, or a combination of all three, blended with fresh lemon juice, onion juice, chopped chives or dill, a tablespoon of vegetable oil, and any of your favorite fresh or dry herbs. The dip should be stiff enough to cling to the vegetables without dripping. There are literally hundreds of recipes for dips. Just use your imagination. Add your seasonings a little at a time, and keep tasting until you have a delightful aromatic blend. For more fun and nutrition, try adding minced olives or clams or a mashed avocado.

You will be surprised at the number of vegetables that can be served: fresh raw carrots, cauliflower, sweet green or red peppers, celery, turnip, small zucchini, cucumber, young asparagus tips, tiny cherry tomatoes, red and white radishes, Belgian endive, mushrooms, Chinese cabbage, Italian finocchio, and—for strictly family gatherings—green onions! The carrots, zucchinis, cucumbers, and peppers should be cut the long way into slim fingers. Cut the cauliflower into flowerets, always leaving a piece of the stem to serve as a handle. Put ice cubes over the vegetables to crisp them before serving and to preserve the vitamins.

Sunlit Food Needs Little Cooking

Fresh garden vegetables have the greatest health and beauty potential when served raw. A raw, fresh salad is a must with every big meal. Cooked vegetables, delicious as they are, should play a secondary role in a high-vitality diet. *If the budget is limited, a good protein dish with a large salad makes an excellent meal.* Of course, there is no reason why you should not also enjoy cooked vegetables. Just remember: the less you cook them, the richer they remain in vitamins and enzymes.

The Chinese, more than any other people, know the art of short-cooking. For centuries they have cooked their vegetables in the quickest and most appetizing manner in a heavy, hot pan. No saturated fats are ever used; instead, they use such oils as soybean, sesame, or poppyseed. Everybody likes short-cooked vegetables simply because they taste much better than the water-soaked, overcooked variety. The big secret in short-cooking is to cut the vegetables in small pieces or slices and place them as quickly as possible in a very hot utensil; and so the vegetable will not burn, put 2 or 3 tablespoons of chicken broth, vegetable water, or just plain water in the pan and drop the finely cut vegetables into this steaming liquid. Keep utensil covered for 2 or 3 minutes; let the steam tenderize the vegetable. When thoroughly tenderized, add a tablespoon of vegetable oil or sunbutter (see index) for each cup of vegetable. Spike with soy sauce, vegetable salt, and any herbs you desire.

Leafy Vegetables

Pick over spinach, beet tops, turnip tops, and all green, leafy vegetables while dry. Then put the greens in a large pan and let the cold water run until greens are clean and crisp. Place them in a hot, heavy cooking utensil. Greens usually contain enough water of their own and do not require added water for short-cooking. Cook, keeping utensil covered for 2 or 3 minutes; then add vegetable oil, sunbutter, or nonhydrogenated margarine. Spike with vegetable salt and herbs.

Golden Carrots

Scrub them until they shine like gold. Then shred them medium (not too fine). Have 2 or 3 tablespoons of chicken broth steaming in hot utensil. Add shredded carrots. Cover for 3 minutes or until tenderized but not soft and soggy. Add a tablespoon of vegetable oil for each cup of carrots, and sprinkle with vegetable salt. These carrots will still be a bit chewy and keep their golden color; and they are unbelievably delicious.

Rose Petal Beets

Select small young beets. Scrub, and shred on medium shredder or grater. Heat a small heavy pan, and add 3 tablespoons of chicken or vegetable broth. When liquid is steaming, add shredded beets. Cover tightly and cook for about 5 minutes, depending on tenderness of beets. Then add sunbutter or vegetable oil, and sprinkle with vegetable salt. Short-cooked beets keep their rose-petal color and have a nutlike flavor all their own.

Easy-to-Digest Cabbage

Shred young white or red cabbage on coarse grater. Heat small heavy utensil and add 3 tablespoons of steaming broth. Place cabbage in pan and keep tightly covered. Young cabbage cooks in 3 to 5 minutes, and is easy to digest. All you add is a little vegetable salt and a bit of sunbutter or vegetable oil.

Delicious Cauliflower

Select a young white cauliflower. Shred on coarse blade. (Shred not only the flower but the whole stem.) Have heavy small utensil steaming with 3 tablespoons of vegetable or chicken broth. Drop in the white shreds and let cook, tightly covered, for about 4 to 6 minutes. They will cook tender but still chewy, and the shreds will keep their appetizing white color. Now add vegetable salt and a bit of sunbutter, and enjoy this new delicious flavor.

Young String Beans

Tender green or yellow beans can be finely shredded lengthwise and placed in small, heavy, hot utensil with 3 tablespoons of steaming broth. Cook tightly covered about 7 minutes. When tender, add vegetable oil or sunbutter and vegetable salt.

Elegant Beans Amandine

Short-cook the youngest and smallest green beans obtainable. In an iron skillet, toast coarsely chopped or slivered almonds to a golden brown. Sprinkle the toasted almonds over the very hot beans and serve at once. Any meal becomes a banquet with such a festive vegetable.

Italian Zucchini

Select small zucchini; do not peel, only scrub with a brush. Slice thin or shred on coarse shredder. Put 3 tablespoons of vegetable or chicken broth in small heavy utensil; when broth steams, add shredded zucchini and cook, tightly covered, for only 3 to 5 minutes. Add vegetable oil or sunbutter and sprinkle with vegetable salt.

Easy Eggplant

Wash but do not peel young, tender eggplant. Shred on coarse shredder. Cook in heavy covered pot in 2 tablespoons of steaming hot vegetable or chicken broth for about 5 minutes. Then add vegetable oil and your favorite seasonings.

Eggplant Toast

Cut unpeeled eggplant into ½-inch slices. Put under slow broiler and toast until golden brown. Spike with vegetable salt. Delicious under poached eggs. A favorite on sophisticated beauty farms.

Delightful Chinese Dishes

Chinese restaurants—even those specializing in spicy regional cuisines, such as Hunanese and Szechuanese—have sprung up everywhere. Chinese cookery requires a maximum of preparation and a minimum of cooking time and fuel. At Don the Beachcomber's in Hollywood there are bowls of neatly sliced and stacked vegetables (celery, bamboo shoots, water chestnuts, spinach, etc.), fresh and crisp, bowls full of sliced lean meats, all in refrigerators within easy reach of the chef. Upon receipt of an order, it takes him only a few seconds to select his ingredients, a skillful blending of meats and vegetables, and within ten or fifteen minutes a delicious meal is ready to serve. Only vegetable oils are used, never any hard fat. When necessary, a small amount of broth is added; seasonings such as soy sauce and vegetable salt are always added last.

Most Chinese recipes require too many special ingredients to make them popular for home cooking. However, there is no reason why we should not include a few Chinese-type recipes to give spice and variety to our meals. Among my favorites (and the simplest to prepare) are Egg Foo Yung, Chicken with Vegetables, Lobster and Vegetables, Pepper Steak, and Chicken and Cucumber. Here are the recipes, which are easy to prepare:

Egg Foo Yung

2½ cups bean sprouts	1 cup finely chopped cooked
Flour	chicken, shrimp, or lobster
3 green onions	5 eggs
6 water chestnuts	Peanut or soya oil
3 ounces mushrooms	

Toss drained bean sprouts in a small amount of flour; slice onions, water chestnuts, and mushrooms very thin; mix chopped meat and vegetables. Beat eggs lightly and stir in mixture of meat and vegetables. Heat oil in heavy skillet. Fry 1 ladleful of batter at a time, using medium heat. Fry each side about 3 or 4 minutes or until golden brown. Place in a warm oven until ready to serve. Add salt and seasoning to taste.

Moo Goo Gai Peen
(Chicken with Mushrooms and Vegetables)

½ pound string beans, cut up	1 cup celery, diced
2 tablespoons oil	1 cup celery cabbage, cut up
1 pound cooked chicken, thinly sliced	1 cup chicken bouillon
	2 tablespoons cornstarch
⅛ pound fresh mushrooms, sliced	2 teaspoons soy sauce
	¼ cup water

Cut string beans into ½-inch pieces and short-cook until tender. Preheat oil in a heavy pan. Add chicken. Add sliced mushrooms and diced celery. Add celery cabbage, cut into ¼-inch pieces. Add chicken bouillon. Cover pan tightly and cook over moderate flame for 5 minutes. Add cooked string beans. Blend together and add cornstarch, soy sauce, and water. Cook for a few more minutes, stirring constantly, until the juice thickens. Add seasoning to taste.

Choy Lung Har
(Lobster and Vegetables)

1 pound green peas	1 cup chicken bouillon
1 cup diced carrots	½ pound lobster meat
2 teaspoons oil	2 tablespoons cornstarch
2 tablespoons onion, finely diced	2 teaspoons soy sauce
1 clove garlic, diced	¼ cup water
½ cup green pepper, diced	Rice
½ cup celery, diced	

Cook shelled peas and diced carrots separately. Preheat oil in a heavy pan; add finely diced onions, garlic, green pepper, and celery. Add chicken bouillon. Cut lobster meat into small pieces and add. Cook over a moderate flame for 5 minutes, stirring constantly. Add cooked peas and carrots. Blend together and add cornstarch, soy sauce, and water. Cook for a few more minutes, stirring constantly until juice thickens. Add seasoning to taste. Serve very hot with fluffy rice.

Pepper Steak

1 pound round steak
1 teaspoon brown sugar
3 tablespoons soy sauce
2 teaspoons soy or peanut oil
1 medium onion, sliced
2 cloves garlic, minced
4 stalks celery, cut in slices
2 green peppers, cut in small squares
1 tablespoon cornstarch
2 tablespoons water
Brown rice

Cut meat into thin slices. Mix with brown sugar and soy sauce. Heat oil in a heavy pan. Add onion and garlic, and cook until onion is golden. Add meat. Cover and cook 8 minutes, or until sauce thickens. Add vegetables; combine cornstarch with water, stir until smooth, and add. Cover and cook until heated through. Serve immediately over brown rice.

Chicken and Cucumber

1 double chicken breast
2½ tablespoons soy sauce
1 small onion, chopped
¾ teaspoon powdered ginger
2 teaspoons oil
½ pound mushrooms, sliced
1 pound fresh peas, shelled
½ cup consommé
½ cucumber, unpeeled
1 tablespoon cornstarch
2 tablespoons water

Cut chicken into thin slices. Mix with soy sauce, onion, and ginger. Heat oil in a pan. Add mushrooms and cook, covered, for 5 minutes. Remove and set aside. Place chicken mixture in pan with peas and consommé. Cover and cook 10 minutes. Cut cucumber in half, lengthwise, then in ¼ inch slices. Combine cornstarch and water and stir until smooth. Combine all ingredients and cook, covered, 5 minutes.

Chinese Fried Rice

3 eggs	½ cup diced cooked chicken, turkey, veal, or lamb
Vegetable oil	1 cup chopped parsley
4 cups cold boiled rice (at least one day old)	2 tablespoons soy sauce
4 chopped scallions	1 teaspoon vegetable salt

Beat eggs. Heat a little oil in skillet. Toss in rice and sauté until hot. Stir and gently press out all the lumps. Add chopped scallions and meat, and mix thoroughly. Stir a hollow in center of the mixture and pour in the eggs. When eggs are semicooked, resume stirring until rice and eggs are blended. Stir in parsley, soy sauce, and salt.

While on the subject of Oriental cooking, we should not overlook the Japanese, who have given the world at least one famous dish—sukiyaki. I have dined at excellent Japanese restaurants in Los Angeles, San Francisco, and New York. One of the best is Miyako, on West Fifty-sixth Street in New York. But sukiyaki is also easily made at home.

Sukiyaki—Japan's National Dish

Heat a heavy iron skillet or wok. When the pan is hot, add 2 or 3 tablespoons of soy oil. Then add meat and chopped vegetables, in equal proportions, to give a good-size serving for each of your guests. The meat should be very thinly sliced lean raw beef or chicken; the vegetables, onions, both Bermuda and green, celery, and spinach. Slice the Bermuda onions thin, and cut the green onions into 2-inch sections. Cut the celery into 2-inch sections and then cut them the long way into strips. Place all ingredients into the pan at the same time. The steam begins to rise immediately and in a few minutes you can see the meat change color and the vegetables begin to soften. At this time you add a small amount of broth and 2 tablespoons of soy sauce, and continue cooking for about 10 minutes. Covering the pan during cooking will speed up cooking time, preserve the color of the vegetables, and prevent loss of vitamin C. The Japanese usually add little squares of soybean curd cheese (tofu) which resembles a thick salty custard; although it is a good source of protein, it is not essential when the sukiyaki contains meat.

24

The Good Carbohydrates

When you load too much coal on a fire, you choke it. And when you load too many empty carbohydrates on your body fire—metabolism—you also choke it. The human body does not know what to do with an excess of foodless starches and sweets, and so it simply deposits them in the form of excess body fat. That's why overrefined empty carbohydrates are great troublemakers. If the two chief offenders, the white-flour products and the white-sugar products, were to be taken out of our supermarkets, there would be a tremendous increase in the health and vitality of our people, and 80 percent of our overweighters would shed their blankets of fat.

However, this does not mean that healthy people should not enjoy the *wholesome* carbohydrates as nature prepares them in our golden grains and sugars. When man does not tamper with these, they are loaded with vitamins, minerals, and enzymes, and can be handled (burned) with ease by any healthy human body.

Here are some recipes prepared with the wholesome natural carbohydrates that you and your family can enjoy with good conscience.

A New Look at Bread

Nothing else can so quickly create a delightful homey atmosphere as the baking of wholesome bread. There was a time when life was less hectic and most homemakers took pride in their own fragrant bread. You may remember, as I do, the aroma of freshly baked bread greeting you when you came home from school. In Sicily, where I am writing this, my cook is now making our own homemade bread, with all the goodness of the grain as it comes from the field. Let me give you a simple version of this delightful 100-percent natural bread. It's easy to make.

Hearty Whole-Wheat Bread

1 package dry yeast (1 ounce)
1 quart potato water or warm milk
1 tablespoon honey
3 pounds fresh whole-wheat flour
1 teaspoon vegetable salt

Place dry yeast with a little potato water and the honey in a warm cup. Put aside for 10 to 20 minutes. Place flour and salt in a large bowl and mix with a big spoon. Little by little, work in the yeast mixture and the rest of the potato water. When well kneaded, pour mixture into 2 or 3 well-oiled bread pans and place in a warm spot. When the dough mixture rises close to the top of the bread pans, bake at 350° F. for 1 hour. This is a hearty, nutritious bread. The potato water helps to keep it firm and moist.

Hearty Whole-Wheat Bread (2)

Here is another delightful bread you should bake for your family:

2½ cups whole-wheat flour
3 tablespoons fresh wheat germ
3 tablespoons soy flour
4 tablespoons powdered skim milk
2 tablespoons brown sugar
1 teaspoon vegetable salt
½ cake compressed yeast (½ ounce)
1 cup lukewarm water
1 tablespoon vegetable oil

Into a large bowl put whole-wheat flour (preferably stone-ground), fresh wheat germ, soy flour, powdered skim milk, brown sugar, and vegetable salt. Dissolve yeast in lukewarm water, and add this to the dry ingredients. Add oil. Mix thoroughly until you have a smooth dough; put it in an oiled bowl, and cover. Let rise in a warm place 1½ hours; punch down, and let rise 20 minutes more. Knead into a compact loaf and put into a large bread pan; cover, and let stand in a warm place. When dough has again risen to top of bread pan, bake for about 40 minutes at 400° F.

El Molino or Elam Bread—Fast and Delicious

If you are too busy or too lazy to follow the above recipes, I suggest you go to your nearest diet and health-food shop and ask for the new El Molino Ready Mix. This is a delightful mixture containing stone-ground whole-wheat flour, unbleached flour, sesame flour, honey, skim milk, brown sugar, and a fast-acting yeast. All you do is add water and bake.

This combination of ground fresh sesame seed and high-protein whole wheat offers you an entirely new experience in bread eating. For real honest-to-goodness bread, I invite you to try this ready mix—nothing could be simpler! Most health and diet shops carry this exciting new product. If yours does not, drop a card to El Molino Mills, City of Industry, California. You might also ask about soy flour, quick-cooked soybeans, soy grits, and the delicious carob flour that this progressive firm introduced to America.

Famous Cornell Bread

1 package dry granular yeast or 1 ounce compressed yeast
¼ cup warm water (lukewarm for compressed yeast)
5 cups unbleached flour
1 tablespoon salt
¼ cup sugar
⅓ cup soy flour
½ cup dry skim milk
¼ cup fresh wheat germ
1 tablespoon vegetable oil
1¾ cups water

Dissolve yeast in ¼ cup water. Combine dry ingredients in mixing bowl. Add dissolved yeast, oil, and water, mixing to blend well. Knead dough until smooth and satiny, then place in well-greased bowl. Cover, and allow to rise in a warm place for about 1½ hours. Punch down by plunging fist into center of dough, then fold over the edges of dough and turn the dough upside down. Cover and allow to rise again for 15 to 20 minutes. Shape into 2 loaves and place in oiled pans. Cover and allow to stand in warm place for about 55 to 60 minutes or until dough rises and fills pans. Bake at 400° F. for 45 minutes.

New Idea—No-Knead Bread

This bread needs no kneading and is a great time-saver. This popular English whole-wheat bread is from Doris Grant's fine book, *Your Bread and Your Life*.

3 pounds whole-wheat flour	4 cups warm water
2 teaspoons salt	2 teaspoons dark molasses
1 ounce fresh yeast	

Mix flour with salt. Mix yeast in a small bowl with 1 cup of water. Let stand for 10 minutes or so, then pour this into the flour with the remaining 3 cups of water and the molasses. Mix well by hand for several minutes until dough feels elastic and leaves sides of bowl clean. Divide dough into three parts and place in three 1-quart bread pans that have been warmed and oiled. Cover pans with a cloth and leave in a warm place to rise by about one third. Bake in a hot oven (about 450° F.) for 35 to 40 minutes.

Hi-Protein Gluten Bread—Easy to Make

1 cake yeast (1 ounce)	2 teaspoons vegetable salt
2 cups lukewarm water	3 cups gluten flour
1 tablespoon vegetable oil	

Dissolve yeast in water and gradually add oil, salt, and gluten flour. Knead until mixture is smooth. Put in oiled bowl. Let rise until light, about 1½ hours. Then punch and knead again. Shape into small loaves and place in oiled pans. Cover; let rise until double in bulk (about 45 minutes). Bake at 400° F. for 40 minutes.

Milwaukee Rye Bread

2 cakes yeast	3 teaspoons vegetable salt
2 cups lukewarm potato water	4 cups rye flour
1 cup riced potatoes, solidly packed	4 cups unbleached wheat flour
	1 tablespoon caraway seed

Dissolve yeast in ¼ cup lukewarm potato water. Add riced potatoes and salt to remaining 1¾ cups lukewarm potato water. Combine and blend the two mixtures. Combine both kinds of flour and caraway seed. Stir dry ingredients into liquid. When dough is no longer sticky to the touch, knead until smooth and elastic on a floured board. Then let rise, in oiled bowl, until doubled in bulk. Punch down, and divide dough into two parts. Knead each another minute or two, and form into loaves. Put into 2 oiled 4½ x 8½ x 2½ inch bread pans. When doubled in bulk, bake at 375° F. about 1 hour.

Swedish Rye Crisps—a Delight for Dieters

2 cups sour milk
½ cup corn oil
½ cup honey

6 cups rye flour
2 tablespoons wheat germ
1 teaspoon vegetable salt

Mix sour milk with oil and honey. Then add flour, wheat germ, and salt. Knead this stiff dough well. Roll out thin on floured board and cut into squares or triangles. Place on cookie sheets and bake at 400° F. for about 12 minutes.

Wheat-Germ Sticks

2 cups whole-wheat flour
1¼ cups fresh milk
½ cup vegetable oil

2 cups fresh wheat germ
1 tablespoon honey
1 teaspoon vegetable salt

Mix and knead all ingredients, then roll dough ¼ inch thick. Cut into sticks about ¼ inch wide and 5 inches long. Place on an oiled cookie sheet. Sprinkle some of the sticks with caraway seeds and others with sesame seeds. Bake at 350° F. about 35 minutes, or until golden brown.

Hi-Protein Muffins

1½ cups soy flour
2 teaspoons baking powder
1½ teaspoons vegetable salt
2 fresh eggs
3 tablespoons brown sugar

1 tablespoon grated orange rind
1 cup milk
1 tablespoon vegetable oil
¼ cup floured raisins
¼ cup floured walnut meats

Sift together flour, baking powder, and salt. Separate eggs; beat yolks until very light and frothy. Beat sugar into the egg yolks, add orange rind, milk, and oil, and mix well. Pour the egg mixture into the dry ingredients and mix. Add raisins and nut meats, and mix thoroughly. Fold in whites, beaten stiff. Pour mixture into small muffin tins and bake in slow oven (300° F.) for about 30 minutes.

Important Note on Baking Powders: Whenever possible, use yeast as a leavening agent in your baking. Yeast adds nourishment. Whenever you must use baking powder, be sure you use one composed of tartaric acid (made from grapes) or phosphates. Get rid of any baking powder that contains aluminum derivatives. If you are unable to procure a wholesome baking powder, let your druggist combine the following:

Potassium bicarbonate	79.5	grams
Cornstarch	56.0	grams
Tartaric acid	15.0	grams
Potassium bitartrate	112.25	grams

Wheat-Germ Muffins

2 fresh eggs
1 teaspoon vegetable salt
1 teaspoon brown sugar
½ cup vegetable oil
1½ cups milk
1½ cups whole-wheat flour
1 cup fresh wheat germ

Separate eggs. Beat yolks; add vegetable salt, brown sugar, and oil. Stir in milk, and add flour and fresh wheat germ. Fold in stiffly beaten egg whites. Bake in hot, oiled muffin tins at 350° F. for about 35 minutes.

Hi-Protein Popovers

¾ cup milk
2 eggs, beaten
¾ cup soy flour
¼ cup gluten flour
Pinch vegetable salt
1 tablespoon wheat germ

Mix milk with eggs. Stir dry ingredients into the milk-egg mixture and mix thoroughly. Pour into well-oiled very hot popover pan or muffin tins. Bake at 450° F. for 30 minutes.

Hi-Protein Beauty-Farm Cake

2 eggs, beaten
1 cup brown sugar
⅓ cup whole-wheat flour
1⅓ cups soy flour
1½ teaspoons baking powder
½ teaspoon vegetable salt
¾ teaspoon cinnamon
1 tablespoon cocoa
⅔ cup milk
⅓ cup vegetable oil

Beat the eggs, gradually adding the sugar; beat until very light. Sift the remaining dry ingredients together, and add to the egg mixture alternately with milk. Stir in oil. Pour into oiled shallow cake tin and bake until done in a moderate (350° F.) oven.

Hi-Protein Waffles

1 yeast cake (1 ounce)
2 cups buttermilk
3 eggs
1 cup fresh wheat germ
1 teaspoon vegetable salt
⅓ cup vegetable oil
1 tablespoon honey
⅓ cup dry skim milk
1¼ cups whole-wheat flour

Put crumbled yeast into warm buttermilk. Separate eggs. To mixture add egg yolks, wheat germ, vegetable salt, oil, and honey. Into these ingredients sift dry skim milk and whole-wheat flour. Mix well, then set bowl in a warm place and let rise for 1 to 2 hours. When bulk has doubled, stir with spoon. Then mix in stiffly beaten egg whites and bake in waffle iron. Serve waffles hot, with honey or maple syrup.

Natural Cereals and Other Grains

How to Cook Cereals While You Sleep

Before retiring, stir ½ cup of your favorite raw cereal—wheat, oats, rye, or buckwheat, preferably cracked—into 2 cups of salted boiling water. Stir for just 3 minutes, then pour into a wide-mouthed thermos bottle. Cork the bottle tightly. Next morning you will be greeted by a hot cereal, ready to be eaten with fresh milk and honey. For even more nourishment, cook cereal in milk instead of water. If fresh milk is not available, simply add ½ cup powdered skim milk to water. Serve with fresh milk and a sprinkle of wheat germ (see below).

Honeyed Wheat Germ

4 cups fresh wheat germ
½ cup honey

Pour wheat germ on large cookie tin and sprinkle with honey (also try maple sugar or molasses). Roast in a 350° F. oven about 15 minutes or until golden brown. Store in a glass jar; and use over hot or cold cereals. Many children who refuse to eat plain wheat germ love this toasted variety.

Kasha, a Special Grain

Kasha, or buckwheat groats, is an almost forgotten grain in America. In Russia it is one of the most important staple foods. It is high in energy and fairly high in protein; but most of all, it is a delicious and welcome change from rice and potatoes. Kasha is easy to cook. The whole kernel takes only about 20 minutes; the cracked ones take only 5 minutes. The Russian method is the simplest and leanest:

1 cup whole buckwheat groats (kasha)	2 cups water (if used for breakfast, otherwise chicken or beef broth)
½ teaspoon vegetable salt	

Use heavy cooking utensil. Stir unwashed buckwheat groats into boiling liquid. Add salt, let boil for 1 or 2 minutes; then cover. Turn heat low and let simmer for 15 minutes, or until all liquid is absorbed. Every grain should be separate. Kasha must never be mushy!

My Favorite Method: Put 2 tablespoons of vegetable oil into heavy skillet. When oil is very hot, stir in 1 cup of buckwheat groats, which have been mixed previously with a raw beaten egg. Add a teaspoon of vegetable salt. Finally add 2 cups of chicken broth, Hauser Broth, or vegetable water. Bring to a boil, then reduce heat; cover tightly and let cook until all liquid is absorbed, stirring occasionally.

Kashaburgers

These inexpensive and delicious kashaburgers make an excellent and different luncheon dish.

½ onion, finely chopped	1 egg, slightly beaten
1½ tablespoons vegetable oil	1 tablespoon chopped nutmeats
2 cups cooked kasha (buckwheat groats)	

Sauté onion in oil to golden brown. Mix with kasha, egg, and nuts. Form into patties and sauté on hot oiled skillet, or drop heaping tablespoonfuls onto skillet. Sauté until golden brown.

Brown Rice—the Easy Way

1 cup natural brown rice 1 teaspoon vegetable salt
5 cups boiling water

Pick over rice and remove any husks and foreign particles. Put in a wire strainer and rinse under cold running water to remove dust. Bring water to boiling point, add rice, and boil briskly for 5 minutes. Turn heat low and simmer for 20 minutes. Turn off heat when the rice is soft, add vegetable salt, and let stand over hot water until any remaining water is absorbed, about an hour. The grains should be whole and fluffy.

Golden Rice Pilaf

6 tablespoons vegetable oil 3 cups fat-free chicken broth
1½ cups brown rice (or broth from chicken
½ teaspoon saffron bouillon cubes)
2 teaspoons vegetable salt ½ cup chopped sunflower seeds

Use a 2-quart heavy saucepan or flameproof casserole. Pour in the oil. When it is hot, stir in the rice; cook, stirring, about 5 minutes. Sprinkle the saffron over the rice, stir well; add the salt, stirring continually. Add the broth and chopped seeds. Bring to a boil. Cover, reduce heat, and cook until the rice is tender and has absorbed the broth, about 15 to 20 minutes.

Potatoes Can Be Good for You

Mashed versus "Smashed" Potatoes

When you peel, cut up, and boil perfectly good potatoes, and then pour off the water in which they have been cooked, and then mash the potatoes, you have what I call "smashed" potatoes, because all the goodness has been "smashed" out. To make nourishing, lean mashed potatoes, simply cook them in their jackets, in a small amount of unsalted water, covered, until all the water is absorbed. Then pull off the thin peeling, sprinkle with 1 tablespoon dry skim milk, a little vegetable salt, and a handful of chopped parsley. Then mash, adding enough liquid skim milk to make them smooth and creamy. Yes, even on a reducing menu, you can occasionally have ½ cup of potatoes cooked this way.

Lighthearted Baked Potatoes

Fragrant, delicate potatoes baked by this recipe need not add ounces to anyone's weight. Select medium-sized baking potatoes. Scrub them thoroughly and remove any blemishes. Wipe dry, then rub skin with a little vegetable oil.

Bake the potatoes on a rack in a moderately hot oven (425° F.) for 40 to 60 minutes, or until the potatoes feel soft when pressed with your towel-protected fingers. Remove the potatoes from the oven and break open the skin immediately to let the steam escape. Blend, for each potato, 1 tablespoon yogurt, ¼ teaspoon vegetable salt, and 1 teaspoon finely cut chives. Scoop out the hot potato from the shells into a bowl, and blend quickly with the yogurt mixture. Return mixture to potato shells. Reheat for a few minutes in a slow oven and serve piping hot.

Potatoes à la Garbo

Scrub large baking potatoes; do not peel. Cut in half and scoop out most of the middle portion, until only about ½ inch of potato is left lining the skin. Rub skins with vegetable oil and bake in very hot oven until brown and crispy. Greta Garbo first served these potatoes to me and I dedicate this recipe to her. If you like a crisp baked-potato skin, you will love these.

Royal Hashed Potatoes

Heat 1 tablespoon vegetable oil in heavy iron skillet. Add 2 cups unpeeled potatoes, boiled and diced, and ¼ cup minced onion. Season with vegetable salt. Then add 3 tablespoons milk and let cook without stirring until browned on the bottom. Fold over like an omelet, and serve garnished with parsley. These were the favorite potatoes of Queen Alexandra of Yugoslavia. We ate them daily during Their Majesties' stay in America, so I respectfully dedicated this recipe to her.

Homemade Potato Chips

You can eat these with a clear conscience. Simply scrub potatoes until they shine. Do not peel, but slice very thin. Spread out thinly on a cookie sheet and sprinkle lightly with vegetable oil and vegetable salt. Place in moderate oven for about 40 minutes, or until potatoes turn into brown chips. Then turn off heat, but leave in for 15 minutes longer to make them extra crisp.

25

Healthy, Healing Vegetable Juices

In Czechoslovakia there was a sanatorium where people with digestive difficulties flocked by the thousands. There I learned about the importance of fresh raw vegetable juices. Around this sanatorium were acres and acres of vegetables, and they were grown on rich organic soil. The head gardener and his assistants collected golden carrots, baskets full of dark-green parsley, young tender spinach leaves, celery and celery roots. From the orchard the men brought ripe red apples, pears, and other fruits of the season. The head nurse, Schwester Karoline, received these vegetables and fruits with great ceremony, and a buzz started in the diet kitchen. The vegetables were first picked clean, then put into a hydrochloric acid solution (see under "Finger Salad and Fresh Juices," in chapter 5), and finally rinsed in ice-cold water to stop the loss of enzymes and vitamins. Carrots and other roots were scrubbed till they shone, and the leaves were cleaned under running spring water. Then, with hand mills, they ground out the juices of these very fresh vegetables. By ten o'clock every morning, each patient in the Carlsbader Sanatorium had his 8-ounce glass of fresh "live" vegetable juice.

I will never forget Schwester Karoline's expression when she talked about vegetable juices. She called them the "blood of the plant." The green magic of chlorophyll, she would say, is the quickest way of healing overfed and undernourished patients. Many were English and Americans, with colitis, ulcers, and liver and gall-bladder difficulties. It was in this sanatorium that, more than forty years ago, I discovered the immense healing and invigorating power of freshly made raw juices. Since then I have recommended a daily pint of fresh vegetable juice to everybody as one of the best safeguards against tiredness and premature aging.

Needless to say, I was happy to see the excitement created all over America when Dr. Cheney, of California, announced that fresh cabbage juice cured ulcers in two weeks' time. His cure was based on giving his patients a quart of fresh cabbage juice or 75 percent cabbage and 25 percent celery juice. This is the first time that fresh vegetable juices were "officially recognized" —but why only cabbage juice or celery juice? *All* fresh juices have marvelous healing power, not only because of their vitamin and mineral content but because of the *"matière vivante"* as Bircher-Benner calls it; and no chemist has yet been able to duplicate this energy. It takes the sun, soil, air, and water, nature's mightiest forces, to produce young growing plants. No wonder the healing potential is so great in these fresh "live" juices.

If you have a specific health problem and are interested in the many health-giving and curative properties of fresh vegetable juice extracts, I suggest you read the book (if you can obtain it) *Vegetable Juices for Health,* by H. E. Kirschner, M.D., who has had years of experience in every phase of nutrition. In this book Dr. Kirschner gives many remarkable case reports of what fresh vegetable juices can accomplish in many so-called hopeless cases.

Another source of over two hundred juice recipes is Shirley Ross's *Nature's Drinks* (Vintage Books). Her book is devoted exclusively to beverages that come straight from the earth, with no chemical dyes, preservatives, or artificial sweetening.

For people in the second part of life, juices are doubly valuable because the chewing of raw vegetables may be a problem, or the raw bulk may be irritating. And, of course, much larger quantities of vegetables can be taken in juice form. Not many people can eat five large carrots, yet a grandmother of ninety-five can easily drink the juice of five carrots. The vitamins and minerals have been extracted from the pulp and are more easily absorbed by the body, and there is no vitamin or mineral loss due to overcooking. Last but not least, vegetable juices are delicious and are therefore the easiest and laziest way to add vitamins, minerals, enzymes, and other as yet undiscovered factors to the daily diet.

How to Make Fresh Vegetable Juices

Wash all vegetables carefully. Do not soak any vegetables in water for a length of time—this will leach out vitamins B and C, which dissolve in water as salt does—but wash them under running cold water. Do not peel carrots and other root vegetables. Instead, scrub them with a stiff brush (the Japanese make an excellent oval brush that is sold in most health-food stores) and cut them in pieces.

If you are buying a new vegetable juicer, buy the most modern one you can find, one that does not vibrate and get out of balance, and one that gives you vegetable juice with some of the vitamin-rich finely suspended microscopic pulp, not just the watery liquid. An efficient juicer is a good investment for the entire family. Many have come on the market since I introduced the drinking of vegetable juices; some are made for bars and some for home use. The one I take with me all over the world weighs only about six pounds. It is easy to operate because it has only four parts. Also—and this is important—if you buy a new device, the juice must not touch tin, lead, or aluminum; it must flow into a bowl of stainless steel, glass, or plastic, which cannot possibly affect the color, taste, or chemistry of the vitamin-charged juices.

When you have scrubbed your vegetables sparkling clean, put them into the juicer and drink your first glassful right from the spout. If you make extra juice, be sure to put it at once on ice and cover tightly to stop enzyme action, or the juice will lose its appetizing color. Never expose fresh vegetable extracts to the air a moment longer than you have to. Work fast!

Drink your juices fresh as they come from the juicer; for maximum benefit, drink two cups each day, and sip them through a straw. Don't gulp them down!

Removing Poisonous Sprays

Insecticides are so widely used now that it is wise to wash all vegetables in the hydrochloric acid solution given in chapter 5. You should be especially careful if you are in Mexico or the Orient, or if you have a sensitivity to certain insect sprays.

Golden Carrot Juice

This is the great favorite with everybody. The dark California carrots are best. Drink this to your heart's content. Remember, a cup of carrot juice is rich in vitamins A, B, and C, plus a good combination of the minerals calcium, iron, and even iodine. Carrot juice helps complexions to glow, helps the eyes, soothes the "inner man" with its vegetable mucilage. But more than anything else, it tastes so good, straight or mixed with practically any other juice.

Carrot Milk Shake

Half a cup of carrot juice with half a cup of milk makes one of the finest "builder-uppers," rich in vitamins and double rich in calcium. It makes an ideal between-meal drink and is a favorite on beauty farms. (Waistline watchers should use skim milk.)

Celery Juice

This is a favorite in England. It is a natural digestive and one of the best appetizers. By all means use some of the dark-green outside stalks; they contain more chlorophyll. But do not use too many of the dark-green leaves; they make the juice too bitter, and they may have been sprayed heavily. Mixing in a few drops of lemon or grapefruit juice adds to the flavor and prevents the juice from turning dark. Celery espresso contains vitamins A, B, C, and some E, also the minerals sodium, potassium, and chlorine. This makes it an ideal cocktail for reducers. Celery juice can be mixed with many other juices; try celery and carrot juice, half and half.

Fresh Beet Juice

Young beets, scrubbed and put through the juicer, make an extremely beautiful wine-red juice; but the taste is less agreeable, and only small amounts of beet juice should be mixed with other juices. Two-thirds pineapple juice and one-third fresh beet juice make a pleasant combination. Try "borscht" in the modern manner: simply add ½ cup of beet juice to 1 pint of milk, heat, and spike with vegetable salt.

Apple Juice

Apple juice is mentioned here because it blends so well with vegetable juices, and apples are plentiful the year around. Nothing can taste better than the juice from fresh ripe apples made by cutting the unpeeled apple into four parts and putting it through a juicer. The juice cannot be compared with ordinary apple juice or cider. It should be called "liquid apples" because it contains the whole aroma and goodness of the apple, including vitamins A and B in fair amounts, vitamin C in good amounts, and minerals, including good amounts of sodium. Fresh apple juice has for years been recommended in gout and rheumatism; but in our program, it should be drunk for its deliciousness. Here's hoping that the apple growers of the Northwest install apple-juicing machines all over the land, the way citrus growers have done. I am willing to bet that all their apples will be sold, once Americans have tasted these "liquid apples."

P.S. Fresh apple juice taken between meals while reducing is a welcome change, and the pectin of apples makes it especially soothing to the "inner person."

Fresh Cabbage Juice

Pick tender young cabbage and cut in slices to fit vegetable juicer. This makes a sweet-tasting, light-green juice, but a few dark-green stalks of celery add flavor and character to cabbage juice. Fresh cabbage juice contains vitamins A, B, and C, which are important healing factors, as well as vitamin "U," as Dr. Cheney calls the healing factor in cabbage juice. I see no reason why cabbage juice cannot be flavored with carrot juice or any other juice to help eliminate the blandness of just cabbage juice. In other words, 75 percent cabbage juice and 25 percent carrot juice (or tomato juice) can give the same results. Cabbage juice, as well as all other vegetable juices, must be made fresh daily and never kept from one day to the next.

Gaylord Hauser Cocktail

Cut up equal amounts of dark-green celery, golden carrots, and red apples and put through your juicer. This contains an abundance of vitamins, minerals, enzymes, and chlorophyll. Three glasses a day of this pleasant combination is your best life and health insurance.

N.B. Always put the apples in *last,* because the pectin clogs up the strainer of your juicer.

Liquid Salads—If Chewing Is a Problem

Liquid salads are an important part of the diet therapy used at the famous Bircher-Benner clinic in Switzerland. Old and young are given two glasses of vegetable juices a day. This "liquid salad" idea is an excellent one to adopt, since many people never completely chew their salads and raw vegetables to get all the food from them.

Let your imagination guide you. Put any combination of vegetables into the juicer. A combination of celery, carrots, and tomatoes tastes delicious, as does a combination of watercress, celery, and tomatoes. Another great favorite is a mixture of celery, apples, and a sprig of parsley. You might even have a "liquid salad bowl" and put head lettuce, a bit of cabbage, celery, a small cucumber, tomatoes, and half a green pepper through the juicer. Spike with a little vegetable salt and a few drops of lemon juice. Such a liquid salad taken *before* a meal is a wonderful way of breaking yourself of overeating.

Eat, Drink, and Be Beautiful!

Distinguished hostesses all over the world now serve at least one cocktail without alcohol for guests who do not wish martinis and for those who watch their waistlines. One of the most elegant parties I ever attended was at the French embassy in Constantinople on the Bosporus. Madame de Saint Hardouin, the lady ambassador, served cool carrot and celery juice and chilled peach and mint cocktails in high-stemmed champagne glasses, side by side with the other cocktails. A king and his queen, many princesses, and diplomats from many lands enjoyed these refreshing drinks and asked for seconds. It is no wonder that Madame de Saint Hardouin was one of the most beautiful women of our time. Her blond hair and skin were the envy of every diplomat's wife. Ily de Saint Hardouin, I am happy to say, has been a long-time friend and student; and because of her, the entire French embassy had the benefit of beauty-full eating.

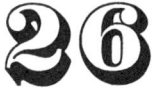

Delightful Desserts

Do Something New with Fresh Fruit

There is no dessert in the whole wide world that can compare with fresh, ripe fruit. Traveling the world over, I am happy to notice that more and more homes and smart restaurants serve fresh fruits at the end of a good meal. In France and Italy fruits are served with the proper flourish. The waiter brings a whole box of beautiful peaches, pears, or melons to your table. Very often each piece of fruit is carefully nested on its own bed of cotton to prevent bruising. You pick the ripest and juiciest fruit, and then proceed to eat it with the proper fork and knife.

I wish more people would acquire the good habit of eating ripe fruits. It is a fine way to train the palate away from gooey desserts. All fruits are excellent; select the ones you like most. For waistline watchers, ripe melon is especially recommended. To make it more flavorsome, squeeze over it lemon or lime juice. Ripe berries of all types—eat them in as natural a state as possible; or do as South Americans do: sprinkle them with orange or pineapple juice, then they won't need any further sweetening.

One of the favorite desserts at my home is a big crystal bowl full of every kind of fresh fruit. You start the bottom layer with ripe strawberries; on the top of those you place a layer of sliced, ripe peaches, then a layer of blueberries, and still another layer of red raspberries, and so on. When the fruits are ripe, they need no sweetening; however, some sweet, fresh orange juice sprinkled over each layer gives added flavor. If the fruits are not sweet enough, sprinkle them with a little mild honey. But never sweeten fruits so much that you drown the natural taste, and never, never sweeten with white sugar.

Lady Mendl's Honey Compote

I learned this secret from the fabulous Lady Mendl's chef, Monsieur Fraise, who has made this compote for kings and queens, dukes, and duchesses. I also have seen Sir Winston Churchill eat the compote with delight.

Select ripe fruit or berries, such as peaches, pears, apricots, strawberries, raspberries, or blackberries. Use them singly, or in combination when a variety are on the market. If the fruits are cut into wedges, they will "cook" more readily. Small ripe peaches or apricots can be used whole or cut in half.

Make a syrup of 1 part honey and 1 part water. When it boils up, pour it over the fresh fruit, cover, and allow to stand until cool; then put compote in refrigerator until serving time. Make just enough syrup to coat the fruit. For variety, add a few slices of lemon or orange and perhaps a sprinkling of cinnamon.

Broiled Grapefruit Caribbean

Half a fresh, ripe grapefruit is always a welcome dessert, but occasionally you might like it broiled. Simply cut ripe grapefruit in half, remove seeds, and cut the sections; but do not cut out the center. Place 1 teaspoon of brown sugar in center, also 1 teaspoon of sherry. Place in broiler pan under a low flame and broil for about 10 minutes. Be sure to put a little water on bottom of pan to prevent burning.

Jamaican Bananas

This picturesque dessert is no more fattening than baked apples. Peel 6 large, ripe bananas, split in half, and place in a shallow baking dish, cut side down. Mix 1 tablespoon sesame oil, ⅓ cup brown sugar, and 2 tablespoons lemon or lime juice, and pour over bananas.

Bake 20 minutes in a slow oven (300° F.), basting several times. Sprinkle with shredded coconut and serve hot.

Pineapple au Kirsch

At Maxim's in Paris, fresh pineapple is served with pomp and circumstance. The headwaiter slices a very ripe peeled pineapple with a long sharp knife. On two paper-thin slices he pours a spoonful of kirsch, and serves the dish with a low bow. We lucky people in the land of plenty can eat pineapple without cutting it so thin, and with or without kirsch (but, of course, no extra sugar).

Pineapple de Luxe

1 ripe pineapple	1 quart orange sherbet
Honey	2 small tangerines

Pare the pineapple, slice, and cut in small cubes. Pour a little honey over the cubes; mix until all the pineapple is coated lightly with honey. Put in a glass dish or china bowl, and chill.

To serve, spoon pineapple cubes and a little of the honey liquid from the bowl into a tall, flared dessert glass, or into a large wineglass. Fill glass with orange sherbet. Garnish with peeled sections of tangerine. Makes 8 or more servings—and always wins compliments.

Fresh Yogurt and Fruit

Fresh yogurt takes the place of cream or whipped cream for people who value their waistline. You can make many attractive dessert combinations. Place ripe sliced peaches in your finest crystal goblets, cover them with a tablespoon or two of yogurt, and sprinkle the top with just a little honey and some finely grated lemon peel.

Raspberries and strawberries look beautiful in crystal glasses and become more delicious when you add fresh yogurt. People who love the taste of thick cream over strawberries or raspberries, as they make them in Paris, say that these yogurt fruit desserts are tops.

Lighthearted Piecrust

The most tasty and flaky crusts can be made with fresh vegetable oils, fragrant whole-wheat flour, and sesame, poppy, or chopped sunflower seeds. Fresh and honeyed fruits of all kinds can be piled high into these tender pie shells. Small individual pie shells also make welcome and elegant desserts without insulting the waistline. To add more nutrition and glamour to fruit pies, before baking the crust sprinkle a tablespoon of your favorite seeds over pie shell and press in.

½ cup sesame oil (or sunflower oil)
⅓ cup cold water
2 cups whole-wheat or unbleached flour
1 teaspoon vegetable salt
1 tablespoon sesame seeds

Mix seasame oil with the water and quickly add flour and salt. Mix as quickly as possible with a fork. Form into a ball and place mixture between two sheets of waxed paper and roll thin. Line pie plate with the crust, sprinkle with seeds, and bake to a light golden brown. Fill crust with your favorite fruit, and top with yogurt if you wish.

Quick Viennese Pie Shell

1 cup whole-wheat flour
½ cup vegetable oil or sunbutter
1 tablespoon honey
1 hard-boiled egg yolk, finely mashed
½ teaspoon vegetable salt
½ teaspoon grated lemon peel

Mix ingredients well. Press on pie plate and chill in refrigerator. Then bake to a golden brown. Let cool. Fill with fresh honeyed fruit. Also makes delightful individual tart shell. So easy to make, and delicious.

Honeyed Wheat-Germ Piecrust

1 cup sifted whole-wheat flour
⅛ teaspoon grated nutmeg
¾ teaspoon vegetable salt
¼ cup vegetable oil
2 tablespoons milk
¼ cup honeyed wheat germ

Sift flour, nutmeg, and vegetable salt together into a mixing bowl. Pour over, all at once, without combining, the oil and milk. Stir all ingredients lightly together. Add honeyed wheat germ, and continue stirring until blended. Form mixture into a ball. Place on a large sheet of waxed paper, flatten slightly, cover with another sheet of waxed paper, and roll out the dough. Remove the top paper. Invert the rolled dough and its bottom paper into a pie pan. Remove the paper. Shape the dough into the pan as usual, trim the edge, and make a decorative rim with thumb and forefinger or by pressing with a fork. Prick bottom of crust well with a fork. Bake in a hot oven (475° F.) 10 minutes, or until golden and crisp.

Let crust cool. Pile high with sliced ruby-red strawberries. Or pour in honey custard (the recipe follows under "Sherbets, Custards, and Other Desserts") to half-fill the crust, and chill; then fill with fresh fruit slices, raspberries, or blueberries. It is also wonderful with fresh plums prepared this way: cut them in half, do not peel; remove stones. Simmer halves in a mixture of equal parts water and honey, to cover, about 7 minutes. Let cool in honey mixture. Then spoon the fruit carefully on the custard filling. I dedicate this delightful dessert to my adorable sister-in-law Mrs. O. R. Hauser, who first served it to me.

You Can Make Gelatin Doubly Nutritious

Since gelatin lacks many of the important amino acids and is an incomplete protein, many nutritionists do not recommend it. However, when gelatin is eaten with a meal containing a complete protein—as in meat, milk, eggs, or cheese—the inferior gelatin protein becomes a valuable and nutritious first-class protein. Therefore, gelatin desserts, when served with a balanced meal, are valuable. Naturally, we use only the pure colorless, unsweetened gelatin, which you can buy by the pound or in packages of convenient envelopes. The highly colored sweet gelatins are mostly sugar and should not be used by intelligent homemakers. For color and flavor, we add pure unsweetened fresh or frozen fruit and vegetable juices. Follow directions on package.

Unsweetened grape juice makes a delightful dish, a doubly nutritious and decorative gelatin dessert. When it is partially set, remove it from the refrigerator and beat it until it is light and foamy. Then pour into a mold that has been rinsed in cold water.

Chill. Serve with fresh milk or a spoonful of honey custard (the recipe follows under "Sherbets, Custards, and Other Desserts).

Orange juice, flavored with a little sherry, makes a golden jelly. For variety's sake, try this orange-sherry gelatin. Whip it as described above; pour it into a mold and chill. Serve garnished with thin sections of fresh orange, and sprinkle with a little coconut. Or pour it into a square pan and chill; when firm, cut in small cubes. Pile the sparkling golden squares into dessert glasses. Garnish with fresh cherries, if available.

Wine Jelly—a Fine Party Dessert

There is an elegant aura about wine jelly. The color captures the sparkle of dinnertable candles, the flavor reminds one of summer and the vineyards of France. Incidentally, it is a nutritious and easy-to-make dessert, and a dieter's favorite.

4 tablespoons unflavored gelatin	Grated peel and juice of 1 lemon
1 cup cold water	
3 cups boiling water	2½ cups sherry, Madeira, or port wine
2 tablespoons honey	
Juice of 1 orange	

Soften gelatin in cold water about 5 minutes. Then add boiling water and honey and stir until gelatin dissolves. Stir in fruit juices and peel, and let cool. (Some cooks strain out the peel after a few minutes.) When the gelatin mixture has cooled, add the wine. Pour into a 2-quart mold that has been rinsed with cold water. Chill until firm. Unmold onto a chilled serving dish. Garnish with grape leaves and small clusters of grapes. Makes 8 to 12 servings.

Sherbets, Custards, and Other Desserts

French Sherbet

1 cup thick yogurt	1 tablespoon lemon juice
½ cup fresh or frozen fruit juice	Vegetable salt
¼ cup honey	2 fresh egg whites

Mix yogurt with fresh or frozen fruit juice. Add honey, fresh lemon juice, and a pinch of vegetable salt, and mix thoroughly. Place mixture in freezing tray and freeze until quite firm. Then remove to a bowl and stir until smooth. Now fold the fresh egg whites, stiffly beaten, into the mixture. Return to freezing tray. Dozens of smooth French yogurt sherbets can be made with the fresh or frozen fruit juices in your market.

Raspberry Sherbet—a Great Favorite

2 teaspoons unflavored gelatin
¼ cup cold water
1 quart fresh or quick-frozen red raspberries
¼ cup lemon juice
1¾ cups water

¾ cup honey
2 egg whites
⅛ teaspoon salt
Few reserved whole berries and fresh mint leaves

Soften gelatin in the ¼ cup cold water. Press the berries through a sieve or ricer, or use a blender. Add lemon juice to the berries, and mix. Combine the 1¾ cups water and the honey in a saucepan and boil 10 minutes. Remove from heat and stir the soaked gelatin into this hot syrup to dissolve. Let syrup cool. Add sieved berries and mix to combine smoothly. Pour into refrigerator tray; chill about 30 minutes. Whip egg whites with salt until they are stiff and stand in peaks when beater is withdrawn. Fold egg whites into the chilled berry mixture. Pour back into refrigerator tray. Freeze for 30 minutes, then beat well. Freeze 3 hours or more, beating the sherbet, at half-hour intervals. Beat once again before serving. Makes 5 to 6 servings. To serve this fragrant frozen dessert, heap it in large wineglasses instead of the usual dessert dishes. Place a geranium or grape leaf under each stemmed glass on dessert plate. Garnish sherbet with a few whole berries and a mint leaf.

Golden Carrot Sherbet

1 quart fresh carrot juice
1 can (6 ounces) frozen orange juice

3 medium bananas
3 tablespoons honey

Place all ingredients in electric blender and mix until very smooth. Pour mixture into refrigerator tray and freeze. Stir several times before serving.

Golden Papaya Ice

1 cup water
1¾ cups honey
1 tablespoon grated lemon peel
⅓ cup lemon juice
2 cups sieved fresh ripe or cooked papaya

Combine water, honey, and lemon peel in a saucepan. Cook over low heat and stir until blended. Then bring to boiling, and boil gently 5 minutes without stirring. Let cool. Add the lemon juice and papaya, and mix well. Pour papaya mixture into a freezing tray. Freeze until firm. Then remove from tray and break up the mixture with a wooden spoon into a large bowl. Beat with electric mixer or hand rotary beater until it is free of lumps, but still of a thick consistency. Return it to freezing tray, and let freeze again. Beat once more before serving; then serve at once. Garnish as desired.

Honey Ice Cream—for Skinnies

2 cups whole milk
¾ cup honey
¼ teaspoon salt
2 eggs
1 cup heavy cream

Scald milk in top of double boiler. Add honey and salt. Beat eggs. Pour scalded milk into egg mixture, and stir until well blended. Return to top of double boiler and cook over hot water for 3 or 4 minutes. Let the mixture cool. Beat cream and fold it into custard mixture. Pour into refrigerator tray and freeze. Stir once or twice during the freezing period.

Golden Honey Custard

4 eggs
½ cup honey
3 cups whole milk
⅛ teaspoon vegetable salt

Separate egg yolks from whites. Beat yolks until lemon-colored, adding honey gradually as you beat. Then add milk gradually, beating the mixture until smooth. Whip egg whites, with the salt, until they are stiff and stand in peaks when the beater is withdrawn. Fold yolk mixture into egg whites. Pour into 6 or 8 individual custard cups. Place the cups in a shallow pan, and add about 1 inch hot water to the pan around the cups. Bake in moderate oven (325° F.) until the custard is firm. This should be in about 1 hour. To test, insert a silver knife blade; if custard does not adhere to the blade, it is ready to be removed from the oven. Let cups cool a little, then chill in refrigerator.

California Apricot Soufflé

¾ pound dried California apricots
5 egg whites

5 tablespoons brown sugar
Vegetable salt

Soak apricots in warm water overnight. Drain and press through sieve, or put in mixer and purée. Beat egg whites until stiff, and beat into them the brown sugar and a pinch of vegetable salt. Fold into apricot purée. Pile lightly into a buttered baking dish, and bake in slow oven (300° F.) until center is firm, about 45 minutes. Served with vanilla or fruit sauce, it makes a festive dessert.

Quick Apricot Whip

1½ cups of slightly cooked dried apricots are folded into 1 cup chilled yogurt, and sprinkled with honey and grated orange peel. Prune whip can be made the same way. Both prune and apricot whip make delicious fillings for individual pie shells.

Molasses Meringue

Beat 2 egg whites until foamy. Then add ⅓ cup molasses to the egg whites and beat until it stands up in peaks. Pile gently on top of pie, and place under broiler until delicately brown.

Plump Juicy Prunes, Apricots, and Raisins without Cooking

Simply wash dried prunes, apricots, or raisins, and place in quart jar. Cover with warm water, 1 tablespoon honey, and 1 tablespoon lemon juice. Cover jar, let stand 24 hours; then enjoy the juiciest, plumpest fruits you ever tasted. Excellent for breakfast or dessert.

27

Coffee or Tea

Coffee for Connoisseurs

We in the Americas have the best coffee beans in the world; but we do not always use them wisely. What was once an aromatic lean beverage has become a sugar-and-cream-laden concoction with which millions of Americans wash down their food. Yes, many thousands of Americans, who otherwise do not overeat, carry twenty or more pounds of excess weight around because of sugar and cream in their coffee. If you are one of these people, here's hoping I can help you break the habit.

Café au Lait

Why not acquire the *café au lait* habit? Thus you get the mild stimulation of fresh coffee plus the nourishment of hot milk; and it requires no sugar at all. Or learn to enjoy a cup of hot freshly brewed coffee as is; you will be surprised at how soon you will enjoy your cup of coffee black. I find that more and more smart people the world over would not think of spoiling the aroma of coffee with cream and sugar.

Caffè Espresso

The fight against the cream and sugar habit is also sweeping Europe. Caffè espresso is the strong black coffee the Italians have enjoyed for many years; even the small restaurants have their espresso machines and serve very small cups of flavorsome black coffee. I was delighted to see this coffee served not only in Italy but also in Germany, the home of the fattening *Schlag*, and in France, the home of sugared chicory coffee. It is common now in good American restaurants to find espresso coffee being served. It is quite strong, but there is so little of it in a serving. Italians claim that its bitters aid digestion. The first time you drink espresso, try a little honey with it, if you wish; then use less and less until you can enjoy the fragrant brew just as it comes out of the steaming machine.

Mint Coffee—a New Delight for Sophisticates

As you enter the new and beautiful Hotel Phoenicia in Beirut, an attendant wearing a fez welcomes you with a steaming hot cup of mint-flavored coffee. The Sheik of Kuwait was so impressed with this gesture of hospitality that he decided to build an elaborate hotel on the Persian Gulf and serve mint coffee to his royal guests. Here is the recipe for this delightful and new coffee treat. Simply add a teaspoon of dried peppermint leaves to finely ground drip coffee. Put in a drip coffee maker and pour on boiling water. (You can increase or decrease the amount of peppermint leaves.) Serve very hot in small cups with honey or brown sugar.

American Coffee

It can be made in many different ways, but I believe that the most flavorsome is drip coffee, made in one of those wonderful porcelain pots. Freshly ground coffee is placed in a filter and boiling water is poured over the coffee and allowed to drip through. This method is also known as filtered coffee—or *café filtre*, as the French call it. The coffee made in a porcelain filter pot (available at any gourmet cookware store) is delicious and acid-free. There is no tin or aluminum to change the delicate flavor of freshly ground coffee. My morning cup of coffee is brought to me in one of these porcelain pots, and it is always fragrant and never bitter. The next best method of making coffee is in the glass vacuum-type of coffee maker, where the freshly boiled water goes just once through the freshly ground coffee and extracts only its aromatic flavor and none of the bitter-tasting acids. Black, fragrant coffee is the dieter's delight, and it can be taken several times a day. Whenever coffee tastes bitter, it has been cooked too long; and that's why millions of people have acquired the fattening sugar and cream habit.

Swiss Coffee

Thousands enjoy this lean and delicious beverage. You simply fill a large cup half full of freshly made coffee, then fill the rest of the cup with hot fortified milk. In Zurich, Switzerland, they pour coffee and milk at the same time; the coffee pot is in one hand and the milk pot in the other. Both streams meet in the cup, and the result is a frothy cup of delicious brew that needs no sweetening. (If you must, add just a little honey.) The extra milk provides added protein, which is so important, especially for breakfast.

Instant Swiss Coffee

If you are in a hurry, you can simplify the whole procedure and make instant Swiss coffee. Simply put 2 to 3 teaspoonfuls of nonfat dry milk and 1 teaspoon of your favorite instant coffee into a cup. Fill the cup with hot water and stir. This is a most pleasant and easy-to-make drink. Nervous and sleepless people should use decaffeinated coffee.

New Orleans Nightcap

If coffee keeps you awake, stir 2 teaspoons of unsulphured molasses into a cup of very hot milk, add a pinch of salt, stir, and drink immediately.

Tea for Connoisseurs

Tea drinkers talk about themselves, and coffee drinkers talk about others—so goes a saying. I don't know if that is so, but I do know that there are two distinct camps—coffee-lovers and tea-lovers. There are many ways to make good coffee, but there is only one way to make good tea. The water should be fresh—it should be "singing," not boiled flat. The pot should be earthenware or porcelain. Metal pots change the flavor, say the real tea connoisseurs. The hot water and tea should steep in the pot for exactly 5 minutes, and no more, to get all the flavor but not the tannic acid from the tea leaves. Such tea is delicious. It can be drunk, hot or iced, to your heart's content. Drink it clear or with lemon; and if you must use a sweetener, try a little honey. *A cup of tea with a teaspoonful of honey taken 30 minutes before dinner is another way to curb a ravenous appetite.*

Tea Variations

With *minted tea*, you can combine the "lift" of regular tea with the fragrance of mint. You simply use two thirds of your favorite tea leaves and one third of dried peppermint leaves. This makes a delicious between-meal or five-o'clock pickup. My friend the lovely Ann Astaire, who lived for many years in England and Ireland, has long enjoyed this tea; she now serves it to her guests. I must say it is a wonderful drink.

Papaya tea, a century-old after-dinner digestive, is becoming more and more popular. The dried papaya leaves contain a digestive enzyme; a mixture of half papaya and half mint tea makes a delicious after-dinner drink to help digestion.

Rose-hip tea is an old standby in the Bircher-Benner Sanatorium in Switzerland. Rose hips are rich in vitamin C, and when steeped for 4 minutes they make a beautiful and flavorsome pink drink.

Strawberry tea, made from the dried leaves of wild strawberries, makes an excellent brew and tastes very much like regular tea. A teaspoon of dried leaves is simmered in boiling water for 3 minutes. Delicious served with milk and honey.

If you are a chronic tea drinker, may I suggest that you acquire the excellent habit of mixing your tea leaves with any one of the above fragrant and healthful herbs—all free of tannic acid.

Tranquilitea

Instead of synthetic tranquilizers and dangerous sleeping tablets, try this century-old recipe. Mix 1 ounce dry peppermint leaves (nature's digestive), 1 tablespoon rosemary leaves (nature's tranquilizer), and 1 teaspoon sage leaves (nature's sleep producer). Mix and keep in tightly closed jar. Use 1 heaping teaspoon of mixture to a cup of boiling water. Let steep for one minute, strain, sweeten with honey, and sip! Amazing tranquilizing effect—without a hangover.

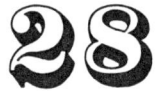

Milk and Milk Foods

Milk, like eggs, contains first-class tissue-building protein. The milk you buy in your market is pasteurized, and homogenized (a process that breaks the fat into smaller globules that won't separate when milk is left standing), and many important elements are lost; but all milk still contains its valuable protein. Casein (milk protein) is considered by nutritionists to be a complete protein because in laboratory experiments it was found to main tain life *and* support growth. Both casein and lactalbumin (also a milk protein) contain a good balance of amino acid. One quart of milk contains about 35 grams of protein. Therefore, if an adult drinks a pint of milk a day, he gets 17½ grams of protein, plus the important calcium.

Milk is an ideal food for fortifying other foods. In some parts of Italy people have learned to cook their spaghetti in milk, thus increasing the low protein value of their spaghetti; and in the Scandinavian countries, cereals are often cooked in milk instead of water. Millions of homemakers here have learned the secret of increasing the protein value of many dishes by using the inexpensive dry powdered skim milk (instant nonfat dry milk). Dry milk should never take the place of fresh milk, but it is ideal for fortifying the watery skim milk; simply add 1 to 1½ cups of dry skim milk to a quart of fresh skim milk. This doubles its protein value and gives you 70 grams of protein, plus calcium, riboflavin, and other needed B vitamins.

Hi-Vi Milk

I recommend Hi-Vi milk as sheer kitchen magic, especially for families who have to economize. Use this good-tasting milk in your coffee, over cereals, and in cream gravies. Always have a bottle in your refrigerator.

Hi-Vi Milk Formula

Combine 1 quart fresh skim milk, 1 to 1½ cups dry skim milk, and 2 tablespoons vegetable oil. Thoroughly mix in blender or with egg beater. Use this formula not only as a beverage but also for cooking purposes and for pouring over cereals.

You may add any healthful flavor to your Hi-Vi milk—one or two tablespoons of dark molasses (rich in iron), one or two tablespoons of carob powder to give a chocolaty flavor, a tablespoon of instant coffee, or a few drops of vanilla extract.

Cream—If You Must

1 cup fresh skim milk   ½ cup dry skim milk
1 tablespoon vegetable oil

Combine all ingredients and mix at high speed in blender. Serve at once.

Fortified Milk for Reducers

Most of the calories are in the cream of milk, but whole milk still has too much fat. It is therefore wise to buy skim milk and fortify it with dry skim milk. In this manner you receive double the amount of protein, calcium, riboflavin, and other vitamins of the B family, in one quart of milk. Such fortified skim milk prevents hunger pains and gives that satisfied feeling when taken with or between meals. I recommend this fortified milk drink to everyone—and for overweighters; it is their best friend. Here is how to make this superfood so that you won't even know it is skimmed milk:

Put a little less than a quart of fresh skim milk into a cocktail shaker or electric mixer and add ½ cup of dried skim milk. Then add 2 tablespoons dried brewers' yeast and 1 tablespoon molasses or honey. Shake well or mix until frothy. Keep on ice and drink to your heart's content during the day. Heat a cup to the simmering point (do not boil) and take as a nightcap for deep, sound sleep. A cup of this fortified milk provides 13.7 grams of protein, and a total of 145 calories. Of that total, 75 calories are derived from lactose. *Many adults do not absorb lactose completely, and what they fail to absorb fails to add weight.*

Famous Milk Lassie

Beat 2 level tablespoons powdered skim milk and 2 teaspoons unsulphured molasses into 1 cup fresh milk. Add 1 teaspoon powdered brewers' yeast. Beat until smooth. Serve cold between meals or hot (but do not boil) before retiring.

Honey-lass

Put 1 teaspoon honey and 1 teaspoon molasses into 1 cup of hot milk. Stir with fork until smooth. Excellent for weight-*gaining* when taken between meals or before retiring.

Hi-Vi Chocolaty Milk (hot or cold)

Unfortunately, the widespread habit of drinking "chocolate milk" is a bad one, especially for youngsters. Recent tests show that the important calcium in chocolate milk is not nearly so well absorbed as it is in plain milk. Therefore, since so many adults and children are already woefully short of calcium, chocolate milk cannot be recommended.

Carob powder, made from the dried fruit of the locust tree (St.-John's-bread of biblical times), has a delightful chocolate-like flavor. One tablespoon of carob powder, beaten into a cup of fortified fresh milk, makes a delightful and nourishing milk drink. It can be served hot or cold. Most diet and health-food shops now have delightful carob powder to make chocolaty drinks instantly.

Cinnamon Milk Shake

Blend 2 tablespoons nonfat dry milk into 1 pint of fluid skim milk and add ¼ teaspoon powdered cinnamon. Shake well and put in refrigerator. Shake again before using.

Nutmeg Milk Shake

To 1 pint fresh skim milk add 2 tablespoons nonfat dry milk and ¼ teaspoon powdered nutmeg. Shake. Keep in refrigerator; shake again before using.

Instant Coffee Milk Shake

Mix 1 teaspoon instant coffee with 1 pint fluid skim milk and 2 tablespoons nonfat dry milk. Shake and refrigerate. Shake again before using.

Orange-Lemon Milk Shake

This is a refreshing combination. Add ½ teaspoon grated orange and lemon peel to 1 pint fresh skim milk, plus 2 tablespoons nonfat dry milk. Shake and refrigerate. Shake again before using.

Molasses Milk Shake

Into 1 pint fluid skim milk, mix 2 teaspoons unsulphured molasses and 2 tablespoons nonfat dry milk. Shake and refrigerate. Shake again before using. This also makes a delicious hot coffee substitute.

Milk Shakes Unlimited

With a little practice, you can make a different mixture for practically every day of the year. Always use the same base: 2 tablespoons nonfat dry milk and 1 pint fluid skim milk. Remember that this gives you 25 grams of good protein. And it has been found that taking milk drinks between meals is the best and surest way to keep the stomach contented and happy.

Hi-Vi Fruit Drinks

Many who are allergic to fresh milk—or just plain don't like it—enjoy the following nutritious mixtures. The addition of dried skim milk, brewers' yeast, wheat germ, and natural fruit sugars make Lucullan drinks. These are rich not only in vitamin C but also in vitamins of the B family, vitamin E, many minerals, and the ever-necessary amino acids. Most of these drinks can be made in a cocktail shaker; but for superb results, you should invest in one of those electric mixers that blend everything into smooth, easier-to-digest liquids. Be inquisitive; try each of the various drinks. Then experiment and create new combinations. But don't overdo, as some health faddists do, and make combinations that taste like hay. There must be pleasure in eating. *We also eat with our eyes, so make everything as attractive and appetizing as possible.* Drink these concentrated mixtures through a straw—and slowly, please. Here are some of my favorite combinations.

Orange Juice Shake

Shake or mix 1 glass orange juice with 2 tablespoons powdered skim milk and 1 tablespoon honey. Mix until smooth and frothy. Drink at once for quick energy.

Pineapple Shake

Put ¼ cup nonfat dry milk and 1 teaspoon honey into a large glass of unsweetened pineapple juice. Beat until frothy. For better nourishment, also add 1 teaspoon brewers' yeast; gradually increase to 1 heaping tablespoon as you become accustomed to the flavor. You can also try this combination with grape juice, loganberry juice, apricot juice, or apple juice.

All-in-One Cocktail—a Meal in a Glass

Pour a glass of pineapple juice or apple juice into your blender. Add 1 tablespoon nonfat dry milk, 1 tablespoon nut kernels, 1 teaspoon wheat germ, 1 teaspoon powdered brewers' yeast, and 1 teaspoon honey. For extra flavor, add 1 tablespoon of berries and a few slices of banana. Mix thoroughly. In one minute you will have a most delicious "building drink"—a meal in a glass! This combination I dedicated to Leopold Stokowski, whose energy seems to increase with each year, after we drank it at a Beverly Hills health bar.

Curvaceous Cocktail

Into 1 cup milk (or 1 cup orange juice) beat 1 egg yolk, 2 teaspoons peanut oil, 1 tablespoon wheat germ, and 1 teaspoon honey. Excellent for weight *gaining* and for repairing leathery, dry skin.

Pineapple Delight

Pour 1 cup unsweetened pineapple juice into an electric blender. Add 2 tablespoons wheat germ, 1 tablespoon nonfat dry milk, and 1 teaspoon honey or molasses. Blend until smooth and creamy; serve at once.

Special Banana Milk for Skinnies

Mix in an electric blender 1 very ripe, almost black banana, 2 tablespoons nonfat dry milk, 1 teaspoon honey, and 1 glass whole milk. This combination, taken with meals, has helped many people *put on* healthy pounds.

Special Formulas for Reducers

Mix 4 tablespoons dried brewers' yeast (celery flavor) with 1 quart canned tomato juice. For additional flavor, add ½ teaspoon vegetable salt, 1 tablespoon lemon juice, and your choice of 1 tablespoon parsley or chives or green onions, or 1 teaspoon caraway seeds. Shake in cocktail shaker, or whip in electric blender, until frothy. Keep in refrigerator. Taken 30 minutes before meals, it prevents overeating.

Mix 1 pint tomato juice, 1 pint sauerkraut juice, 4 tablespoons dried brewers' yeast, and a pinch of caraway seeds if you like. Keep in refrigerator. Excellent as a first course or between-meals snack.

Mix 1 pint tomato juice, 1 pint yogurt, dash of vegetable salt, and 2 tablespoons dried brewers' yeast. Shake in cocktail shaker or mix in blender until smooth. Keep in refrigerator.

Mix 1 teaspoon dried brewers' yeast into a glass of unsweetened grapefruit juice.

Note: Since dried brewers' yeast is such a wonder food, try to increase the amount to a tablespoonful. In France people take brewers' yeast before meals to help satisfy enormous appetites.

Make Your Own Anticholesterol Buttermilk

A newly discovered secret about buttermilk is that it is an anticholesterol drink. It is rich in protein, calcium, and vitamin B_2. Cool buttermilk is a tasty between-meals drink. Here's how to make your own:

Pour ½ cup of buttermilk into a quart bottle of warm (not hot) fresh milk from which ½ cup has been removed, and let stand in a nondrafty place overnight. When milk has thickened, shake bottle and place in refrigerator. (Save ½ cup for the next batch.)

Homemade Kefir

This cultured milk drink is enjoyed by millions who do not possess refrigerators. You can find kefir at health-food and diet shops. Simply place some kefir grains in a quart of fresh milk. Let stand overnight. The next day you will have a delightful milk drink. Many who do not like sweet milk enjoy this tart kefir milk. Be sure to strain out the kefir grains and save them for the next batch.

Protein Whipped Cream

With ordinary skim milk you can make a delectable and protein-rich whipped cream to be used over your favorite desserts. Try it on berries and apricots and over fruit pies:

1 cup skim milk	½ teaspoon vanilla
1 tablespoon pure gelatin	Pinch salt
1 tablespoon honey	

Warm milk, and dissolve gelatin in it. Add honey, vanilla extract, and salt. Whip to consistency of whipped cream. Use at once.

Yogurt Means Long Life

Through the ages, yogurt has played an important part in the diets of many people. The Armenians call yogurt *mahdzoon*. The Yugoslavs call it *kiselo mleko*, and King Peter assured me that there were hundreds of centenarians in his country who thrived on it. The Russians love their yogurt with black bread; they call it *yagyrt*. The French eat quantities of yogurt with *fraises des bois*, and call it *yaourt*. In Sardinia it is called *gioddu;* in India, *dadhi;* in Egypt, *lebenraib*. But in any language, yogurt always means long life.

Whether there are so many one-hundred-year-olds in the Balkans because they love yogurt is debatable. But what interests us most is that although milk in itself is a good food, in the form of yogurt it becomes nutritionally superior in many respects. The important protein in yogurt is partially *predigested* by the yogurt bacteria, and the calcium in the milk lactic acid is easier to digest. The valuable bacteria in yogurt, living in the intestines, help break down milk sugar into lactic acid; and many of the bacteria that cause gas and fermentation are destroyed. Yogurt also lowers the level of cholesterol in the blood. See page 161. These are some of the reasons why many people who are allergic to sweet milk can enjoy yogurt without difficulties. Even more important, according to Warner Laboratories, which has done so much yogurt research, the bacteria in yogurt synthesize or manufacture valuable B vitamins; so the person who daily uses yogurt has a built-in vitamin B factory in his intestines. For this reason, many doctors now recommend yogurt after antibiotic treatments have destroyed many friendly and valuable bacteria.

How to Make Real Yogurt

The easiest way to make yogurt is with one of the new home yogurt-makers. Just follow the simple instructions. Or, if you want to "do it yourself," heat 1 quart of fresh skim milk carefully until it is hot, but do not boil. This is important—boiling kills the *Lacto bacillus bulgaricus*. Into this hot, but *not* boiling milk, you stir 1 cup of nonfat dry milk, plus 3 tablespoons of fresh yogurt. Pour this mixture into a wide-mouthed thermos jar, cover, and let it stand overnight. It takes from 4 to 6 hours for yogurt to become solid. The next morning, remove top of thermos and place the yogurt in refrigerator.

Yogurt Cocktail

Put 1 cup yogurt and 2 cups tomato juice in a shaker. Spike with a pinch of caraway seeds and a pinch of vegetable salt. Add 2 pieces of ice, and shake well. This is excellent for nondrinkers at cocktail parties.

Morning-After Yogurt

Mix ½ cup yogurt with ½ cup thick tomato juice; spike with pinch of vegetable salt and a few drops of fresh lemon juice. This is an excellent pickup for the morning after and does much more good than a Bloody Mary. It is also a delicious appetizer and between-meals lift.

Cholly Breakfast Yogurt

For a delicious and nutritious drink, mix equal amounts of tomato juice and yogurt. Add a sprinkling of vegetable salt and paprika, or a pinch of your favorite herb. Blend well and serve chilled. This delicious mixture keeps well when refrigerated. It is excellent for Sunday breakfast or as an appetizer before dinner. I recommend this combination highly and dedicate it to Count Cassini, a yogurt enthusiast who frequently drinks it for breakfast.

Fruit-Juice Yogurt

Mix 1 tablespoon frozen orange, pineapple, or Concord-grape juice concentrate with 1 cup fresh yogurt.

These make delightful and nutritious breakfast or between-meal drinks, each one giving about 10 grams of first-class protein. Any frozen fruit concentrate can be used, provided it is unsweetened.

Delightful Cucumber Relish

1 cucumber
1½ cups yogurt

1 tablespoon fresh chopped dill
or 1 teaspoon dried dill
Vegetable salt

Chop the cucumber finely and add it to the yogurt. Add the chopped dill and vegetable salt, and stir. Chill before serving. Makes an excellent appetizer, relish, or salad.

Green Yogurt Dressing

Add a handful of chopped greens—parsley, chives, fresh mint, green-onion tops, watercress, or green peppers—to a cup of yogurt. Use the greens singly or in any combination that appeals to you.

Yogurt Spring Salad

1 cup yogurt
1 tablespoon chopped fresh mint
1 clove garlic

2 cucumbers (sliced thin)
Vegetable salt
3 red radishes (sliced thin)

Add the mint and garlic (put through a press) to the yogurt. Stir well. Add cucumber slices and vegetable salt. Garnish with radish slices.

Yogurt Cream Pie—for Skinnies

1 cup yogurt
1 large package cream cheese
(8 ounces)

1 tablespoon honey
½ teaspoon vanilla extract

Combine all ingredients and whip to the consistency of whipped cream. Pour into a baked pie shell and put in refrigerator until it sets. Sprinkle with honeyed wheat germ and/or grated lemon peel before serving.

Yogurt Cream Cheese

This creamy cheese, based on a French recipe, is a protein food. You will find many uses for it because it is made from yogurt. It also is friendly to the "inner man." Here is how to make your own:

Simply dump a cup of yogurt (bought or homemade) into a piece of muslin or thick cheesecloth and let it hang above your sink overnight. Next morning you will find a white ball of the tenderest, creamiest cheese you ever ate. To give the cheese more savor and flavor, add a pinch of vegetable salt or a pinch of brown sugar to the yogurt before placing it in the muslin bag. For sandwiches, salads, and dips, add Roquefort cheese to taste.

APPENDIX

INDEXES

The New 1973 Recommended

FOOD AND NUTRITION BOARD NATIONAL ACADEMY
RECOMMENDED DAILY DIETARY

Designed for the maintenance of good nutrition

	(YEARS) From Up to	WEIGHT (kg)	WEIGHT (lbs)	HEIGHT (cm)	HEIGHT (in)	ENERGY (kcal)[2]	PROTEIN (g)	FAT-SOLUBLE VITAMINS			
								VITAMIN A ACTIVITY (RE)[3]	(IU)	VITAMIN D (IU)	VITAMIN E ACTIVITY (IU)[5]
Infants	0.0–0.5	6	14	60	24	kg x 117	kg x 2.2	420[4]	1,400	400	4
	0.5–1.0	9	20	71	28	kg x 108	kg x 2.0	400	2,000	400	5
Children	1–3	13	28	86	34	1300	23	400	2,000	400	7
	4–6	20	44	110	44	1800	30	500	2,500	400	9
	7–10	30	66	135	54	2400	36	700	3,300	400	10
Males	11–14	44	97	158	63	2800	44	1,000	5,000	400	12
	15–18	61	134	172	69	3000	54	1,000	5,000	400	15
	19–22	67	147	172	69	3000	52	1,000	5,000	400	15
	23–50	70	154	172	69	2700	56	1,000	5,000		15
	51+	70	154	172	69	2400	56	1,000	5,000		15
Females	11–14	44	97	155	62	2400	44	800	4,000	400	10
	15–18	54	119	162	65	2100	48	800	4,000	400	11
	19–22	58	128	162	65	2100	46	800	4,000	400	12
	23–50	58	128	162	65	2000	46	800	4,000		12
	51+	58	128	162	65	1800	46	800	4,000		12
Pregnant						+300	+30	1,000	5,000	400	15
Lactating						+500	+20	1,200	6,000	400	15

[1] The allowances are intended to provide for individual variations among most normal persons as they live in the United States under usual environmental stresses. Diets should be based on a variety of common foods in order to provide other nutrients for which human requirements have been less well defined.

[2] Kilojoules (KJ) = 4.2 x kcal.

[3] Retinol equivalents.

[4] Assumed to be all as retinol in milk during the first six months of life. All subsequent intakes are assumed to be one-half as retinol and one-half as β-carotene when calculated from international units. As retinol equivalents, three-fourths are as retinol and one-fourth as β-carotene.

Dietary Allowances

OF SCIENCES–NATIONAL RESEARCH COUNCIL ALLOWANCES,[1] Revised, 1973

of practically all healthy people in the U.S.A.

WATER-SOLUBLE VITAMINS							MINERALS					
ASCOR-BIC ACID (mg)	FOLA-CIN[6] (μg)	NIA-CIN[7] (mg)	RIBO-FLAVIN (mg)	THIA-MIN (mg)	VITA-MIN B$_6$ (mg)	VITA-MIN B$_{12}$ (μg)	CAL-CIUM (mg)	PHOS-PHORUS (mg)	IODINE (μg)	IRON (mg)	MAG-NESIUM (mg)	ZINC (mg)
35	50	5	0.4	0.3	0.3	0.3	360	240	35	10	60	3
35	50	8	0.6	0.5	0.4	0.3	540	400	45	15	70	5
40	100	9	0.8	0.7	0.6	1.0	800	800	60	15	150	10
40	200	12	1.1	0.9	0.9	1.5	800	800	80	10	200	10
40	300	16	1.2	1.2	1.2	2.0	800	800	110	10	250	10
45	400	18	1.5	1.4	1.6	3.0	1200	1200	130	18	350	15
45	400	20	1.8	1.5	1.8	3.0	1200	1200	150	18	400	15
45	400	20	1.8	1.5	2.0	3.0	800	800	140	10	350	15
45	400	18	1.6	1.4	2.0	3.0	800	800	130	10	350	15
45	400	16	1.5	1.2	2.0	3.0	800	800	110	10	350	15
45	400	16	1.3	1.2	1.6	3.0	1200	1200	115	18	300	15
45	400	14	1.4	1.1	2.0	3.0	1200	1200	115	18	300	15
45	400	14	1.4	1.1	2.0	3.0	800	800	100	18	300	15
45	400	13	1.2	1.0	2.0	3.0	800	800	100	18	300	15
45	400	12	1.1	1.0	2.0	3.0	800	800	80	10	300	15
60	800	+2	+0.3	+0.3	2.5	4.0	1200	1200	125	18+[8]	450	20
60	600	+4	+0.5	+0.3	2.5	4.0	1200	1200	150	18	450	25

[5] Total vitamin E activity, estimated to be 80 percent as α-tocopherol and 20 percent other tocopherols.

[6] The folacin allowances refer to dietary sources as determined by Lactobacillus casei assay. Pure forms of folacin may be effective in doses less than one-fourth of the RDA.

[7] Although allowances are expressed as niacin, it is recognized that on the average 1 mg of niacin is derived from each 60 mg of dietary trypotophan.

[8] This increased requirement cannot be met by ordinary diets; therefore, the use of supplemental iron is recommended.

GENERAL INDEX

adrenal glands, 130, 136–7, 249
Aebersold, Dr. Paul G., 8
age, see longevity
Ageless Youth, 324
alcohol, 156–7
alcoholism, 139, 272
Alcoholism: The Nutritional Approach, 272
Alexandra, Queen, 376
Alieva, Dr. O. K., 324
All-American Coed, The, 67
allergies, 126–9, 350
allowance, dietary, 412–13
aluminum, 58
Alvear Palace Hotel, 87
amblyopia, 183
Ameche, Don, 9
American Cider Book, The, 311
American Dieticians' Ass'n, 109
American Journal of Physiology, 121
American Speech and Hearing Ass'n, 186
amino acids, 4, 17, 27, 109, 121, 126, 138–9, 169, 196, 350, 399
Anatomy of Melancholy, The, 291
anemia, 54–6, 58, 121–2
apples, 305–10
arachidonic acid, 4
Arden, Elizabeth, 146, 204, 242
arsenic, 59
arteries, hardening of, 24, 41–2, 44, 113, 158–64, 166, 273–5, 324
arteriosclerosis, see arteries
arthritis, 111, 129–30
ascorbic acid, see vitamin C
Aslander, Dr. Alfred, 188
Astaire, Adele, 86, 255–6, 262, 326
Astaire, Ann, 255–6, 397
atherosclerosis, see arteries
Atkins, Dr. Robert C., 114
Atkinson, Dr. Donald T., 181–2
avocado, 32; see also recipe index

Bailey, Herbert, 50
baldness, see hair
Banting, 287–90
Barker, Dr., 136
Barton, Clara, 260
Baruch, Bernard, 176
Bates, Dr. William H., 183–4
baths, 207–12, 232, 240, 313
Bauer, Dr., 147
bean sprouts, 347–8
beauty farms, 218, 227–34, 237, 242–244; kitchen for, 232–3; names and addresses of, 243–4
Beery, Wallace, 9
Berg, Ragnar, 76
Bergman, Ingrid, 150
Bergson, Henri, 253
between-meals, 67, 73–5, 117, 125, 153–4, 228, 239–40; for reducing, 295, 297, 308–9; for elimination diet, 315–19
biotin, 3, 42, 124, 350
Bircher-Benner, 5, 47, 379, 383
Biskind, Drs., 131
blackheads, treatment of, 221–2
Blackwell, Earl, 89
blood sugar, 60–1, 125; low, 113–17, 129, 137; diet for, 139–40
Bloom, Dr. Walter Lyon, 322
body, makeup and care of, 7–8, 10, 93–6
bone meal, and teeth, 188–9
bones, 93–6, 157–8, 187
Bortz, Dr. Edward, 254
Brady, Dr. William, 130, 164, 324
breakfast, 60–3, 73–6, 117, 153, 227, 238–9; for reducing, 293–4, 296, 302, 308–9; for elimination diet, 315, 317–18
brewers' yeast, see yeast, brewers'
Briggs, Dr., 289
bromine, 59
brown spots, 221

Bruch, Dr. Hilda, 324
Buchinger, Dr., 321-2
Burton, Robert, 291
Bykov, Dr. K. M., 304

calcium, 4, 26, 47-8, 72, 120; function of, and foods for, 28-9, 52-4, 152-3, 399, 401; deficiencies of, 55-6; and nervousness, 124-5; and arthritis, 129; and menopause, 131; and sex glands, 139; and sleep, 152-153; and bones, 157-8, 187; for teeth, 169, 186-7, 191, 326; and eyes, 182-3; for hair color, 222; and teen-agers, 270
calories, 3, 7, 15, 23, 27, 69, 156-7, 324; and reducing, 69, 288-91, 298
Cameron, Dr. A. J., 183
cancer, 117-18, 200
capillaries, 168-9, 195-6, 303
carbohydrates, 3, 7, 15, 21-3, 124, 235 323, 367; and reducing, 288-90, 292-7, 301, 303; *see also* sugar
Carlson, Dr. Anton J., 325
Castle, Irene, 85
cataract, 181-3
Cavendish, Lord Charles, 256
cellular therapy, 175-6
cellulite, 303
Centre Gayelord Hauser, 88, 298
cereals, 234-5
Chaplin, Charlie, 176
Cheney, Dr., 379, 383
children, diet for, 265-70
chin, double, 218-19
chlorine, function of, 57-8
cholesterol, 23-4, 41-2, 44, 48, 51, 65, 120-1, 185, 273, 275, 304, 324-325, 341; and arteries, 159-62, 166, 273, 275
choline, 3, 38, 41-4, 113, 121, 160-2, 185, 194, 222, 349-50
chromium, 4
Church, Dr. A. S., 325
Churchill, Winston, 143, 176, 386
circulatory system, 101-3
Claire, Ina, 145
Cleopatra, and skin care, 215-16
cobalt, 4, 58
Coca, Dr. Arthur F., 128
Coller, Dr., 136
Colony Club, 261
constipation, 171-5, 297, 313, 324; *see also* elimination
copper, 55, 121-2
cortisone, 137
cosmetics, 202-5, 223
Cott, Dr. Allan, 140

Culpepper, Dr., 225
Cummings, Bob, 176

Dahl, Arlene, 217
Dam, Henrik, 312
Davis, Adelle, 221
Davis, Bette, 9
Deane, Martha, 292
Delafield, Ann, 146, 204, 326
Devrient, Dr., 279
diabetes, 112-13, 137, 176
diet, 4-12, 15-32, 60-75, 77-90; vitamins and, 33-51, 109-11, 124-5; minerals and, 51-9, 124-5; protein and, 60-2, 109-11; and infections, 112; and illnesses, 113-17, 120, 122, 130, 132-40, 159, 162-8; high-vitality, 112, 142, 148; and elimination, 172-3, 315-20; and eyes, 179-84; for hearing, 185; and teeth, 186-7, 189, 191; and hair, 191-4, 222; and skin, 195-8; and beauty, 205; Garbo and, 249; for children, 265-70; men and, 271-82; of Presidents, 280, 282; reducing, 285-7, 293-7, 298-309; *see also* food, meals, *and* menus
Diet for a Small Planet, 17
Dietrich, Marlene, 150
digestion, 169-71
digestive system, 97-100
DiMaggio, Joe, 205
dining out, 84-90
dinner, 67-9, 74-5, 117, 154, 229-30, 239-40; for reducing, 295-7, 302-303, 308-9; for elimination diet, 316-19
Diocles, 63
diphtheria, and vitamin C, 110
Dr. Atkins' Diet Revolution, 114
Dodds, Sir Charles, 288-9
Dougherty, Pat, 85
Drobil, Dr. Rudolf, 204
Duncan, Dr. G., 322

Eat and Grow Beautiful, 262
eating, ways of, 11, 98-9, 169-70, 290-2, 297; *see also* food *and* dining out
Eating for Good Health, 291
Eddy, Dr. Walter, 110
eggs, 350-1
Eighty-Year-Old Doctor's Secrets of Positive Health, An, 130
elimination, 172, 174-5, 307, 313-20; *see also* constipation
Elizabeth II, Queen, 326

Ellene, Madame, 218–19
endocrine glands, 132–3, 137
exercise, 9–10, 146–51, 208, 227, 231, 240, 324–5; bicycle, 123; and arthritis, 130; for eyes, 183–4; for teeth, 189; for hair, 192–3; for facial muscles, 202–4; for men, 274; and reducing, 304–6; *see also* stomach lift *and* yoga
eyeglasses, 184
eyes, 33, 179–84, 220–1, 226

face, 201–5
fasting, sanatoriums for, 320–2
fatigue, 142
fats, 7, 15, 325, 340–1; hard, 16, 23–24, 160, 273, 275, 324; vegetable, 23–5; and reducing, 290, 295, 296, 299; *see also* oils
fatty acids, 4, 23, 51, 266
feet, 205–6
Ferry, Mrs. Edgar, 259
fish, 79, 341
fluorine, 187, 189
flush, quick salt-water, 174–5
folic acid, 3, 42
Folk Medicine, 237
Fontana, Mme, 87
Fontanne, Lynn, 150
foods, natural, 4, 11–12, 15; enjoyment of, 10–12, 69, 76–7, 291–2; wonder, 11, 26–32, 163, 172, 346–8, 350; tampering with, 11, 15, 33, 57; protein, list of, 18–20; for vitamins and minerals, 34–45, 48–57, 110–11, 152–3, 349–50; and illnesses, 124, 129, 135; taboo, 234–7, 300; and sex, 277–8
Ford, Gerald, 280, 282
forgetfulness, 125–6
Fraise, Monsieur, 262, 386
French, and reducing, 298–303
Freud, Sigmund, 285
Freyberg, Dr., 136
Friedel, Dr. Herman, 323
Friedmen, Dr. Meyer, 164
fruits, 11, 82–3, 305, 316, 385–6

gallstones, 24, 120–1
Gandhi, Mahatma, 257
Garbo, Greta, 145, 150, 205, 249, 326
Gesichts-Gymnastik, 204
Gilbreth, Dr. Lillian M., 259–60
Gish, Lillian, 205
glands, *see under names of*
Glenard, Dr. Roger, 120
glutamic acid, 126
Goddard, Paulette, 327

Godfrey, Arthur, 205
Gofman, Dr. J. W., 160
goiter, 56, 134
Goto, Dr. Schichiro, 312–13
Grace, Princess, 327
Graham, Martha, 205
Grant, Cary, 326
Grant, Doris, 370
Gyorgy, Dr. Paul, 266

hair, 191–4, 274; graying of, 136, 194, 222; superfluous, 213; loss of, 166, 276–7
Harden, Dr. Eugene B., 234–5
Hauser, Gayelord, 5–6, 259
Hauser's Daily Requirement (HDR), 37–8
Hawkins, Dr. David, 140–1
Hayes, Helen, 86
health care, preventive, 8
hearing, 185
heart disease, 23–4, 44, 50, 159–60, 163–8, 324; diet and, 162–4; prevention of, 164; American men and, 272–6
Heiser, Dr. Victor, 174
hemophilia, 168
Henie, Sonja, 9
herbs, natural, as laxative, 175
Herodicus, 171
Herrmann, Dr., 160
Hertz, Dr. R., 130
Hewitt, Edward R., 44
Hillman Hospital, 31
Hindhede, 5
Hippocrates, 5, 181, 353
Hoffer, Dr. Abram, 140
Holmes, Oliver Wendell, 260
honey, 22, 174, 278
Hope, Bob, 326
hormones, 30–1, 133, 135–7, 139, 248–249, 276
Horwitt, Dr. M. K., 325
husband, how to cook, 281
Hutschnecker, Dr. Arnold, 250
Hutton, Lauren, 264
Huxley Institute for Bisocial Research, 141
Hydro-Spray, 220–1
Hyman, Dr. Harold Thomas, 273–4
hyperthyroidism, 134
hypoglycemia, *see* blood sugar, low
hypothyroidism, 133
infections, 108–12
inositol, 3; functions of, and foods for, 38, 41–4, 349; and hardening of arteries, 113, 160–2; and hearing, 185

insulin, 112–14, 137
intestines, 99–100
Introduction to Cellular Therapy, 176
iodine, 4, 55, 324; function of, and foods for, 56, 341; and arthritis, 130; and thyroid, 134–5; and hair, 192–3; and skin, 197; for children, 267; and sea food, 312
iron, 4, 26; function of, and foods for, 27, 31–2, 54–6; and illnesses, 121–122, 130–1; and skin, 196; and sex, 278
isoleucine, 4

Jack and Charlie's "21" Club, 86
Jacobson, Dr. Michael, 235
Japanese, and health and longevity, 311–13
Jarvis, Dr. D. C., 221, 225, 237
Jenny, Dr. Edouard, 306
Johnson, Lyndon, diet of, 280, 282
Jordan, Dr. Sara M., 248
juices, fresh, 81–2, 310–11, 378–80
Jung, Dr. Carl, 254

Kalsø, Anna, 206
Kannel, Dr. William, 159
Karoline, Schwester, 378–9
Karputhala, Princess, 262
Kavinoky, Dr. N. R., 131
Kekwik, Dr., 290
Keys, Dr. Ancel, 307, 310
kidney disease, 118–19
King, Dr., 110
Kinsell, Dr. Laurance W., 325
Kirschner, Dr. H. E., 379
Kneipp, Father, 5, 207
Kondo, 312
Kopetsky, Dr. Samuel J., 185
Kraines, Dr. S. H., 248
Kumer, Dr. Leo, 217

Laird, Dr. Donald, 146
Lamb, Dr. Lawrence E., 282
Lambert, Mr. and Mrs. Joe, 354
Lane, Lydia, 326
Langford, Frances, 67
Lappe, Frances Moore, 17
Laszlo, Dr. Erno, 197
laughter, 248–9
Laughton, Charles, 9
Laurie, Annie, 210
Lawrence, Mary Wells, 264
Lawton, Dr. George, 255
laxatives, 172–5
lecithin, 43–5, 324, 350, and hardening of arteries, 159, 162, 165–8
Lee, Dr. Royal, 326

Lefort, Colette, 298
Lehmann, Dr. G, 325
Lenclos, Ninon de, 260
leucine, 4
Liebman, Dr. Joshua L., 254
linoleic acid, 4, 24–5, 121, 325
linolenic acid, 4
liver, and sex glands, 130–1; value of, nutritionally, 332–3
longevity, 5–11, 33, 132, 171, 311–13
Loos, Anita, 86, 327
love, 132, 250–2, 269–70
Low Fat Diet, The, 324
Low-Fat Way to Health and Longer Life, The, 44
Lubowe, Dr. Irwin, 191
luncheon, 64–6, 74–5, 117, 153, 228, 239; for reducing, 294–5, 296–7, 302–3, 308–9; for elimination diet, 315, 317–19
Lust, Dr. Benedict, 210
lysine, 4

MacFadden, Bernarr, 259
Macomber, 139
magnesium, 4, 58, 152
Managing Your Mind, 248
manganese, 4, 58
Manger Pour Être Belle, 180
Mann, Dr. George V., 161
Manners, Lady Diana, 262
Marbury, Elizabeth, 261
margarine, 24–5
Martin, Dr. Lillian J., 258–9
maturity, 252–5
Maugham, Somerset, 176
Maxim's, 88–9, 387
Mayer, Dr. Jean, 306
Mayo Clinic, 8, 135
Mayr, Dr., 81
McCarrison, Sir Robert, 191
McCollum, Dr. E. V., 174
McCormick, Dr. W. J., 155
McKay, Dr., 133
Mead, Dr. Margaret, 69, 324
Meade, Julia, 327
meals, planning and preparing of, 60–75, 331–2; *see also* menus
meat, 78–9, 305, 332
meats, organ, 332, 335
megavitamin therapy, 139–41
Mendl, Elsie de Wolfe, 145, 260–3, 386
menopause, 131–2, 136
Menshikov, Dr., 304
mental disturbances, 124–6, 139
Menton, Dr., 110

Index | 419

menus, 73–5; for low blood sugar, 117; for sleep, 153–4; for *your* day, 238–240; for reducing, 288, 293–7, 302–303, 308–9; for elimination diet, 317–19
Mercurio, menu at, 86–7
mercury, 59
metabolism, 49, 114, 133–5, 156–7, 248, 288–9, 299–301, 304–6, 324
Metchnikoff, 170
methionine, 4, 43–4, 185
Meyerson, Anna, 88
milk, 305, 399; powdered skim, 17, 18, 28–9, 109, 399; fortified, 20, 28–9, 125, 129, 153–4, 400–1; cultured, 29; and glutamic acid, 126; for calcium, 152–3; and digestion, 170; for eyes, 226; chocolate, 401–2
Miller, Dr. Fred D., 186
minerals, 4, 7, 11, 15, 17, 27, 51, 58–59, 73; daily needs of, 4, 412–13; for hardening of arteries, 167; and skin, 196; in apple, 307; and sea food, 312; *see also individual names of, and* trace minerals
Minot, Dr. George R., 122
Mirror, Mirror on the Wall, 217
molasses, 31–2, 131, 152, 174
moles, 213
molybdenum, 4
Morehouse, Dr. Lawrence E., 274
Moreton, Dr. J. R., 159–60
Morgan, Anne, 145
Morrison, Dr. Lester M., 44, 159–60, 324
Moses, Grandma, 259
Mueller, Dr. Erich A., 147
Murray, Alan E., 205
muscles, 96–7; facial, 201–4
myxedema, 133

Nature's Drinks, 379
near-sightedness, 182–3
Necheler, Dr., 160
needs, daily, 3–4, 412–13
nervous system, 106–7, 125
nervousness, 124–5
neuritis, and focal infections, 112
New Guide to Intelligent Reducing, 285
New York State Journal of Medicine, 114
Newburgh, Dr., 136
niacin, 3, 27, 35–8, 124–5, 307
nickel, 59
Niehans, Dr. Paul, 176
Nixon, Richard M., diet of, 280
nutrients *and* nutrition, *see* diet
Nutrition and Alcoholism, 156

obesity, 23–4, 76–7, 113, 133, 139, 304, 306, 322; and diabetes, 113–114; and bones, 158; *see also* reducing
Oedipus at Colonus, 260
oil, vegetable, 3, 64–6, 324–5, 358; coconut, 23, 25; "cold-pressed," 24–25, 299–300, 324, 358; crude, 25; sunflower, 25–6, 358; fish-liver, 35, 153, 266, 268; and hair, 191–4; for skin, 215–18; and health, 275; safflower, 357–8; *see also* fats
Open Door to Health, 186
Orentreich, Dr. Norman, 276–7
Orthomolecular Psychiatry: Treatment of Schizophrenia, 141
Orton, Vrest, 311
Osmond, Dr. Humphrey, 140
Over the Tea Cups, 260
overweight, *see* obesity

Page, Dr. Melvin E., 326
pancreas, 136–8
pantothenic acid, 3, 40, 136, 194
papaya leaves, 78
para-aminobenzoic acid, 3, 194, 222
Paracelsus, 5
participation, 250
Pauling, Dr. Linus, 45, 140–1
Pawan, Dr., 290
pellagra, 163
Pennington, Dr., 290
People, 5, 9–10, 252, 255, 263
Pfeiffer, Dr. Carl, 140
Pfister, Dr. Alfred, 176
phenylalanine, 4
philosophy of life, 247–51
phlebitis, 112
phosphorus, 4, 48, 49, 125; function of, and foods for, 52–3, 341; and bones, 157–8, 187; and teen-agers, 270
photophobia, 181
pimples, treatment of, 221
pituitary gland, 135–7, 249
plaque, 187–8
plastic surgery, 213–15
Plummer, Dr. W. A., 133
Pollack, Dr. Herbert, 323
Pope Pius XII, 176
potassium, 4, 57
Preminger, Marion, 257
presbyopia, 179
Price, Dr. Weston A., 191
prostate gland, 278–9
proteins, 7, 9, 15, 26, 55, 332; needed quantity of, 3, 16–19, 109, 412–13; importance and use of, 16–20; "life-

proteins (cont'd)
saving," 17; foods for, 18–20, 27–9, 340–1, 343, 347–52, 399, 401; for salads, 66; tablets for, 73; and illness, 109–11, 120–1, 123, 126–7, 129, 138–9, 164; and digestion, 169; and elimination, 173; and hearing, 185; and hair, 191–3; and skin, 196; and muscle tone, 218; and teenagers, 270; and sex, 278; and reducing, 288, 293–7, 299–301, 303, 323; Japanese and, 311
psycho-cosmetics, 202–3
psychosomatic difficulties, 128–9
Pulse Test, The, 128
Pump Room, menu at, 85
pyorrhea, 190–1
pyrodoxine, 3, 39, 125, 152, 160–2
pyruvic acid, 21

Quigley, Dr. D. T., 323

Ramanones, Countess of, 264
reducing, 285–327, 400–1, tips for, 322–3; comments on, 323–7; drinks for, 405; *see also* diet, fasting, *and* weight chart
relaxation, 6, 9, 142–7, 208, 256, 262, 325; and varicose veins, 123; eating and, 169–70; of eyes, 183–4; and hair, 193
respiratory system, 103–6
Restaurant Caprice, menu at, 88
restaurants, 84–90
Reynolds, Adeline De Walt, 9–10, 139
riboflavin, 3; sources of, 27–9, 31, 36–37, 179, 350, 399, 401; function and daily need of, 35–6; and sex problems, 131; and eyes, 179, 181; and skin, 197; in apple, 307
Rinse, Dr. J., 165–8
Rodin, Auguste, 265
Rollier, Dr. Auguste, 211
rose hips, 47
Rosenman, Dr. Ray, 165
Ross, Dr. Harvey M., 139–40
Ross, Shirley, 379
Rossi, Dr., 160
Rothschild, Philippe de, 88
Russians, and reducing, 303–6

Saint Hardouin, Madame Ily de, 89, 384
salad, 64–6, 77–8, 81, 305; and reducing, 301
salt, 57–8
sanatoriums, for fasting, 320–2

Sandburg, Carl, 23, 292
sauna, facial, 219–20
schizophrenia, 139–40
Schweitzer, Dr. Albert, 257–8
Scripps Clinic, 8
scurvy, 169
seaweeds, 312
seeds, 18, 189, 279
Seely, Dr., 165
selenium, 4
sex, and food, 277–8
sex glands, 130–1, 133, 138–9
sexual problems, 130–2
Sherman, Dr. Henry C., 7, 33–4, 45
Sherrell, Dr., 133
shoes, 205–6
Shute, Drs., 50, 123, 161
silicone injections, 215
silver, 59
sinusitis, 112
skin, 34, 194–205; care and protection of, 198–201, 215–20; lines and wrinkles in, 201–3, 219
Slaughter, Dr. Frank, 202
sleep, 144, 151–4; dry bath for, 210
Slenderness through Psychology, 323
Smith, Dr. Russel, 140
smoking, 155–6, 159, 162
sodium, 4, 57–8
Sophocles, 260
soya products, 17–18, 346–7, 349
soybean, virtues of, 44, 346–7
Spain, Dr. David M., 273
spices, 278
Spies, Dr. Tom, 31
sports, 148
starches, *see* carbohydrates
Stare, Dr. Frederick, 291
Steiner, Dr., 160
Stewart, Dr. Bronte, 24
Stewart, James, 9
Stokowski, Leopold, 145, 249, 404
stomach, 99, 292
stomach lift, 10, 97, 146–7, 149–50, 173, 208, 212, 240
sugar, 16, 21–2, 30–1, 36, 54, 69, 234–236, 326; and diabetes, 113; and cereal, 234–5; *see also* carbohydrates *and* sweets
sun, and skin, 198–201
sunbaths, for infants, 267
Superlevure, 301–3
Swanson, Gloria, 90, 176
sweets, 22–3, 235–6, 308, 323; *see also* carbohydrates
Swiss, apple diet of, 306–10
Swiss Fruit Association, 306

Index | 421

Sydenstricker, Dr., 124
Szent-Györgyi, 168

Taverna della Fenice, menu in, 89–90
tea, laxative, 175
teeth, 111, 186–91, 326; cosmetic dentistry for, 189–90; infection of, 190–191
Tender Loving Cooking, 332
tenderizers, 78
Thetford, E. S., 248
thiamine, 3, 27, 30–1, 35–7, 112, 124–125, 131, 134–5, 307
Thoreau, Henry, 295
threonine, 4
thyroid gland, 56, 58, 133–4, 136, 192, 197
thyroxine, 56, 133–4
tin, 58
Tintera, Dr. John W., 114
Tiralla, Professor, 106,
Titian, 260
tonic, Swiss vinegar-milk, 175
trace minerals, 4, 27, 58–9
Truman, Harry S., 282
tryptophan, 4
"21" Club, 86
Type A Behavior and Your Heart, 165

urinary troubles, 119–20

valine, 4
varicose veins, 122–3
Vegetable Juices for Health, 379
vegetables, 17–18, 20, 29–81, 237, 267, 311–12, 323; for elimination diet, 316; cooking, 360–1
vinegar, kinds of, 65
Verchow, Dr. Rudolf, 63
vitamin A, 3, 33–4, 56; and eyes, 33, 179–81; sources of, 34–5, 110, 179, 181–2, 347, 350; and skin, 34, 196–197; and illness, 109–10, 119–20; and sexual problems, 130; and pancreas, 138; and sex glands, 138–9; and bones, 157–8; and teeth, 187, 191; for children, 266, 270; in apple, 307
vitamin B₁, *see* thiamine
vitamin B₂, *see* riboflavin
vitamin B₆, *see* pyridoxine
vitamin B₁₂, 3, 45, 122
vitamin C, 3, 33, 56; function and sources of, 45–7, 110–11, 179, 182, 347; and illness, 109–12, 120, 123, 129; and sex glands, 138; and smoking, 155–6; and bones, 157–8; and capillaries, 168–9; for teeth, 169, 187, 191; and eyes, 179, 181–2; and skin, 196; and children, 266–7, 270; and sex, 271; and reducing, 303; in apples, 307, 310
Vitamin C and the Common Cold, 45
vitamin D, 3, 125; function, sources, and requirements of, 48–9, 52–4, 153, 179; and arthritis, 130; and sleep, 152; and bones, 158; and eyes, 179, 182–3; and teeth, 187, 189, 191; and children, 266, 268
vitamin E, 3, 30, 41, 325, 358; function of, foods for, and daily requirements of, 49–51; and varicose veins, 123; and sexual problems, 130–1; and sex glands, 138; and the heart, 160–1, 276; for brown spots, 221
Vitamin E—Your Key to a Healthy Heart, 50
vitamin "F," 51, 216–17, 326
vitamin K, 4, 51, 312–13
vitamin P, 168–9
vitamins, 7, 11, 15, 17, 73, 167; daily need of, 3–4, 33–4, 412–13; homemade, 347–8
vitamins, B-complex, 3, 21, 26, 35, 38, 56, 163; sources of, 27, 31, 36–45, 163, 347, 350, 399, 401; and illnesses, 113, 121–2, 124, 126, 129–130; and sexual problems, 130–1; and sex glands, 138; and drinking, 156; and arteries, 160–2; and the heart, 163–4; and digestion, 169; and elimination, 172–3; and eyes, 181; and hair, 193–4; and skin, 196–7; and children, 267, 270; and sex, 278; *see also individual B vitamins*
Vivekananda, 105

walking, 147, 150–1, 228–9, 240–1, 305
Walters, Barbara, 263–4
Way to Health and Longevity, A, 312
weight chart, 293
Welch, Raquel, 264
West, Dr. Charlotte, 324
West, Mae, 327
Weyhbrecht, Dr. Hans, 203
wheat germ, 17, 18, 20, 30–1, 126, 129, 131, 163, 174, 267–8, 275–6, 324; beauty mask of, 223
Whipple, Dr. G. H., 121
White, Dr. Paul Dudley, 324–5
White, Stanford, 261
White House Diary, A, 280

Wilder, Dr. Russell, 135
Will to Live, The, 250
Williams, Mrs. Harrison, 262
Williams, Dr. Roger J., 131, 134, 156, 271–2
Windsor, Duchess of, 262
Wright, Frank Lloyd, 259

Years Between 75 and 90, The, 44
yeast, brewers', 17, 18, 20, 27–8, 124, 126, 129, 131, 162–3, 174, 185, 267, 301, 322, 324
yeasts, food, 27–8, 174, 197, 268

yoga slant boards, 10, 76, 123, 145–6, 149, 204, 212, 229, 231, 240
yogurt, 20, 29–30, 174, 233, 323, 406–407; and menopause, 131; and calcium, 158; and arteries, 161; and digestion, 170
Your Bread and Your Life, 370
your day, 237–42
Yudkin, Dr. John, 235
Yurka, Blanche, 145

zinc, 4, 58, 279
Zukor, Dr., 81

RECIPE INDEX

appetizers, 349–50, 359–60
apple: Bircher muesli, 310
 five-minute dessert, 311
 juice, 310–11, 382
 sauce, raw, 311
 Swiss milk, 310
apricots: prunes, and raisins, 393
 soufflé, California, 393
 whip, 393
avocado: broth, quick, 354
 dressing, 359

baking powder, formula for, 372
bananas: Jamaican, 386–7
 milk, 404
beans: oven-baked, 345
 quick-baked, 345
 string, 362
beauty aids, 209, 215–26, 232
beef: Budapest goulash, 337
 burger, 336–7
 burger, German, 338
 picadillo, 338
 steak, broiled, 336
 steak, pepper, 365
 Stroganoff, 337
beet juice, fresh, 382
beets, rose petal, 361
Bircher apple muesli, 310
bluefish, baked, 342
breads: Cornell, 369
 Elam or El Molino, 369
 gluten, hi-protein, 370
 no-knead, 370
 rye, 370–1
 rye crisps, 371
 whole-wheat, 368–9
breakfast, quick pep, 351

broth: Giuseppe's nutritious, 354
 Hauser, 353
 quick avocado, 354
 Swiss, 71
brown rice, 375
butter, sun, 26

cabbage, easy-to-digest, 362
 juice, 383
cake, hi-protein beauty-farm, 372–3
carob powder, 401–2
carrots: golden, 361
 juice, golden, 381
 loaf, golden, 344
 milk shake, 381
 sherbet, golden, 391
cauliflower, delicious, 362
celery: juice, 381–2
 loaf, 344–5
cereals, cooking of, 373
cheese spread, Hi-Vi, 72
chicken: and cucumber, 365
 liver, 334
 with mushrooms and vegetables, 364
 oven-fried, 340
 roast, with stuffing, 339
 sauce for, 339–40
Chinese dishes, 363–6
choy lung har, 364–5
Cleopatra's oil, 218
cocktails: without alcohol, 384
 all-in-one, 404
 curvaceous, 404
 Gaylord Hauser, 383
 yogurt, 407
coffee: American, 395–6
 café au lait, 394
 caffè espresso, 395

Index | 423

coffee (*cont'd*)
  instant milk shake, 402
  mint, 395
  Swiss, 239, 396
  Swiss instant, 396
compote, honey, Lady Mendl's, 386
cosmetics, *see* beauty aids *and individual names of*
custard, golden honey, 392–3
cream, 400
  protein whipped, 406
cream cheese, yogurt, 409
cucumber relish, delightful, 408

desserts, 311, 372–3, 381, 385–93, 408–9
dressings, salad, 358–9
drinks, for reducers, 404–5
  see also individual names of

eat-and-run drink, 71
eggs: Foo Yung, 364
  pancake, Henrici's, 351
  snack, Hi-Vi, 72
  tonic, German, 351
eggplant: easy, 363
  toast, 363
eye opener, million-dollar, 70

face astringent, 224
fish, 341–3, 364
fruit: 310, 385–7, 393
  drinks, 403–4
  washing of, 82
  and yogurt, 387

gelatin, 389–90
goulash, Budapest, 337
grapefruit, broiled, Caribbean, 386

halibut, steaks, sesame, 341–2
hand lotion, 224
Hauser: broth, 353
  cocktail, 383
  herbal rinse, 224–5
Hi-Protein: beauty-farm cake, 372–3
  gluten bread, 370
  muffins, 371
  popovers, 372
  waffles, 373
Hi-Vi: bomb, 71
  booster, 71
  cheese spread, 72
  chocolaty milk, 71, 401
  egg snack, 72
  fruit drinks, 403–4
  golden drink, 71
  menus, 73–5

milk, 20, 28–9, 70, 400
honey: compote, Lady Mendl's, 386
  custard, 392–3
  ice cream, 392
  lass, 401
  honeyed wheat germ, 373–4

ice cream, honey, 392

juice: fruit, 310–11, 382
  vegetable, 380–4

kasha, 374
kashaburgers, 374
kefir, 405

lamb, sauce for, 340
liver: broiled, 333
  calf's, with avocado, 335
  chicken, 334
  loaf, 334
  sautéed, 333–4
  tonic, 334–5
lobster: tails, broiled, 342–3
  and vegetables, 364–5

marmalade, rose-hip, 47
mayonnaise, 359
meatless dishes, 343–6
meats, 333–8, 364
menus, *see under General Index*
meringue, molasses, 393
milk: chocolaty, 71, 401–2
  fortified, 401
  Hi-Vi, 20, 28–9, 70–1, 401
  lassie, 401
  pads, 226
  soy, 349
  Swiss apple, 310
milk shakes: carrot, 381
  cinnamon, 402
  instant coffee, 402
  molasses, 402
  nutmeg, 402
  orange-lemon, 402
  unlimited, 403
mineral bath, 232
molasses: meringue, 393
  milk shake, 402
moo goo gai peen, 364
muffins: hi-protein, 371
  wheat germ, 372

nightcap: New Orleans, 396
  tranquilizing, 72, 154
nut loaves: pecan, 343
  savory, 344
  walnut, 343

oil bath, 209
orange juice shake, 403
orange-sherry gelatin, 390

pancake, Henrici's egg, 351
pepper steak, 365
pie, yogurt cream, 408–9
pie shell, quick Viennese, 388
piecrust: honeyed wheat-germ, 388–9
  lighthearted, 388
pilaf, golden rice, 375
pineapple: au kirsch, 387
  delight, 404
  de luxe, 387
  shake, 403–4
popovers, hi-protein, 372
potatoes: baked, 376
  chips, 377
  Garbo, 376
  hashed, 376
  mashed, 375–6
poultry, 399–40, 364–5
  sauce for, 339–40
prunes, apricots, and raisins, 393

quick pep breakfast, 351

raisins, apricots, and prunes, 393
rice: brown, 375
  Chinese fried, 366
  pilaf, golden, 375
  wild, 346
rose water, 223–4
rose-hip: marmalade, 47
  tea, 397
Russian wonder cream, 222–3

salad dressings, 358–9, 408
salads: 355–8
  combination, 357
  finger, 81
  liquid, 383–4
  lunch, 64–6
  spring, yogurt, 408
salmon steaks, with herbs, 342
saltimbocca, 87
sauces: 339–40
  basting, beauty-farm, 339–40
shakes: juice, 403
  milk, 351, 381, 402–3
sherbet: French, 390
  papaya, golden, 392
  raspberry, 391
soufflè, California apricot, 393

soups: lemon, Silemi, 354
  potage au crème, 352
  potage Hippocrates, 352–3
soy: grits, 349
  milk, 349
  treats, tasty, 349–50
soybeans: oven-baked, 348
  quick baked, 348
  sprouts, 347–8
steak: broiled, 336
  pepper, 365
string beans: elegant Amandine, 362
  young, 362
stuffing, poultry, 339
sukiyaki, 366
sunbutter, 26

tea: minted, 397
  papaya, 397
  rose-hip, 397
  strawberry, 397
  Tranquillitea, 398
  tonic, hi-potency, 334–5

veal: picadillo, 338
  saltimbocca, 87
  sauce for, 340
vegetables: 344–8, 352–3, 359–63
  preparation of, 79–82
vinegar: cosmetic, 225
  Swiss herb, 358

waffles, hi-protein, 373
wheat germ: honeyed, 373–4
  mask, 223
  muffins, 372
  piecrust, 388–9
  sticks, 371
whip, apricot, 393
wild rice: nut burgers, 346
  quick, 346
wine jelly, 390

yogurt: cholly breakfast, 407
  cocktail, 407
  cream cheese, 409
  cream pie, 408–9
  cucumber relish, 408
  and fruit, 387
  fruit-juice, 408
  Hi-Vi, 72
  morning-after, 407
  salad dressing, 359, 408
  spring salad, 408

zucchini, Italian, 362